Helicobacter Pylori in Human Diseases

Helicobacter Pylori in Human Diseases

Edited by Emma O'Neill

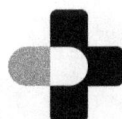

AMERICAN
MEDICAL PUBLISHERS
www.americanmedicalpublishers.com

American Medical Publishers,
41 Flatbush Avenue,
1st Floor, New York,
NY 11217, USA

Visit us on the World Wide Web at:
www.americanmedicalpublishers.com

ISBN: 978-1-63927-142-9

Cataloging-in-Publication Data

Helicobacter pylori in human diseases / edited by Emma O'Neill.
    p. cm.
Includes bibliographical references and index.
ISBN 978-1-63927-142-9
1. Helicobacter pylori infections. 2. Helicobacter pylori. 3. Pathology.
4. Diseases. 5. Medicine. I. O'Neill, Emma.
RC840.H38 H45 2022
616.330 14--dc23

Table of Contents

Preface

This book has been a concerted effort by a group of academicians, researchers and scientists, who have contributed their research works for the realization of the book. This book has materialized in the wake of emerging advancements and innovations in this field. Therefore, the need of the hour was to compile all the required researches and disseminate the knowledge to a broad spectrum of people comprising of students, researchers and specialists of the field.

Helicobacter pylori is a gram-negative microaerophilic bacterium that is found in the stomach. It is associated with gastric ulcers, chronic gastritis, duodenal ulcers and stomach cancer. Almost 85% of the people infected by H. pylori do not experience symptoms and complications. Acute cases of infection may present themselves as an acute gastritis with nausea or abdominal pain. These symptoms may progress into chronic gastritis, nonulcer dyspepsia, nausea, stomach pains, bloating, belching and black stool. Infection with H. pylori is also associated with colorectal cancer and colorectal polyps. The testing for H. pylori may be done using both invasive and non-invasive methods. Stool antigen tests, blood antibody tests, carbon urea breath tests and endoscopic biopsy are the methods for detecting infections with H. pylori. Rising antibiotic resistance has also increased the demand for alternate therapeutic strategies, such as vaccinations. The standard first-line therapy for H. pylori infections consist of proton-pump inhibitors and antibiotics. This book includes some of the vital pieces of work being conducted across the world, on various topics related to Helicobacter pylori infection. It provides significant information on H. pylori to help develop a good understanding of its role in human diseases. The book is appropriate for students seeking detailed information in this domain as well as for experts.

At the end of the preface, I would like to thank the authors for their brilliant chapters and the publisher for guiding us all-through the making of the book till its final stage. Also, I would like to thank my family for providing the support and encouragement throughout my academic career and research projects.

Editor

Low prevalence of *H. pylori* Infection in HIV-Positive Patients in the Northeast of Brazil

Andréa BC Fialho[1], Manuel B Braga-Neto[1], Eder JC Guerra[2], André MN Fialho[1], Karine C Fernandes[1], Juliana LM Sun[1], Christianne FV Takeda[2], Cícero IS Silva[1], Dulciene MM Queiroz[3], Lucia LBC Braga[1*]

Abstract

Background: This study conducted in Northeastern Brazil, evaluated the prevalence of *H. pylori* infection and the presence of gastritis in HIV-infected patients.

Methods: There were included 113 HIV-positive and 141 age-matched HIV-negative patients, who underwent upper gastrointestinal endoscopy for dyspeptic symptoms. *H. pylori* status was evaluated by urease test and histology.

Results: The prevalence of *H. pylori* infection was significantly lower ($p < 0.001$) in HIV-infected (37.2%) than in uninfected (75.2%) patients. There were no significant differences between *H. pylori* status and gender, age, HIV viral load, antiretroviral therapy and the use of antibiotics. A lower prevalence of *H. pylori* was observed among patients with T CD4 cell count below $200/mm^3$; however, it was not significant. Chronic active antral gastritis was observed in 87.6% of the HIV-infected patients and in 780.4% of the control group ($p = 0.11$). *H. pylori* infection was significantly associated with chronic active gastritis in the antrum in both groups, but it was not associated with corpus chronic active gastritis in the HIV-infected patients.

Conclusion: We demonstrated that the prevalence of *H. pylori* was significantly lower in HIV-positive patients compared with HIV-negative ones. However, corpus gastritis was frequently observed in the HIV-positive patients, pointing to different mechanisms than *H. pylori* infection in the genesis of the lesion.

Background

Helicobacter pylori infection is the major etiologic factor of chronic gastritis and peptic ulcer in the general population. Gastrointestinal (GI) symptoms are frequent among patients infected with human immunodeficiency virus (HIV) and with acquired immunodeficiency syndrome (AIDS) [1,2] However, the role of *H. pylori* infection in the GI tract mucosa of HIV patients is not well defined [3]. Some studies suggested that interactions between the immune/inflammatory response, gastric physiology and host repair mechanisms play an important role in dictating the disease outcome in response to *H. pylori* infection, suggesting that the host's immune competence might be an important issue in *H. pylori* infection [4,5].

Data in regard to the prevalence of *H. pylori* infection in HIV-infected population are controversial. Some reports have shown that the rate of the infection in

HIV-positive patients is remarkably low when compared with the general population [6,7]. Conversely, other studies have not found similar results [8-10].

It is well known that the immune deficiencies caused by HIV give rise to many different gastrointestinal opportunistic infections, such as cytomegalovirus (CMV) infection and fungal esophagitis [11,12]. However, there are few studies evaluating the gastric mucosa of patients co-infected by *H. pylori* and HIV [13-15].

Therefore, the aim of this study was to evaluate the prevalence of *H. pylori* infection, risk factors associated with the infection, as well as the macroscopic and microscopic alterations of the gastric mucosa of HIV-infected patients in a high *H. pylori* prevalence area in Northeastern, Brazil.

Methods

The study was approved by the Ethical Committee of Research of the University of Ceará, and informed consent was obtained from each patient. This prospective cross-sectional study was carried out at the Hospital

* Correspondence: lucialib@terra.com.br
[1]Clinical Research Unity - Department of Internal Medicine - Federal University of Ceará, Fortaleza, Ceará, Brazil
Full list of author information is available at the end of the article

São José, a major referral center for assistance of
HIV-infected individuals in the city of Fortaleza, Ceará,
Brazil. From May 2001 to April 2003, 113 HIV-positive
patients who underwent upper gastrointestinal endoscopy for dyspeptic symptoms were included in the
study. The control group was composed by 141
HIV-negative patients who were undergoing upper gastrointestinal endoscopy for investigation of dyspeptic
symptoms at the University Hospital Walter Cantideo,
Fortaleza, Ceara, Brazil. Patients and age matched controls (interval of 10 years) were enrolled at the same
period. All patients gave written informed consent to
participate in the study and answered a questionnaire
about symptoms and consumption of medications,
including acid secretion inhibitors and antibiotics six
months before endoscopy. In the HIV-positive patient
group, data regarding the risk factors for HIV infection
and antiretroviral therapy were also obtained. Total
T CD4 cell count and HIV viral load were accepted as
valid if the blood sample for their determination had
been taken within 1 month before or after the entrance
in the study.

Upper gastrointestinal endoscopy
Gastro-endoscopy was performed with Olympus video
endoscopes (Olympus Optical Co, Ltd. GIF TYPE V) in
the standard manner. Fragments of the gastric mucosa
were obtained from the five sites recommended by the
Houston-updated Sydney system for classification of
gastritis and to evaluate the presence of spiral microorganism stained by Giemsa [16]. Two fragments from the
lesser curvature of the gastric antrum and two from the
lesser curvature of the lower gastric body were obtained
for urease test. The activity of chronic gastritis was
classified as mild, moderate and marked based on the
number of neutrophil infiltration. The specimens were
fixed in 10% formalin, embedded in paraffin wax, and
5-mm sections were stained with hematoxylin and eosin
for histology and with Giemsa staining to evaluate
H. pylori status.

Exclusion criteria included age below 18 years old or
above 80 years old, other serious medical problems, or
previous treatment for H. pylori infection. H. pylori
status was determined by the rapid urease test and histology (Giemsa staining) and was considered negative
when both tests were negative.

Statistical Analysis
Data were analyzed using the software SPSS (version 10.0,
Chicago, IL). Chi square test with Yates' correction or
Fischer's exact test were used to compare results among
the different groups. Significance was accepted at P values
below 0.05.

Results
Two hundred and fifty four subjects were included: 113
HIV-infected patients and 141 age-matched controls. The
mean age of HIV infected patients was 36.0 years (range,
21-70 years) and 61.9% (70/113) were male. The mean age
of the control group was 39.7 years (range 18-76 years)
and 36.2% (51/141) were male. Most of the symptoms of
HIV-positive patients were nonspecific, such as diarrhea,
dyspepsia, abdominal pain, nausea, vomiting, odynophagia
or dysphagia. The frequency of diarrhea, odynophagia, and
dysphagia was significantly higher in HIV-positive group
compared with the controls ($P < 0.05$).

Macroscopic lesions in the HIV-infected group
included, widespread esophageal candidiasis (32.7%;
37/113), esophageal ulcers (7.9%; 9/113) and candidiasis
plus esophageal ulcers (1.7%; 2/113). *Cryptosporidium*
was found in the gastric mucosa of two HIV-infected
patients. Table 1 shows the endoscopic gastric mucosal
findings in HIV-positive and HIV-negative dyspeptic
patients. Corpus gastritis was significantly more frequently observed in the dyspeptic HIV-positive than in
HIV-negative patients.

The overall prevalence of H. pylori infection was significantly lower (p < 0.001) in HIV-infected patients
(37.2%; 42/113) when compared with the controls
(75.2%; 106/141); and did not increase with age (p =
0.73). Of note, the infection prevalence in the oldest
group did not differ between HIV-positive and HIV-
negative patients. The prevalence of H. pylori infection
in the HIV-positive patients and controls according to
the age is shown in Figure 1.

In the HIV-positive group, there was no significant
difference between H. pylori status and gender, age, HIV
viral load, antiretroviral therapy and the use of antibiotics and H2-blocker. Only 4 patients referred the use of
proton pump inhibitors (PPI). A non-significant lower
prevalence of H. pylori infection was observed in the
patients with T CD4 cell count below 200 (Table 2).

**Table 1 Endoscopic findings of the gastroduodenal
mucosa of dyspeptic HIV-positive and negative patients**

Endoscopic findings	HIV + (n = 113)	HIV - (n = 141)	Total	p-value
	N (%)	N (%)	N	
Normal	0 (18.0)	30 (22.0)	50	0.57
Antral gastritis	44 (38.9)	41 (29.1)	85	0.10
Corpus Gastritis	42 (37.2)	25 (12.1)	67	<0.001
Pangastritis	3 (2.7)	0	3	0.05
Gastric erosion	16 (14.2)	27 (19.2)	43	0.29
Gastric ulcer	2 (1.7)	3 (2.1)	5	0.83
Duodenitis	5 (4.4)	2 (1.4)	7	0.15
Duodenal erosion	3 (2.7)	2 (1.4)	5	0.84

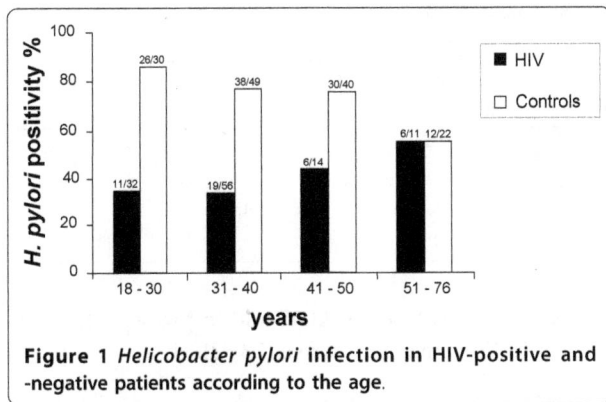

Figure 1 *Helicobacter pylori* infection in HIV-positive and -negative patients according to the age.

The gastric mucosa histological results are shown in Table 3. Chronic active antral gastritis was observed in 87.6% (99/113) of the HIV-infected patients and in 80.1% (113/141; p = 0.11) of the control group. *H. pylori* infection was significantly associated with the presence of chronic active antral gastritis in both groups (p = 0.03 and p < 0.001, respectively). No significant difference (p = 0.89) was also observed between the groups in respect to the frequency of chronic active corpus gastritis (53.1% in the HIV-positive patients and 53.9% in the HIV-negative patient). However, the *H. pylori* infection did not associate with chronic active corpus gastritis in the HIV-positive patients (p = 0.15), but high association was observed

Table 2 Covariates associated with *H. pylori* infection in HIV-positive patients

Variables	H. pylori + N (%)	Total	p-value
Gender			
Female	17 (39.5)	43	0.68
Male	25 (35.7)	70	
CD4 count			
≤200	17 (28.8)	59	0.06
>200	25 (46.3)	54	
Viral load			
<100.10^3	30 (42.8)	71	0.11
≥100. 10^3	12 (27.9)	42	
Antibiotics			
No	23 (44.2)	52	0.15
Yes	19 (31.1)	61	
Use of H2-blocker			
No	31 (38.3)	76	0.25
Yes	11 (16.6)	37	
Antifungic therapy			
No	36 (40.5)	87	0.09
Yes	6 (29.7)	26	
Antiretroviral therapy HAART			
No	12 (38.3)	42	0.15
Yes	30 (16.6)	71	

in the HIV-negative ones (p < 0.001). Additionally, in the HIV-negative group, the degree of gastritis was also associated with *H. pylori* infection, being the presence of the microorganism more frequently observed in the more marked (50%, 40/80) than in moderated (10%, 2/20) gastritis. Atrophy/intestinal metaplasia was observed less frequently in the gastric corpus of HIV-positive (6.2%, 7/113) than in the gastric corpus of HIV-negative (9.9%, 14/141) patients, but the differences were not significant (p = 0.27).

Discussion

The prevalence of *H. pylori* infection was lower in the HIV-positive group than in the age-matched controls. The low prevalence of *H. pylori* infection we observed in the HIV-positive patients differs profoundly from that previously reported (82.0%) in HIV-negative adults from a poor urban Community in the same city (Fortaleza; Brazil) [17]. A similar result has been observed in a cross-sectional study in Southeastern Brazil that evaluated the prevalence of *H. pylori* infection in 528 HIV-infected patients (32.38% of *H. pylori* positivity) [18]. Studies from East countries, where *H. pylori* infection is highly prevalent such as Taiwan [19] and China [20] also demonstrated a lower *H. pylori* infection prevalence (17.3% and 22.1%, respectively) in HIV-infected than in non-infected (63.5% and 44.8%, respectively) patients. Conversely, studies from Argentina and from India showed similar *H. pylori* infection prevalence in HIV-infected and non infected patients [13,21,22].

It has to be emphasized that *H. pylori* infection was diagnosed by histology and urease test in all patients. The results were concordant with those obtained by the evaluation of *H. pylori* specific *ure*A gene in the paraffin imbedded gastric tissue from a subgroup of patients (data not shown) and both HIV-positive and -negative patients belong to the same low-income population. As above mentioned, the prevalence of *H. pylori* infection in a similar population from Fortaleza in respect to the socio-economical level is high [17]. It is well known that *H. pylori* infection is mainly acquired during childhood and that once acquired it is life-long lasting [1]. Therefore, we may hypothesize that the HIV-infected patients we studied had been exposed to the bacterium early in life and most of them became infected, but loose the infection after acquired HIV infection. Alternatively, the *H. pylori* gastric load might be decreased in the HIV-positive patients leading to *H. pylori* infection misdiagnosis. Explanations include decreased gastric acid secretion predisposing to gastric colonization by other microorganisms that might compete with *H. pylori*, the use of either antibiotics or PPI and, as suggested in other studies, the low count of T CD4 cells in AIDS patients [6,21,23,24].

Table 3 Association between the frequency of *H. pylori* infection and antral and corpus active gastritis in HIV-infected patients and controls

	HIV-positive (n = 113)		HIV-negative (n = 141)		*p*-value
	HP+ (n = 42)	HP- (n = 71)	HP+ (n = 106)	HP- (n = 35)	
Chronic active antral gastritis	41 (97.6%)	58 (81.7%)	105 (99.1%)	8 (22.9%)	0.15
	p = 0.03		p < 0.001		
Chronic active corpus gastritis	26 (61.9%)	34 (47.9%)	69 (65.1%)	7 (20.0%)	0.89
	p = 0.15		p < 0.001		

It has been suggested that T CD4 cells play a role in inducing or perpetuating tissue and epithelial damage that may facilitate *H. pylori* colonization [25]. In this study, HIV-positive patients were stratified according to the T CD4 cell counts above or below 200 cells/mm3 and a tendency of lower prevalence of *H. pylori* infection was observed in the group of patients with T CD4 cell count of 200 or below.

Hypochlorhydria has been described in HIV-positive patients [23]. Previous studies have shown that HIV-positive patients with overt AIDS have significantly increased serum levels of gastrin and pepsinogen II compared with HIV-positive patients without overt AIDS [26]. Hypochlorhydria may provide a less suitable environment for *H. pylori* and predispose to overgrowth of other bacteria [27]. Inhibition of *H. pylori* by competition with other opportunistic pathogens such as Cytomegalovirus via unknown mechanisms has been also suggested [23,28]. The intragastric environment may be also modified by previous use of PPI. In this study; however, only four HIV-positive patients were under PPI therapy. The frequent usage of antibiotics for treatment or prophylaxis against opportunistic infections in patients at an advanced stage of HIV infection might explain the low prevalence of *H. pylori* infection in the patient group. However, the antibiotics most commonly used in AIDS patients are not always efficacious against *H. pylori*. Furthermore, low *H. pylori* eradication ratio is observed with the use of mono therapy, even with clarithromycin that has a good anti-*H. pylori* activity [29].

An interesting finding observed in this study was the presence of active chronic gastritis in the gastric body of HIV-positive patients independently of the *H. pylori* positivity, in agreement with the studies of Welage et al.; Marano et al., and Mach et al. [23,30,31], which; however, was not observed by others [6,32]. Otherwise, in this study, the *H. pylori* status was significantly associated with the presence of active chronic gastritis in the antral gastric mucosa of HIV-positive and -negative patients. Taking together the data, it is possible that different mechanisms participate in the development of corpus chronic active gastritis in HIV-positive patients. Therefore, other microorganisms such as Cytomegalovirus or

some drugs used to treat AIDS and to prevent opportunistic infections may play a role [18,33].

Conclusion

Although the prevalence of *H. pylori* infection in HIV-positive patients was lower than in HIV-negative ones, the presence of chronic active gastritis was similarly high either in HIV-positive or -negative patients, which points to the possibility that other mechanisms than *H. pylori* infection are involved in the genesis of corpus gastritis in HIV positive patients.

Author details
[1]Clinical Research Unity - Department of Internal Medicine - Federal University of Ceará, Fortaleza, Ceará, Brazil. [2]Laboratory of Bacteriology Research - Federal University of Minas Gerais, Belo Horizonte, Minas Gerais, Brazil. [3]São José Hospital, Fortaleza, Ceará, Brazil.

Authors' contributions
EG: participated in the conception, performed the endoscopies, and helped writing the manuscript. MB and ABN participated in the statistical analysis, interpretation and critical writing of the manuscript. AMN: participated in implementation of the study, data collection, database management and statistical analysis. CT and CS: participated in design and implementation of the study. KC, JS and IS: participated in implementation of the study, data collection IM: statistical analysis, interpretation and writing the manuscript. DQ: performed critical writing and reviewing LB: participated in conception, design, implementation, coordination of the study and critical writing and reviewing. All authors have read and approved the final manuscript.

Competing interests
The authors declare that they have no competing interests.

References
1. Peterson WL: **Helicobacter pylori and peptic ulcer disease.** *N Engl J Med* 1991, **324:**1043-1048.
2. Dooley CP, Cohen H, Fitzgibbons PL: **Prevalence of *Helicobacter pylori* infection and histologic gastritis in asymptomatic persons.** *N Engl J Med* 1989, **321:**1562-1566.
3. Romanelli F, Smith KM, Murphy BS: **Does HIV infection alter the incidence or pathology of *Helicobacter pylori* infection?** *AIDS Patient Care and STDs* 2007, **21(12):**908-919.
4. Bamford KB, Fan X, Crowe S: **Lymphocytes in the human gastric mucosa during *Helicobacter pylori* have a T helper cell 1 phenotype.** *Gastroenterology* 1998, **114:**482-492.
5. Moran AP, Svennerholm AM, Penn CW: **Pathogenesis and host response of Helicobacter pylori.** *Trends Microbiol* 2002, **10(12):**545-7.
6. Edwards PD, Carrick J, Turner J, Lee A, Mitchell H, Cooper DA: **Helicobacter pylori-associated gastritis is rare in AIDS: antibiotic effect or a**

consequence of immunodeficiency? *Am J Gastroenterol* 1991, **86**:1761-1764.

7. Francis ND, Logan RP, Walker MM, Polson RJ, Boylston AW, Pinching AJ, Harris JR, Baron JH: **Campylobacter pylori in the upper GI tract of the patients with HIV-1 infection.** *J Clin Pathol* 1990, **43**:60-2.

8. Sud A, Ray P, Bhasin D, Wanchu A, Bambery P, Singh S: **Helicobacter pylori in Indian HIV infected patients.** *Trop Gastroenterol* 2002, **23(2)**:79-81.

9. Olmos M, Araya V, Pskorz E, Quesada EC, Concetti H, Perez H, Cahn P: **Coinfection: Helicobacter pylori/human immunodeficiency virus.** *Dig Dis Sci* 2004, **49**:1836-39.

10. Alimohamed F, Lule GN, Nyong'o A, Bwayo J, Rana FS: **Prevalence of Helicobacter pylori and endoscopic findings in HIV seropositive patients with upper gastrointestinal tract symptoms at Kenyatta national hospital, Nairobi.** *East Afr Med J* 2002, **79**:226-231.

11. Francis ND, Boylston AW, Roberts AH, Parkin JM, Pinching AJ: **Cytomegalovirus infection in gastrointestinal tracts of patients infected with HIV-1 or AIDS.** *J Clin Pathol* 1989, **42**:1055-1064.

12. Dieterich DT, Wilcox CM: **Diagnosis and treatment of esophageal diseases associated with HIV infection. Practice Parameters Committee of the American College of Gastroenterology.** *Am J Gastroenterol* 1996, **91**:2265-2269.

13. Sud A, Ray P, Bhasin D, Wanchu A, Bambery P, Singh S: **Helicobacter pylori in Indian HIV infected patients.** *Trop Gastroenterol* 2002, **23(2)**:79-81.

14. Battan R, Raviglione MC, Palagiano A, Boyle JF, Sabatini MT, Sayad K, Ottaviano LJ: *Helicobacter pylori* **infection in patients with acquired immune deficiency syndrome.** *Am J Gastroenterol* 1990, **85**:1576-1579.

15. Lim SG, Lipman MC, Squire S, Pillay D, Gillespie S, Sankey EA, Dhillon AP, Johnson MA, Lee CA, Pounder RE: **Audit of endoscopic surveillance biopsy specimens in HIV positive patients with gastrointestinal symptoms.** *Gut* 1993, **34(10)**:1429-32.

16. Dixon MF, Path FRC, Genta RM, Yardley JH, Correa P: **Classification and grading of gastritis. The updated Sydney system. International workshop on the histopathology of gastritis, Houston 1994.** *Am J Surg Pathol* 1996, **20**:1161-81.

17. Rodrigues MN, Queiroz DM, Rodrigues RT, Rocha AM, Braga Neto MB, Braga LL: **Helicobacter pylori infection in adults from a poor urban community in northeastern Brazil: demographic, lifestyle and environmental factors.** *Braz J Infect Dis* 2005, **9(5)**:405-10.

18. Werneck-Silva AL, Prado IB: **Dyspepsia in HIV-infected patients under highly active antiretroviral therapy.** *J Gastroenterol Hepatol* 2007, **22(11)**:1712-1716.

19. Chiu HM, Wu MS, Hung CC, Shun CT, Lin JT: **Low prevalence of Helicobacter pylori but high prevalence of cytomegalovirus associated peptic ulcer disease in AIDS patients: Comparative study of symptomatic subjects evaluated by endoscopy and CD4 counts.** *J Gastroenterol Hepatol* 2004, **19(4)**:423-428.

20. Fu-Jing LV, Xiao-Lan Luo, Meng Xin, Rui Jin, Ding Hui-Guo, Shu-Tian Zhang: **A low prevalence of H pylori and endoscopic findings in HIVpositive Chinese patients with gastrointestinal symptoms.** *World J Gastroenterol* 2007, **13(41)**:5492-5496.

21. Olmos M, Araya V, Pskorz E, Quesada EC, Concetti H, Perez H, Cahn P: **Coinfection: Helicobacter pylori/human immunodeficiency virus.** *Dig Dis Sci* 2004, **49**:1836-39.

22. Alimohamed F, Lule GN, Nyong'o A, Bwayo J, Rana FS: **Prevalence of Helicobacter pylori and endoscopic findings in HIV seropositive patients with upper gastrointestinal tract symptoms at Kenyatta national hospital, Nairobi.** *East Afr Med J* 2002, **79**:226-231.

23. Welage LS, Carver PL, Revankar S, Pierson C, Kauffman CA: **Alterations in gastric acidity in patients infected with human immunodeficiency virus.** *Clin Infect Dis* 1995, **21**:1431-8.

24. Lichterfeld M, Lorenz C, Nischalke HD, Scheurlen C, Sauerbruch T, Rockstroh JK: **Decreased prevalence of Helicobacter pylori infection in HIV patients with AIDS defining diseases.** *Z Gastroenterol* 2002, **40**:11-4.

25. Bontems P, Fabienne R, Van Gossum A, Cadranel S, Mascart F: *Helicobacter pylori* **modulation of gastric and duodenal mucosal T cell cytokine secretions in children compared with adults.** *Helicobacter* 2003, **8(3)**:216-226.

26. Fabris P, Pilotto A, Bozzola L, Tositti G, Soffiatis G, Manfrin V: **Serum pepsinogen and gastrin levels in HIV-positive patients: relationship with CD4+ cell count and Helicobacter pylori infection.** *Aliment Pharmacol Ther* 2002, **16**:807-11.

27. Lake-Bakaar G, Quadros E, Beidas S, Elsakr M, Tom W, Wilson DE, Dincsoy HP, Cohen P, Straus EW: **Gastric secretory failure in patients with the acquired immunodeficiency syndrome (AIDS).** *Ann Intern Med* 1988, **109**:502-4.

28. Shaffer RT, LaHatte LJ, Kelly JW, Kadakia S, Carrougher JG, Keate RF, Starnes EC: **Gastric acid secretion in HIV-1 infection.** *Am J Gastroenterol* 1992, **12**:1777-80.

29. Peterson WL, Graham DY, Marshall B, Blaser MJ, Genta RM, Klein PD, Stratton CW, Drnec J, Prokocimer P, Siepman N: **Clarithromycin as monotherapy for eradication of Helicobacter pylori: a randomized, double-blind trial.** *Am J Gastroenterol* 1993, **88**:1860-4.

30. Marano B, Smith F, Bonanno C: **Helicobacter pylori prevalence in acquired immunodeficiency syndrome.** *Am J Gastroenterol* 1993, **88(5)**:687-690.

31. Mach T, Skwara P, Biesiada G, Cieśla A, Macura : **Morphological changes of the upper gastrointestinal tract mucosa and Helicobacter pylori infection in HIV-positive patients with severe immunodeficiency and symptoms of dyspepsia.** *Med Sci Monit* 2007, **13(1)**:14-19.

32. Skwara P, Mach T, Tomaszewska R: **Morphological changes of gastric mucosa in HIV-infected patients.** *HIV&AIDS Review* 2002, **2**:47-51.

33. Rossi P, Rivasi F, Codeluppi M, Catania A, Tamburrini A, Righi E, Pozio E: **Gastric involvement in AIDS associated cryptosporidiosis.** *Gut* 1998, **43**:476-77.

2

Long-term follow up *Helicobacter Pylori* reinfection rate after second-line treatment: bismuth-containing quadruple therapy versus moxifloxacin-based triple therapy

Min Soo Kim[1], Nayoung Kim[1,2]*, Sung Eun Kim[1], Hyun Jin Jo[1], Cheol Min Shin[1], Young Soo Park[1,2] and Dong Ho Lee[1,2]

Abstract

Background: The increasing trend of antibiotic resistance requires effective second-line *Helicobacter pylori* (*H. pylori*) treatment in high prevalence area of *H. pylori*. The aim of our study was to evaluate the reinfection rate of *H. pylori* after second-line treatment that would determine the long-term follow up effect of the rescue therapy.

Methods: A total of 648 patients who had failed previous *H. pylori* eradication on standard triple therapy were randomized into two regimens: 1, esomeprazole (20 mg b.i.d), tripotassium dicitrate bismuthate (300 mg q.i.d), metronidazole (500 mg t.i.d), and tetracycline (500 mg q.i.d) (EBMT) or 2, moxifloxacin (400 mg q.d.), esomeprazole (20 mg b.i.d), and amoxicillin (1000 mg b.i.d.) (MEA). At four weeks after completion of eradication therapy, *H. pylori* tests were performed with ^{13}C urea breath test or invasive tests. In patients who maintained continuous *H. pylori* negativity for the first year after eradication therapy, *H. pylori* status was assessed every year. For the evaluation of risk factors of reinfection, gender, age, clinical diagnosis, histological atrophic gastritis or intestinal metaplasia were analyzed.

Results: The recrudescence rate of the EBMT was 1.7% and of the MEA group 3.3% ($p = 0.67$). The annual reinfection rate of *H. pylori* of EBMT was found to be 4.45% and the MEA group 6.46%. Univariate analysis (Log-rank test) showed no association with any clinical risk factor for reinfection.

Conclusions: The long-term reinfection rate of *H. pylori* stayed low in both of bismuth-containing quadruple therapy and moxifloxacin-based triple therapy; thus reinfection cannot affect the choice of second-line treatment.

Keywords: *Helicobacter pylori*, Reinfection, Quadruple, Moxifloxacin, Second-line

Background

Helicobacter *pylori* (*H. pylori*) is a common pathogen of the gastric mucosa. It is estimated that at least 50% of the world's human population has *H. pylori* infection [1]. Since the majority of patients with *H. pylori* infection do not have any related clinical disease, routine screening is not considered [2]. However, as the current evidence suggests that *H. pylori* play a major role in peptic ulcer disease, gastric MALT lymphoma and in gastric cancer [3], screening and treatment in these diseases are recommended in several guidelines [2,4-7]. In addition, European guidelines recommend eradicating *H. pylori* infection in first-degree relatives of patients with gastric cancer, in long term NSAIDS or acid suppression users and in patients with functional dyspepsia [4]. According to these guidelines, public health efforts toward eradication will be more effective in *H. pylori* high prevalence areas. Naturally, it is expected that increasing use of antibiotics must lead

* Correspondence: nayoungkim49@empas.com
[1]Department of Internal Medicine, Seoul National University Bundang Hospital, Seongnam, Gyeonggi-do, South Korea
[2]Department of Internal Medicine and Liver Research Institute, Seoul National University College of Medicine, Seoul, South Korea

to increased resistance of antibiotics. Currently, the most commonly used initial treatment is a triple regimen combining a proton pump inhibitor (PPI) with two antibiotics (clarithromycin and amoxicillin/or metronidazole) for the eradication of *H. pylori* [2,4-7]. Although this regimen has been shown to be effective in numerous clinical trials, the most recent data show that the eradication rate has declined to less than 80% worldwide, largely related to development of resistance to clarithromycin [8]. In Korea, the recent eradication rate of this regimen was less than 80% in a long-term follow up study (≥ 5 years) [9,10]. Therefore, this decreasing eradication rate requires effective second-line treatment. Many clinicians have been using second-line therapy with bismuth-containing quadruple therapy or including fluoroquinolone antibiotics such as levofloxacin and moxifloxacin.

In this situation, reinfection of *H. pylori* will determine the long-term effect of the eradication therapy for *H. pylori*. If a regimen shows a high reinfection rate, then this eradication therapy should be avoided or strictly used only when absolutely indicated for *H. pylori* eradication. We reported the long-term annual reinfection rate of *H. pylori* in standard PPI-based triple therapy to be 3.51% per year in Korea [11]. Now that second-line therapy is frequently used there is increasing interest regarding the reinfection and recrudescence rates after rescue therapy. However, there are few reports regarding the reinfection rate of *H. pylori* after quadruple therapy [12] and none for quinolone based triple therapy. From this background the aim of our study was to evaluate the reinfection rate of *H. pylori* after two kinds of second-line treatment over a long-term follow up period.

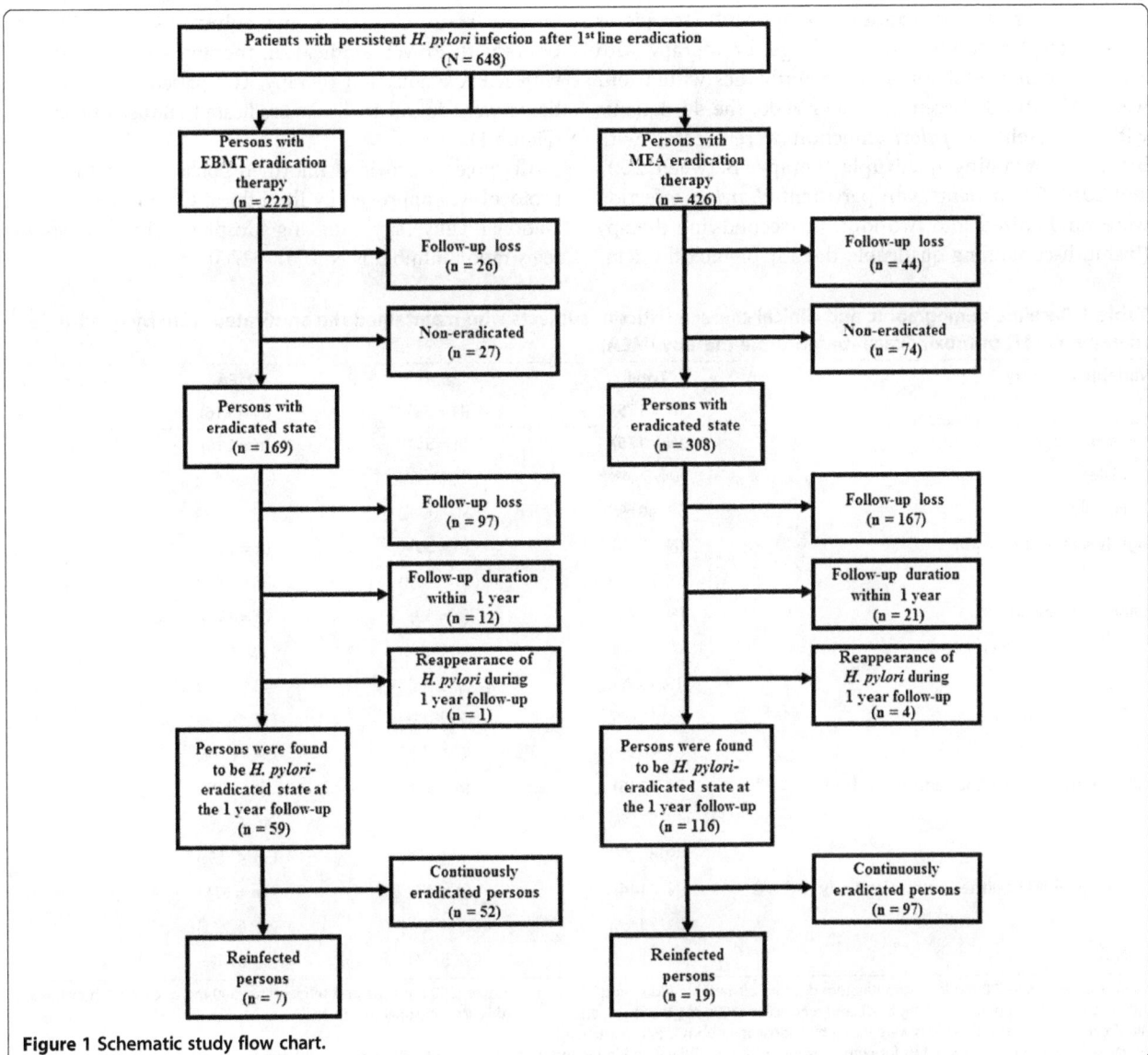

Figure 1 Schematic study flow chart.

In addition, we investigated the risk factors for reinfection after this second-line treatment.

Methods

Study population

The schematic flow of this study is shown in Figure 1. This was a prospective study performed between 2003 and 2010 at Seoul National University Bundang Hospital in Korea. A total of 648 patients with persistent *H. pylori* infection after first-line treatment (PPI-based triple therapy) were enrolled. PPI-based triple therapy included PPI (standard dose), amoxicillin 1 g, and clarithromycin 500 mg, all twice daily, for 7 days. Patients were considered persistent *H. pylori* infection if ^{13}C-urea breath test (UBT) or invasive *H. pylori* test (Giemsa histology, CLO test, culture) were positive despite PPI-based triple therapy. Patients were excluded from the study if they had a history of renal or hepatic impairment, previous gastric surgery, pregnancy or lactation, therapy with steroids or non-steroidal anti-inflammatory drugs, or therapy with a proton pump inhibitor (PPI) or antibiotics within four weeks of entry. Between 2003 and 2006, the 44 patients with persistent *H. pylori* infection were treated with bismuth-containing quadruple therapy. Between 2007 and 2010, 604 patients with persistent *H. pylori* infection were randomized into two kinds of second-line therapy (bismuth-containing quadruple therapy or moxifloxacin-based triple therapy). However, if the patient preferred one regimen, after sufficient information for side effect and eradication rate of each regimen a change was permitted. Finally, 222 patients were treated for 14 days with esomeprazole 20 mg b.i.d, tripotassium dicitrate bismuthate 300 mg q.i.d, metronidazole 500 mg t.i.d, and tetracycline 500 mg q.i.d (EBMT) as second-line treatment regimen for *H. pylori* infection. 426 patients were treated for 14 days with moxifloxacin 400 mg q.d, esomeprazole 20 mg b.i.d, and amoxicillin 1000 mg b.i.d (MEA) as second-line treatment regimen for *H. pylori* infection. At four weeks after completion of the second-line treatment, *H. pylori* eradication was evaluated by ^{13}C-UBT or invasive tests. Invasive tests were performed in the patients in whom follow up endoscopic examination was necessary for peptic ulcer, adenoma or gastric cancer. *H. pylori* negative status after eradication was defined as a negative ^{13}C-UBT or all negative of Giemsa stain, CLO test, and culture. Among 222 patients with EBMT eradication therapy and 426 patients with MEA eradication therapy, 169 patients and 308 patients were found to be in eradicated status, respectively (Figure 1).

All subjects provided informed consent, and the study protocol was approved by the Ethical Committee at Seoul National University Bundang Hospital. ClinicalTrials.gov registration number is NCT01792700.

Table 1 Baseline demographic and clinical characteristics of subjects who maintained the eradicated state by quadruple therapy (EBMT) or moxifloxacin-based triple therapy (MEA)

Variable category	Total (N = 175)	EBMT (N = 59)	MEA (N = 116)	p-value[*]
Gender	(N = 175)	(n = 59)	(n = 116)	
Male	(104, 59.4%)	(35, 59.3%)	(69, 59.5%)	0.98
Female	(71, 40.6%)	(24, 40.7%)	(47, 40.5%)	
Age (years) (mean ± SD)	(N = 175)	(n = 59)	(n = 116)	0.67
	(56.6 ± 9.4)	(56.1 ± 9.3)	(56.8 ± 9.5)	
Clinical diagnosis	(N = 175)	(n = 59)	(n = 116)	
Early gastric cancer	(40, 22.9%)	(11, 18.6%)	(29, 25.0%)	0.06
Dysplasia	(19, 10.9%)	(3, 5.1%)	(16, 13.8%)	
Peptic ulcer disease	(34, 19.4%)	(17, 28.8%)	(17, 14.7%)	
Chronic gastritis	(82, 46.9%)	(28, 47.5%)	(54, 46.6%)	
Histological AG in either antrum or body	(N = 116)	(n = 37)	(n = 79)	
Yes	(67, 57.8%)	(21, 56.8%)	(46, 68.7%)	0.88
No	(49, 42.2%)	(16, 43.2%)	(33, 41.8%)	
Histological IM in either antrum or body	(N = 144)	(n = 47)	(n = 97)	
Yes	(84, 58.3%)	(23, 48.9%)	(61, 62.9%)	0.11
No	(60, 41.7%)	(24, 51.1%)	(36, 37.1%)	

EBMT: esomeprazole (20 mg b.i.d), tripotassium dicitrate bismuthate (300 mg q.i.d), metronidazole (500 mg t.i.d), and tetracycline (500 mg q.i.d); *MEA*: moxifloxacin (400 mg q.d.), esomeprazole (20 mg b.i.d), and amoxicillin (1000 mg b.i.d.); *AG*, atrophic gastritis, *IM*, intestinal metaplasia.
All of early gastric cancer patients were cured by endoscopic submucosal dissection.
*p-value for Pearson chi-square test for comparison of categorical data, and independent samples t-test for comparison of age.

Invasive *Helicobacter pylori* test (Giemsa histology, CLO test, and culture) and histology

To determine the presence of current *H. pylori* infection, 10 biopsy specimens were taken from the gastric mucosa at each endoscopy (two biopsy specimens each from the greater curvature of the antrum and body, and three each from the lesser curvature of the antrum and body). Among them, four biopsy specimens (one each from the greater curvature and lesser curvature of the antrum and body) were fixed in formalin, and used for determination of *H. pylori* infection by Giemsa staining. Another four specimens from the four gastric mucosa areas mentioned above were used for *H. pylori* culturing. The remaining two specimens from the lesser curvature of the antrum and body were used for the rapid urease test (CLO test; Delta West, Bentley, Australia).

Four of the biopsy specimens used for determination of *H. pylori* infection were also used for histological evaluation. These specimens were examined for the presence of gastric atrophy and intestinal metaplasia by H&E staining. The presence of atrophy on any of four specimens was diagnosed as gastric atrophy, and the same method was applied to intestinal metaplasia. The definition of atrophy is the loss of appropriate glands including both metaplastic and non-metaplastic atrophy. Both metaplastic and non-metaplastic atrophy can be allocated to one of three grades of severity using grading criteria modeled on those suggested by the original and the updated Sydney System [13].

[13]C-urea breath test

Patients fasted for 4 h before testing. Then, 100 mg of ^{13}C-urea powder (UBiTkit; Otsuka Pharmaceutical,

Table 2 Baseline demographic and clinical characteristics of study subjects depending on reinfection

Variable category	EBMT				MEA			
	Total (59, 100%)	Reinfected group (7, 11.9%)	Continuously eradicated group (52, 88.1%)	p-value*	Total (116, 100%)	Reinfected group (19, 16.4%)	Continuously eradicated group (97, 83.6%)	p-value*
Gender	(N = 59)	(n = 7)	(n = 52)		(N = 116)	(n = 19)	(n = 97)	
Male	(35, 59.3%)	(4, 57.1%)	(31, 59.6%)	0.816	(69, 59.5%)	(12, 63.2%)	(57, 58.8%)	0.353
Female	(24, 40.7%)	(3, 42.9%)	(21, 40.4%)		(47, 40.5%)	(7, 36.8%)	(40, 41.2%)	
Age (mean ± SD)	(N = 59)	(n = 7)	(n = 52)		(N = 116)	(n = 19)	(n = 97)	
	(56.1 ± 9.3)	(59.9 ± 9.8)	(55.6 ± 9.2)		(56.8 ± 9.5)	(56.7 ± 9.4)	(56.8 ± 9.6)	
20-29	(1, 1.7%)	(0, 0.0%)	(1, 1.9%)	0.306	(1, 0.9%)	(0, 0.0%)	(1, 1.0%)	0.479
30-39	(1, 1.7%)	(0, 0.0%)	(1, 1.9%)		(3, 2.6%)	(0, 0.0%)	(3, 3.1%)	
40-49	(13, 22.0%)	(2, 22.2%)	(11, 21.2%)		(21, 18.1%)	(6, 31.6%)	(15, 15.5%)	
50-59	(21, 35.6%)	(1, 14.3%)	(20, 38.5%)		(40, 34.5%)	(5, 26.3%)	(35, 36.1%)	
60-69	(20, 33.9%)	(3, 42.9%)	(17, 32.7%)		(42, 36.2%)	(6, 31.6%)	(36, 37.1%)	
70-79	(3, 5.1%)	(1, 14.3%)	(2, 3.8%)		(8, 10.5%)	(2, 10.5%)	(6, 6.2%)	
80-89	(0, 0.0%)	(0, 0.0%)	(0, 0.0%)		(1, 0.6%)	(0, 0.0%)	(1, 1.0%)	
Clinical diagnosis	(N = 59)	(n = 7)	(n = 52)		(N = 116)	(n = 19)	(n = 97)	
Early gastric cancer	(11, 18.6%)	(0, 0.0%)	(11, 21.2%)	0.198	(29, 25.0%)	(7, 36.8%)	(22, 22.7%)	0.77
Dysplasia	(3, 5.1%)	(1, 14.3%)	(2, 3.8%)		(16, 13.8%)	(3, 15.8%)	(13, 13.4%)	
Peptic ulcer disease	(17, 28.8%)	(4, 57.1%)	(13, 25.0%)		(17, 14.7%)	(3, 15.8%)	(14, 14.4%)	
Chronic gastritis	(28, 47.5%)	(2, 28.6%)	(26, 50.0%)		(54, 46.6%)	(6, 31.6%)	(48, 49.5%)	
Histological AG in either antrum or body	(N = 37)	(n =6)	(n = 31)		(N = 79)	(n = 14)	(n = 65)	
Yes	(21, 56.8%)	(5, 83.3%)	(16, 51.6%)	0.113	(46, 58.2%)	(9, 64.3%)	(37, 56.9%)	0.575
No	(16, 43.2%)	(1, 16.7%)	(15, 48.4%)		(33, 41.8%)	(5, 35.7%)	(28, 43.1%)	
Histological IM in either antrum or body	(N = 47)	(n = 6)	(n = 41)		(N = 97)	(n = 15)	(n = 82)	
Yes	(23, 48.9%)	(4, 66.7%)	(21, 51.2%)	0.193	(61, 62.9%)	(8, 53.3%)	(53, 64.6%)	0.52
No	(24, 51.1%)	(2, 33.3%)	(20, 48.8%)		(36, 37.1%)	(7, 46.7%)	(29, 35.4%)	

EBMT: esomeprazole (20 mg b.i.d), tripotassium dicitrate bismuthate (300 mg q.i.d), metronidazole (500 mg t.i.d), and tetracycline (500 mg q.i.d); *MEA*: moxifloxacin (400 mg q.d.), esomeprazole (20 mg b.i.d), and amoxicillin (1000 mg b.i.d.); *AG*, atrophic gastritis; *IM*, intestinal metaplasia.
All of early gastric cancer patients were cured by endoscopic submucosal dissection.
* P-value for Log-rank test.

Table 3 Reinfection and recrudescence rate of *Helicobacter pylori*

Variable category	E B M T group	M E A group	p-value[*]
Recrudescence	(n = 60)	(n = 120)	
Yes	1 (1.7%)	4 (3.3%)	0.67
No	59 (98.3%)	116 (96.7%)	
Reinfection	(n = 59)	(n = 116)	
Yes	7 (11.9%)	19 (16.4%)	0.43
No	52 (88.1%)	97 (83.6%)	

EBMT: esomeprazole (20 mg b.i.d), tripotassium dicitrate bismuthate (300 mg q.i.d), metronidazole (500 mg t.i.d), and tetracycline (500 mg q.i.d); *MEA*: moxifloxacin (400 mg q.d.), esomeprazole (20 mg b.i.d), and amoxicillin (1000 mg b.i.d.).
* P-value for Pearson chi-square test or Fisher's exact test for comparison of categorical data.

Tokyo, Japan) was dissolved in 100 mL water and administered orally; a second breath sample was collected 20 min later. The collected samples were analyzed using an isotope-selective, non-dispersive infrared spectrometer (UBiT-IR300; Otsuka Pharmaceutical). The cutoff value used for *H. pylori* eradication was 2.5‰.

Follow-up of *H. pylori* tests

All of the eradicated patients received gastroscopy with invasive tests (modified Giemsa stain and CLO test) not only from greater and lesser curvature of antrum but also from body after 1 year. If any one of these tests were positive then the patient was regarded as recrudescence case. After this time the patients were followed up for one year with gastroscopy with invasive tests. However, when the patients preferred ^{13}C-UBT or wanted to receive the gastroscopy every other year it was also accepted because the Korea government national health

insurance program recommends biannual endoscopy instead of one year.

Statistical analysis

The annual reinfection rate (percentage per year) of *H. pylori* was calculated as (total number of infected patients/ cumulative observation years for all patients) X 100.

SPSS for Windows (version 18.0; SPSS, Inc., an IBM Company, Chicago, Illinois, USA) was used for all statistical analyses. Categorical variables were analyzed using the Pearson chi-square test or Fisher's exact test, and continuous variables were analyzed using independent samples *t*-test. The risk of *H. pylori* reinfection with time was estimated using the Kaplan-Meier method. To determine the risk factors for reinfection, we used the log-rank test. Null hypotheses of no difference were rejected if *p*-values were less than 0.05.

Results

Patient characteristics

Among eradicated 169 patients in the EBMT group and eradicated 308 patients in the MEA group, 59 patients and 116 patients maintained *H. pylori*-negative status continuously for one year, respectively (Figure 1). Specifically, 110 patients dropped out in the EBMT group and 192 in the MEA group for the following three reasons: 97 patients in the EBMT group and 167 in the MEA group for not returning for gastroscopy or ^{13}C-UBT after treatment, 12 in the EBMT group and 21 in the MEA group for follow-up duration within 1 year, 1 patient in the EBMT group and 4 in the MEA group for reappearance of *H. pylori* during 1 year follow-up. Finally, 59 patients and 116 patients in each group

Table 4 Annual reinfection rate of *Helicobacter pylori*

	Follow up period	No. of patients	Mean no. of *H. pylori* test	No. of reinfected patients	Patient-years (yr)	Annual reinfection rate (%)
	1 ≤ year <2	23	1.39	3	33.08	9.07
E	2 ≤ year <3	18	2.22	3	42.25	7.10
B	3 ≤ year <4	5	2.00	0	16.58	0
M	4 ≤ year <5	8	2.63	0	34.67	0
T	5 ≤ year <6	3	6.00	1	16.58	6.03
	6 ≤ year <7	1	5.00	0	6.5	0
	7 ≤ year <8	1	5.00	0	7.5	0
	Total	**59**	**2.05**	**7**	**157.17**	**4.45**
	1 ≤ year <2	39	1.36	8	54.12	14.78
M	2 ≤ year <3	37	2.05	8	91.75	8.72
E	3 ≤ year <4	30	3.67	1	104.58	0.96
A	4 ≤ year <5	10	3.80	2	43.33	4.62
	Total	**116**	**2.31**	**19**	**294.08**	**6.46**

EBMT: esomeprazole (20 mg b.i.d), tripotassium dicitrate bismuthate (300 mg q.i.d), metronidazole (500 mg t.i.d), and tetracycline (500 mg q.i.d); *MEA*: moxifloxacin (400 mg q.d.), esomeprazole (20 mg b.i.d), and amoxicillin (1000 mg b.i.d.).

maintained *H. pylori*-negative continuously at one year. The demographic and clinical characteristics of two study groups, who maintained *H. pylori*-negative continuously at one year after the EBMT or MEA therapy, are summarized in Table 1. Gender, the mean age of the patients, clinical diagnosis, atrophic gastritis, and intestinal metaplasia of the two were similar. The enrolled early gastric cancer patients were cured by endoscopic submucosal dissection and follow-up was continuously performed regularly. During long-term follow-up patients in the EBMT or in the MEA group were divided into two groups: reinfected group and continuously eradicated group. The demographic and clinical characteristics of the reinfected and continuously eradicated group are summarized in Table 2. In the EBMT group and

MEA group, there was no significant evidence that re-infection of *H. pylori* was related with gender, the mean age of the patients, clinical diagnosis, atrophic gastritis, and intestinal metaplasia. The *H. pylori* recrudescence and reinfection rates are shown in Table 3. One patient in the EBMT group and four patients in the MEA group, who were *H. pylori* positive again at 1 year follow-up, were assigned to recrudescence cases. The rate was calculated at 1.7% (1/60) for the EBMT group and 3.3% (4/120) for the MEA group, and these percentages were not significantly different ($p = 0.67$). During long-term follow-up 1 year after eradication *H. pylori* reappeared in 7 (11.9%) of EBMT group and in 19 (16.4%) of MEA group and these percentages were not significantly different depending on each rescue treatment ($p = 0.43$). Among the

Table 5 Baseline characteristics of study subjects

Variable category	Total (175, 100%)	Reinfected group (26, 14.9%)	Continuously eradicated group (149, 85.1%)	p-value[*]
Gender	(N = 175)	(n = 26)	(n = 149)	
Male	(104, 59.4%)	(16, 61.5%)	(88, 59.1%)	0.75
Female	(71, 40.6%)	(10, 38.5%)	(61, 40.9%)	
Age (years) (mean ± SD)	(N = 175)	(n = 26)	(n = 149)	
	(56.6 ± 9.4)	(57.6 ± 9.4)	(56.4 ± 9.5)	
20-29	(2, 1.1%)	(0, 0.0%)	(2, 1.3%)	0.47
30-39	(4, 2.3%)	(0, 0.0%)	(4, 2.7%)	
40-49	(34, 19.4%)	(8, 30.8%)	(26, 17.4%)	
50-59	(61, 34.9%)	(6, 23.1%)	(55, 36.9%)	
60-69	(62, 35.4%)	(9, 34.6%)	(53, 35.6%)	
70-79	(11, 6.3%)	(3, 11.5%)	(8, 5.4%)	
80-89	(1, 0.6%)	(0, 0.0%)	(1, 0.7%)	
Clinical diagnosis	(N = 175)	(n = 26)	(n = 149)	
Early gastric cancer	(40, 22.9%)	(7, 26.9%)	(33, 22.1%)	0.74
Dysplasia	(19, 10.9%)	(4, 15.4%)	(15, 10.1%)	
Peptic ulcer disease	(34, 19.4%)	(7, 26.9%)	(27, 18.1%)	
Chronic gastritis	(82, 46.9%)	(8, 30.8%)	(74, 49.7%)	
Histological AG in either antrum or body	(N = 116)	(n = 20)	(n = 96)	
Yes	(67, 57.8%)	(14, 70.0%)	(53, 55.2%)	0.14
No	(49, 42.2%)	(6, 30.0%)	(43, 44.8%)	
Histological IM in either antrum or body	(N = 144)	(n = 21)	(n = 123)	
Yes	(84, 58.3%)	(10, 47.6%)	(74, 60.2%)	0.20
No	(60, 41.7%)	(11, 52.4%)	(49, 39.8%)	
Regimen	(N = 175)	(n = 26)	(n = 149)	
EBMT	(59, 33.7%)	(7, 26.9%)	(52, 34.9%)	0.23
MEA	(116, 66.3%)	(19, 73.1%)	(97, 65.1%)	

EBMT: esomeprazole (20 mg b.i.d), tripotassium dicitrate bismuthate (300 mg q.i.d), metronidazole (500 mg t.i.d), and tetracycline (500 mg q.i.d); *MEA*: moxifloxacin (400 mg q.d.), esomeprazole (20 mg b.i.d), and amoxicillin (1000 mg b.i.d.); *AG*, atrophic gastritis; *IM*, intestinal metaplasia.
All of early gastric cancer patients were cured by endoscopic submucosal dissection.
[*] P-value for Log-rank test.

reinfected persons no one was belonged to the same household.

Long-term follow-up and reinfection rate

The mean duration of follow-up of 59 patients in the EBMT group and 116 in the MEA group was 31.9 months (range: 18–90 months) and 30.4 months (range: 18–59 months). The mean number of *H. pylori* tests per patient was found to be 2.05 tests for the EBMT group and 2.31 tests for the MEA group (Table 4). Reinfection with *H. pylori* occurred in 7 of 59 patients of EBMT group (11.9%) and in 19 of 116 patients of MEA group (16.4%) sporadically during the follow-up period. The calculated total annual reinfection rate was found to be 4.45% (7/157.17 patient years X 100) for EBMT and 6.46% (19/294.08 patient years X 100) for MEA.

Risk factors for reinfection

When the reinfected group (n = 26) and continuously eradicated group (n = 149) were compared in terms of demographic information and clinical characteristics, no statistical differences were found by univariate analysis (Log-rank test), in both groups (Table 5). Specially, there was no significant evidence that reinfection of *H. pylori* is related with eradication regimen (*p* = 0.23) (Figure 2).

Discussion

We performed a prospective study to investigate reinfection rate of *H. pylori* in patients who had been successfully treated with second-line therapy after an initial failure to

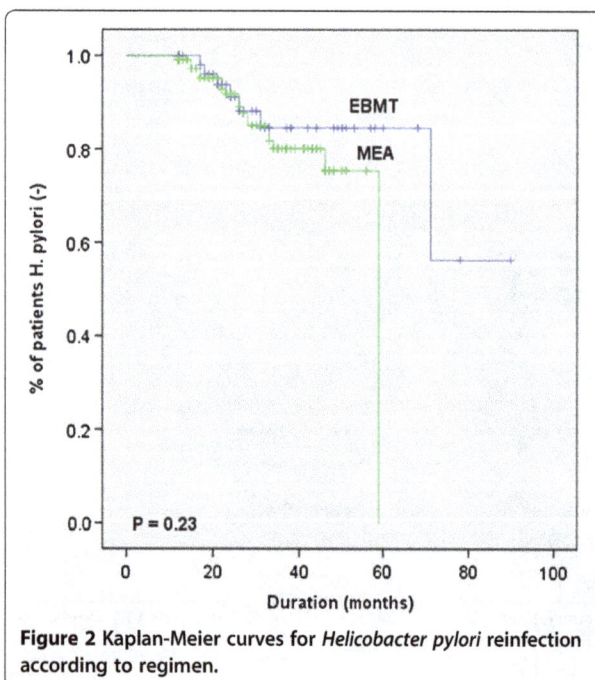

Figure 2 Kaplan-Meier curves for *Helicobacter pylori* reinfection according to regimen.

eradicate *H. pylori*. To the best of our knowledge, this is the first report comparing the reinfection rate of EBMT and MEA therapy.

Reinfection is defined as an infection with a new strain of *H. pylori* that is different from the original strain after complete eradication, while recrudescence is a relapse of original strain, which was temporarily suppressed by eradication therapy [14,15]. The recurrence rates of *H. pylori* decrease with time and decline sharply after the first year, and beyond the first year, recurrence rates come close to the rate of natural acquisition of *H. pylori* infection in adulthood [14,16,17]. From these reports the confirmation of continuous *H. pylori* negativity for the first year after eradication therapy has been accepted as complete eradication [18-20]. Therefore, in our study, reinfection was defined as the situation where tests for *H. pylori* infection, after continuous *H. pylori* negativity for the first year after eradication therapy, become positive again at a later stage. In addition, patients, who become *H. pylori* positive again during 1 year follow-up were classified as recrudescence cases. We could not perfectly distinguish between recrudescence of an original strain and reinfection because DNA analysis of the strain using molecular fingerprinting techniques was not performed. However, this definition is supported by data obtained using DNA analysis that the cause of *H. pylori* recurrence after first year is reinfection [14].

In the previous study, we reported that annual reinfection in patients received standard PPI-based triple eradication therapy in Korea was 3.51% and the recrudescence rate 4.9% [11]. This result was similar to the mean annual reinfection rate (3.4%), calculated from the studies performed in developed countries [16]. The increase in antimicrobial resistance with the standard triple therapy has led to an increase of alternative therapy. However, there are few reports regarding the reinfection of *H. pylori* in patients received second-line therapy. In 2006, our group reported the annual reinfection rate after second-line therapy (EBMT) during 1996–2004, at 6.0% per patients-years in Seoul, Korea [12]. In the present long-term follow-up study for up to 90 months we investigated the reinfection rate of EBMT and MEA therapy, performed during 2003–2010 in Gyeonggi province near Seoul, and those rates are 4.45% for EBMT and 6.46% for MEA per year. When eradication has truly been successful, reinfection is associated with the risk of re-exposure to *H. pylori*. Relatively low reinfection rates might be related to the decrease in prevalence of *H. pylori* infection [21] and the recent improvement of sanitation conditions in Korea. In addition, when the reinfection rate of these two kinds of rescue therapy were compared, there was no significant difference (*p* = 0.43). Therefore, we suggest that reinfection cannot affect the choice of second-line treatment.

In our study, recrudescence rate in the EBMT group and MEA group was found to be 1.7% and 3.3%, which appears slightly lower than reported after initial eradication with standard PPI-based triple regimen (4.9%) [11]. This result might be related to the decreasing trend in eradication rate of standard triple therapy in Korea. That is, the eradication rate of per protocol (PP) analysis decreased up to 75.9% in 2006 [9]. Some studies reported that the recurrence of *H. pylori* infection more frequently occurred in patients treated with a low efficacy regimen than in those treated with a high efficacy regimen, as a result of recrudescence of the organism after temporary suppression, not elimination [14,16,22,23]. In the previous studies, the PP eradication rates were reported at 77.2% for the 7- and 93.6% for the 14 day EBMT regimen [24], and 83.8% for the 7-, 82.6% for the 10- and 79.9% for the 14 day MEA regimen [25]. Our lower recrudescence rate might be related to the higher efficacy of the EBMT and MEA regimens. In addition, there was no difference in the recrudescence rate between EBMT and MEA regimen (*p* = 0.67).

Limited information exists regarding risk factors for reinfection of *H. pylori*. Candidate risk factors include younger age [26,27], infection of close contacts [14,28], dental plaque [29,30], and contaminated endoscopic equipment [14,16,31]. Other studies did not identify any factors predictive of *H. pylori* reinfection [32-34]. In the previous study, we reported that male gender and low income were significantly associated with reinfection of *H. pylori* by multivariate analysis [11]. However, the current study did not identify any predictive factors concerning *H. pylori* reinfection in the EBMT group and MEA group.

This study is the first study with large sample size and a long-term follow-up period in the investigation of reinfection rate of *H. pylori* in patients who had been successfully treated with second-line therapy after an initial failure to eradicate *H. pylori*. However, our study has limitations. First, recrudescence cases could be included in the reinfection cases. Theoretically the fingerprinting should be performed for the differentiation of reinfected and recrudescence. However, we did not perform DNA analysis to identify the strains. In clinical practice, it is not easy to perform DNA analysis. Secondly, despite our efforts to enroll all patients, many patients dropped out from this study, and refused to receive *H. pylori* tests every year, especially when there was no gastrointestinal symptom.

Conclusions

In summary, in Korea, the long-term reinfection rate of *H. pylori* stayed low in both bismuth-containing quadruple therapy and moxifloxacin-based triple therapy; thus reinfection cannot affect the choice of second-line treatment.

Competing interests
The authors have no competing of interests to declare.

Authors' contributions
KN- designed the study and performed the major role of collecting patients; KMS- collected patients' data and wrote the manuscript; KSE- collected patients' data and was involved in editing the manuscript; JHJ- collected patients' data and were involved in editing the manuscript; SCM- collected patients' data and were involved in editing the manuscript; PYS- collected patients' data and were involved in editing the manuscript; LDH- collected patients' data and was involved in editing the manuscript. All authors read and approved the final manuscript.

Acknowledgments
This work was supported by a grant from the National Research Foundation of Korea funded by the Korean Government (2012R1A1A3A04002680) and partly supported by the Seoul National University Budang Hospital Research fund (grants no 02-2010-014). MRCC of Seoul National University Hospital was consulted about the statistical analysis of the present manuscript.

References
1. Go MF: **Review article: natural history and epidemiology of Helicobacter pylori infection**. *Aliment Pharmacol Ther* 2002, 16(Suppl 1):3–15.
2. Chey WD, Wong BC: **American College of Gastroenterology guideline on the management of Helicobacter pylori infection**. *Am J Gastroenterol* 2007, **102:**1808–1825.
3. McColl KE: **Clinical practice. Helicobacter pylori infection**. *N Engl J Med* 2010, **362:**1597–1604.
4. Malfertheiner P, Megraud F, O'Morain CA, Atherton J, Axon AT, Bazzoli F, Gensini GF, Gisbert JP, Graham DY, Rokkas T, *et al*: **Management of Helicobacter pylori infection–the Maastricht IV/ Florence Consensus Report**. *Gut* 2012, **61:**646–664.
5. Fock KM, Katelaris P, Sugano K, Ang TL, Hunt R, Talley NJ, Lam SK, Xiao SD, Tan HJ, Wu CY, *et al*: **Second Asia-Pacific Consensus Guidelines for Helicobacter pylori infection**. *J Gastroenterol Hepatol* 2009, **24:**1587–1600.
6. Asaka M, Kato M, Takahashi S, Fukuda Y, Sugiyama T, Ota H, Uemura N, Murakami K, Satoh K, Sugano K: **Guidelines for the management of Helicobacter pylori infection in Japan: 2009 revised edition**. *Helicobacter* 2010, **15:**1–20.
7. Kim N, Kim JJ, Choe YH, Kim HS, Kim JI, Chung IS: **[Diagnosis and treatment guidelines for Helicobacter pylori infection in Korea]**. *Korean J Gastroenterol* 2009, **54:**269–278.
8. Graham DY, Fischbach L: **Helicobacter pylori treatment in the era of increasing antibiotic resistance**. *Gut* 2010, **59:**1143–1153.
9. Chung JW, Lee GH, Han JH, Jeong JY, Choi KS, Kim do H, Jung KW, Choi KD, Song HJ, Jung HY, *et al*: **The trends of one-week first-line and second-line eradication therapy for Helicobacter pylori infection in Korea**. *Hepatogastroenterology* 2011, **58:**246–250.
10. Chung WC, Lee KM, Paik CN, Lee JR, Jung SH, Kim JD, Han SW, Chung IS: **[Inter-departmental differences in the eradication therapy for Helicobacter pylori infection: a single center study]**. *Korean J Gastroenterol* 2009, **53:**221–227.
11. Kim MS, Kim N, Kim SE, Jo HJ, Shin CM, Lee SH, Park YS, Hwang JH, Kim JW, Jeong SH, *et al*: **Long-term Follow-up Helicobacter Pylori Reinfection Rate and Its Associated Factors in Korea**. *Helicobacter* 2013, **18:**135–142.
12. Cheon JH, Kim N, Lee DH, Kim JM, Kim JS, Jung HC, Song IS: **Long-term outcomes after Helicobacter pylori eradication with second-line, bismuth-containing quadruple therapy in Korea**. *Eur J Gastroenterol Hepatol* 2006, **18:**515–519.
13. Rugge M, Correa P, Dixon MF, Fiocca R, Hattori T, Lechago J, Leandro G, Price AB, Sipponen P, Solcia E, *et al*: **Gastric mucosal atrophy:**

interobserver consistency using new criteria for classification and grading. *Aliment Pharmacol Ther* 2002, **16**:1249–1259.

14. Zhang YY, Xia HH, Zhuang ZH, Zhong J: **Review article: 'true' re-infection of Helicobacter pylori after successful eradication–worldwide annual rates, risk factors and clinical implications.** *Aliment Pharmacol Ther* 2009, **29**:145–160.

15. Cameron EA, Bell GD, Baldwin L, Powell KU, Williams SG: **Long-term study of re-infection following successful eradication of Helicobacter pylori infection.** *Aliment Pharmacol Ther* 2006, **23**:1355–1358.

16. Gisbert JP: **The recurrence of Helicobacter pylori infection: incidence and variables influencing it. A critical review.** *Am J Gastroenterol* 2005, **100**:2083–2099.

17. Peitz U, Hackelsberger A, Malfertheiner P: **A practical approach to patients with refractory Helicobacter pylori infection, or who are re-infected after standard therapy.** *Drugs* 1999, **57**:905–920.

18. Bell GD, Powell KU: **Helicobacter pylori reinfection after apparent eradication–the Ipswich experience.** *Scand J Gastroenterol Suppl* 1996, **215**:96–104.

19. Hildebrand P, Bardhan P, Rossi L, Parvin S, Rahman A, Arefin MS, Hasan M, Ahmad MM, Glatz-Krieger K, Terracciano L, *et al*: **Recrudescence and reinfection with Helicobacter pylori after eradication therapy in Bangladeshi adults.** *Gastroenterology* 2001, **121**:792–798.

20. Soto G, Bautista CT, Roth DE, Gilman RH, Velapatino B, Ogura M, Dailide G, Razuri M, Meza R, Katz U, *et al*: **Helicobacter pylori reinfection is common in Peruvian adults after antibiotic eradication therapy.** *J infect Dis* 2003, **188**:1263–1275.

21. Yim JY, Kim N, Choi SH, Kim YS, Cho KR, Kim SS, Seo GS, Kim HU, Baik GH, Sin CS, *et al*: **Seroprevalence of Helicobacter pylori in South Korea.** *Helicobacter* 2007, **12**:333–340.

22. Xia HX, Talley NJ, Keane CT, O'Morain CA: **Recurrence of Helicobacter pylori infection after successful eradication: nature and possible causes.** *Dig Dis Sci* 1997, **42**:1821–1834.

23. Seo M, Okada M, Shirotani T, Nishimura H, Maeda K, Aoyagi K, Sakisaka S: **Recurrence of Helicobacter pylori infection and the long-term outcome of peptic ulcer after successful eradication in Japan.** *J clin Gastroenterol* 2002, **34**:129–134.

24. Lee BH, Kim N, Hwang TJ, Lee SH, Park YS, Hwang JH, Kim JW, Jeong SH, Lee DH, Jung HC, *et al*: **Bismuth-containing quadruple therapy as second-line treatment for Helicobacter pylori infection: effect of treatment duration and antibiotic resistance on the eradication rate in Korea.** *Helicobacter* 2010, **15**:38–45.

25. Yoon H, Kim N, Lee BH, Hwang TJ, Lee DH, Park YS, Nam RH, Jung HC, Song IS: **Moxifloxacin-containing triple therapy as second-line treatment for Helicobacter pylori infection: effect of treatment duration and antibiotic resistance on the eradication rate.** *Helicobacter* 2009, **14**:77–85.

26. Gomez Rodriguez BJ, Rojas Feria M, Garcia Montes MJ, Romero Castro R, Hergueta Delgado P, Pellicer Bautista FJ, Herrerias Gutierrez JM: **Incidence and factors influencing on Helicobacter pylori infection recurrence.** *Rev Esp Enferm Dig* 2004, **96**:424–627.

27. Shimizu T, Yarita Y, Kaneko K, Yamashiro Y, Segawa O, Ohkura R, Taneike I, Yamamoto T: **Case of intrafamilial Helicobacter pylori reinfection after successful eradication therapy.** *Pediatr Infect Dis J* 2000, **19**:901–903.

28. Gisbert JP, Arata IG, Boixeda D, Barba M, Canton R, Plaza AG, Pajares JM: **Role of partner's infection in reinfection after Helicobacter pylori eradication.** *Eur J Gastroenterol Hepatol* 2002, **14**:865–871.

29. Karczewska E, Konturek JE, Konturek PC, Czesnikiewicz M, Sito E, Bielanski W, Kwiecien N, Obtulowicz W, Ziemniak W, Majka J, *et al*: **Oral cavity as a potential source of gastric reinfection by Helicobacter pylori.** *Dig Dis Sci* 2002, **47**:978–986.

30. Kilmartin CM: **Dental implications of Helicobacter pylori.** *J Can Dent Assoc* 2002, **68**:489–493.

31. Sugiyama T, Naka H, Yachi A, Asaka M: **Direct evidence by DNA fingerprinting that endoscopic cross-infection of Helicobacter pylori is a cause of postendoscopic acute gastritis.** *J Clin Microbiol* 2000, **38**:2381–2382.

32. Feydt-Schmidt A, Kindermann A, Konstantopoulos N, Demmelmair H, Ballauff A, Findeisen A, Koletzko S: **Reinfection rate in children after successful Helicobacter pylori eradication.** *Eur J Gastroenterol Hepatol* 2002, **14**:1119–1123.

33. Leal-Herrera Y, Torres J, Monath TP, Ramos I, Gomez A, Madrazo-de la Garza A, Dehesa-Violante M, Munoz O: **High rates of recurrence and of transient reinfections of Helicobacter pylori in a population with high prevalence of infection.** *Am J Gastroenterol* 2003, **98**:2395–2402.

34. Thong-Ngam D, Mahachai V, Kullavanijaya P: **Incidence of Helicobacter pylori recurrent infection and associated factors in Thailand.** *J Med Assoc Thai* 2007, **90**:1406–1410.

3

Low Helicobacter pylori primary resistance to clarithromycin in gastric biopsy specimens from dyspeptic patients of a city in the interior of São Paulo, Brazil

Rodrigo Buzinaro Suzuki[1,2], Rodrigo Augusto Basso Lopes[1], George Arouche da Câmara Lopes[1], Tin Hung Ho[1] and Márcia Aparecida Sperança[1,2*]

Abstract

Background: Clarithromycin, amoxicillin, and a pump proton inhibitor are the most common drugs recommended as first-line triple therapy for *H.pylori* treatment, which results in eradication rates close to 80%, varying regionally, principally due to emergency cases and increases of clarithromycin resistant strains. Nucleotide substitutions at the *H. pylori* domain V of the 23S rRNA fraction are involved in the macrolide resistance and the A2142G and A2143G mutations are predominant in clinical isolates worldwide including in Brazil. As *H. pylori* culture is fastidious, we investigated the primary occurrence of *H. pylori* A2142G and A2143G rDNA 23S mutations using a molecular approach directly on gastric biopsies of dyspeptic patients consecutively attended at Hospital das Clinicas of Marilia, São Paulo, Brazil.

Methods: Biopsy specimens obtained from 1137 dyspeptic patients, were subjected to histopathology and *H. pylori* diagnosis by histology and PCR. PCR/RFLP assay was used to detect A2142G and A2143G point mutations at domain V of the *H. pylori* 23S rDNA associated with clarithromycin resistance. Through the developed assay, a 768 bp PCR amplicon corresponding to1728 to 2495 bp of the 23S *H. pylori* rDNA is restricted with M*boll* for A2142G mutation detection and with B*sal* for A2143G mutation detection. Occurrence of 23S rDNA A2142G results in two DNA fragments (418 and 350 bp) and of 23S rDNA A2143G results in three DNA fragments (108, 310 and 350pb), due to a conserved B*sal* restriction site.

Results: The PCR method used to diagnose *H. pylori* presented sensitivity, specificity and accuracy of 77,6%, 79,3% and 78,6%, respectively, compared to histology, the gold standard method for *H. pylori* diagnosis used in our routine. Prevalence of *H.pylori* with clarithromycin resistant genotypes was 2,46%, with predominance of A2143G 23S rDNA point mutation.

Conclusions: The PCR/RFLP assay was a rapid and accurate *H.pylori* diagnostic and clarithromycin resistance determination method useful for routine practice. As prevalence of primary resistance of *H.pylori* to clarithromycin due to A2142G and A2143G mutations remains low in Marilia, the standard clarithromycin containing triple therapy is still valid.

Keywords: *Helicobacter pylori*, Clarithromycin resistance, *Helicobacter pylori* 23S rDNA, Gastric diseases, Nucleic acid based diagnostic

* Correspondence: marcia.speranca@ufabc.edu.br
[1]Department of Molecular Biology, Marilia Medical School, Marilia, São Paulo, Brazil
[2]Center of Natural and Human Sciences, Universidade Federal do ABC, Santo André, São Paulo, Brazil

Background

It is widely accepted that *Helicobacter pylori*, a Gram negative microaerophylic bacterium, is involved in several clinical digestive tract conditions such as chronic gastritis, peptic and duodenal ulcers, gastric cancer and lymphoproliferative disorders [1]. Treatment of *H. pylori* infection results in ulcer healing and in a reduction of the risk of gastric cancer and lymphoma [2,3].

Once the bacterium *H. pylori* is detected in altered gastric mucosa, the indicated treatment consists of a triple antibiotic regimen including methronidazol, clarithromycin, amoxicillin, tinidazole, tetracycline and fluoroquinolones associated with a pump proton inhibitor such as omeprazol, lansoprazol or pantoprazol [4-6]. *H. pylori* eradication rates with a number of combined agents and regimens are close to 80% [7-9], varying from country to country and regionally, within countries [10]. Several factors contribute to this low rate of *H. pylori* healing including the inefficiency of the antibiotic penetration in the gastric mucosa, inactivation of the antibiotic by the acid secretion of the stomach [11], lack of the patient compliance [12] and principally, emergency cases and increasing *H. pylori* antibiotic resistant strains [13]. Thus, regional *H. pylori* resistance surveillance is of great importance for test and treatment strategies.

In Brazil, a country of continental dimensions, the majority of practicing clinicians employ the classical triple regimen composed of clarithromycin, amoxicillin and a proton pump inhibitor for seven days as first line therapy to overcome *H. pylori* infection [5,14]. This regimen has been proved to become inefficient worldwide, mainly as a result of the emergence and increase of *H. pylori* strains resistant to clarithromycin, which reduces the bacterium treatment efficiency from 55% to 100% [15-18]. Among Brazilian localities, *H. pylori* clarithromycin resistance presents high prevalence, varying from 7-16% in adults [19-22] and 27% in children [23]. Accordingly, considering the clinical importance of primary *H. pylori* resistance to clarithromycin, its prevalence should be considered before choosing eradication regimens [24].

Determination of *H. pylory in vitro* susceptibility to antibiotics can be performed by standard techniques such as the agar diffusion, agar dilution and broth microdilution methods and the E-test. However, because of the slow growth and the particular requirements of *H.pylori* culture, this approach is not reliable for use in most routine clinical laboratories, principally in developing countries. Hence, molecular tests targeting *H. pylori* resistance associated gene mutations directly from gastric biopsy specimens have the potential for use in large scale studies [25-29].

The molecular mechanism involved in clarithromycin resistance consists of mutations in the sequence of the *H. pylori* domain V of the 23S rRNA fraction which is involved in the peptiltransferase ribosome binding site preventing the ligation of the macrolide to the rRNA [30]. The major characterized point mutations are A to G at positions 2142 and 2143, A to C at 2142 [31-33], A to T at 2144 [34], T to C at 2717 [35] and C to A at 2694 [36]. The A2142G and A2143G mutations are predominant in clinical isolates worldwide including in Brazil [21,37-40]. Thus, in order to perform a large scale investigation of clarithromycin primary resistance directly from biopsy specimens of 1137 patients attended at the Hospital das Clínicas of Marilia, a city in the interior of São Paulo, Brazil, we developed a polymerase chain reaction associated with restriction fragment length polymorphism (PCR-RFLP) assay to detect the A2142G and A2143G nucleotide substitutions at domain V of the *H. pylori* 23S rDNA.

Methods

Patients

1137 adult patients resident in Marilia city, São Paulo State of Brazil, aged 19 to 91 years, who had consecutively undergone esophagogastroduodenoscopy (EGD) for upper abdominal pain or dyspeptic symptoms from February 2003 through December 2006 at the gastroenterology outpatient clinic of the Hospital das Clínicas of Marília Medical School, were enrolled in this study.

Endoscopy and biopsies

The EGD was accomplished by fibroendoscope (GIF-XP20, GIF-XQ20) or video-endoscope (GIF-100) both from Olympus, Shinjuku-ku, Tokyo, Japan. Gastric or duodenal ulcer diagnostic was defined by endoscopy and two fragments of the antrum were collected to perform the rapid urease and histopathological tests. The biopsy used for the rapid urease test was further submitted to DNA extraction. The protocol used is in agreement with the Helsinki Declaration and was approved by the Ethical Committee in Human Research from Marilia Medical School, under reference number 388/01. In the Ethical Committee approved research protocol a written informed consent from each patient included in this study was waived as all gastric biopsy samples analyzed were the same biopsies used routinely for urease rapid test as part of the gastroenterology outpatient service of the Hospital das Clinicas of Marilia Medical School and thus, no specific patient intervention was necessary for the enrollment in this proposed study. Accordingly, waiver of the written informed consent did not adversely affected the rights and welfare of the subjects included in this research, and also the confidentiality of the patients identity was guaranteed.

Histology

One antral specimen was fixed in formol solution at 10% and embedded in paraffin. Sections were Giemsa stained for *H. pylori* evaluation and were stained with hematoxilin and eosin for assessment of histopathologic alterations [41].

Polymerase chain reaction, restriction and sequencing analysis

The same biopsy used for the rapid urease test was submitted to DNA extraction with the employment of the GFx DNA extraction kit purchased from Amersham/Pharmacia Biotech, following the manufacturer's instructions. DNA was quantified in agarose gel electrophoresis using the Invitrogen, Grand Island, New York, USA, low mass ladder and 50-100ug of total DNA were used in the PCR reactions with the oligonucleotides: Hp23Sr6 sense (5′ CACACAGGTAGATGAGATGAGTA3′) and Hp23Sr7 antisense (CACACAGAACCACCGGATCACTA3′), which amplified a fragment of 768pb corresponding to the domain V of the *H. pylori* 23S rDNA (Figure 1). To overcome the problems of extensive genetic polymorphism for precise PCR detection of *H.pylori*, the oligonucleotide construction was performed after a comparative analysis of the 23S rDNA from *H.pylori* and related organisms available at Genebank on MegAlign Lasergene software. PCR condition was 94°C 5′ followed by 40 cycles of 94°C 30″/60°C 30″/72°C 30″ and one cycle at 72°C 7′, with a total volume of 25 µl containing 1× PCR buffer, 200 µM dNTPs, 2,0 mM $MgCl_2$, 1 µM of each oligonucleotide,

1,25 U Taq DNA Polimerase Platinum Brazil (Invitrogen). In all PCR reactions a negative and a positive control were used corresponding to, respectively, sterile water and *H. pylori* PCR positive gastric biopsies. The amplified fragments were digested with *MboII* and B*saI* (New England Biolabs). These enzymes distinguish mutations in the *H. pylori* domain V of the 23S rDNA at the positions 2142 and 2143, respectively. In the presence of A2142G mutation the resulting restriction DNA fragments are of 418 bp and 350 bp and in the presence of A2143G mutation the resulting fragments are of 108, 310 e 350 bp. As a control of *MboII* digestion we used a PCR amplified DNA fragment of 601 bp corresponding to the *Leishmania major* chitinase gene that contains a restriction site for *MboII*. A conserved B*saI* restriction site at the 768 bp PCR amplicon is the positive control for digestion with this enzyme producing DNA fragments of 108 and 660 bp in the absence of A2143G mutation. The products of PCR reactions and restriction analysis were resolved in 1,5% agarose gels, stained with ethidium bromide and photographed under UV light. 23S rDNA 768 bp PCR amplicons from four gastric biopsies (two positive and two negative for *H. pylori* histologic test) with clarithromycin sensitive *MboII* and B*saI* restriction pattern, and from ten gastric biopsies with clarytromycin resistant *MboII* (three samples) and B*saI* (seven samples) restriction patterns were submitted to

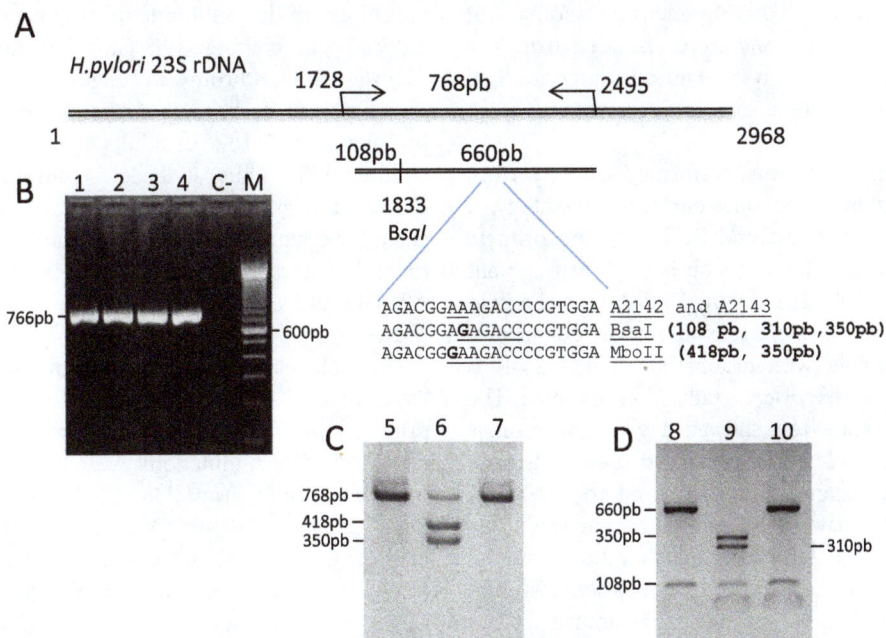

Figure 1 Molecular diagnosis of *Helicobacter pylori* by PCR and RLFP detection of the domain V of the 23S rRNA mutations A2142G and A2143G responsible for clarithromycin resistance. A. Representation of the *H. pylori* 23S coding gene (Genbank:HPU27270), position of the primers used for PCR and of the A2142 and A2143 from fraction V of the 23S rDNA, size of the fragments obtained with restriction enzymes Bsal and *Mboll* in PCR fragments containing the mutations A2142G and A2143G, and internal Bsal restriction site of the 768 bp amplicon, are indicated. **B, C** and **D.** Agarose gel stained with ethidium bromide containing a PCR diagnostic analysis, restriction analysis of the 768pb amplicon with *Mboll* and Bsal, respectively. 1–10 correspond to different human biopsy specimens; C-, negative control of PCR, M-100 bp ladder purchased from Invitrogen. Sizes of the DNA fragments are indicated on the left or right of each gel figure.

sequencing with DyeTM Terminator v3.0 cycle Sequencing Ready Reaction kit and an ABI-3100 machine purchased from Applied Biosystem, according to the manufacturer's instructions. Nucleotide sequence determination was performed in duplicate and comparative analysis was carried out by basic nucleotide BLAST alignment [42].

Statistical analysis

H. pylori diagnostic tests were evaluated by calculating sensitivity, specificity and accuracy employing histology as the gold standard.

Results and discussion

This is the first Brazilian large scale study on *H. pylori* diagnosis and clarithromycin resistance directly from biopsy specimens of 1137 consecutive patients submitted to upper gastroscopy, over a four year period, in a city in the interior of São Paulo, Brazil.

Gastric disease outcome of all patients enrolled in this study attended at the gastroenterology outpatient clinic of Hospital das Clínicas of Marília was investigated by endoscopy and histopathology. Endoscopic finds of peptic or duodenal ulcer disease (PUD) was present in 123 patients. Different degrees of chronic gastritis (CG) were observed by histopathology in 706 patients and normal gastric mucosa, associated or not to gastroesophageal reflux disease (GERD) was found in 290 patients. Eighteen patients were diagnosed as having adenocarcinoma (15) and MALT lymphoma (3) and were excluded from the study. Epidemiological analysis, clinical outcome and *H. pylori* prevalence of these samples were recently published [43].

Detection of *H. pylori* was performed directly from biopsy specimens by three different tests: histology, a household rapid urease test and PCR with the primers Hp23Sr6/r7 which amplify a 768 bp bacterium fragment of the domain V of the 23S rDNA. Histology is the gold standard *H.pylori* diagnostic test employed in our clinical routine which together with histopathological analysis is used to decide for *H. pylori* eradication therapy. The household rapid urease test showed a very low positive predictive value for *H. pylori* associated gastric diseases and a high discrepancy when compared to histology; consequently these data were excluded from the study (data not shown). The 23S rDNA PCR method detected *H. pylori* in 488 gastric biopsies specimens where histology was positive for 451 biopsies samples. Comparative analysis of the PCR assay performed with the Hp23Sr6/r7 with histology showed sensitivity, specificity and accuracy of 77,6%, 79,3% and 78,6%, respectively (Table 1). As both tests were performed on a single and different biopsy and *H. pylori* infection presents a focal characteristic of infection [44,45], accuracy of 78,6% is acceptable for a trustworthy diagnostic test. It can be demonstrated by consistence of the

H.pylori detection by PCR and histology employed in CG (53,1% and 52,7%, respectively) and PUD (61,2% and 62,6%, respectively) patients (Table 1). PCR detected *H.pylori* in 12,75% in patients with normal gastric mucosa while histology was positive for only 0,8% of the samples. These results can be explained by the more sensitive characteristic of the acid nucleic based method. In order to improve the diagnosis of *H.pylori* some authors suggest the analysis of multiple biopsies [44]. In order to confirm the specificity of the PCR fragments obtained, amplicons from two samples with histologic test for *H. pylori* positive and two samples with histologic test for *H. pylori* negative were sequenced. BLASTN analysis of all four biopsy amplified PCR fragments with the 23S rDNA *H. pylori* specific primers [Genbank:KF680642, Genbank:KF680643, Genbank:KF680644 and Genbank:KF680645] revealed identity of 100% with the 23S rDNA referent to different strains of *H. pylori*. Accordingly, the developed PCR assay is rapid and accurate and can be used as a practical method for the detection of *H.pylori* infection.

Antibiotic treatment of gastric diseases is recommended when *H. pylori* diagnosis is positive and the bacterium classic eradication therapy composed of clarithromycin, amoxicillin and a pump proton inhibitor is prescribed. The chosen therapy present a high failure of *H.pylori* eradication rate in areas where resistance to clarithromycin is higher than 15%, probably in response to the widespread use of this antibiotic for respiratory tract infection, especially in children [9]. Global primary resistance of *H. pylori* to clarithromycin ranges from 1 to 29% [46]. In Brazil, several studies reported a clarithromycin resistance prevalence of 7-16% in adults [19,20,22,47] and 27% in children [23]. Thus, in order to improve the empirical choice of *H.pylori* associated disease therapy, we investigated the regional rate of *H.pylori* clarithromycin resistance through detection of the major related point mutations, A2142G and A2143G at domain V of the *H. pylori* 23S rDNA.

Thus, all 488 *H.pylori* PCR positive samples were analyzed by RFLP of the 768 bp PCR fragment obtained with primers Hp23Sr6/7 with the restriction enzymes MboII and BsaI, with detect mutations A2142G and A2143G at domain V of the *H. pylori* 23S rDNA, respectively (Figure 1). Only 12 samples (2,46%) showed the mutated restriction pattern, three (25%) harboring A2142G mutation, seven (58,3%) A2143G and one sample (8,7%) showed both rDNA point mutations in the PCR 23S rDNA 768 bp fragment. One sample showed partial digestion with the enzyme MboII (Figure 1). The point mutations A2142G and A2143G of the amplicons obtained from three [Genbank: KF680646, Genbank:KF680647 and Genbank:KF680647] and seven [Genbank:680649, Genbank:680650, Genbank:680651, Genbank:680652, Genbank:680653, Genbank:680654 and Genbank:680655] different biopsies samples, respectively,

Table 1 Clinical outcome and comparison of *H. pylori* diagnostic methods

	PUD (n = 123)			CG (n = 706)			N (n = 290)			
	His+	His-		His+	His-		His+	His-		T
PCR+	63	13	76	286	89	375	1	36	37	488
PCR-	14	33	47	86	245	331	1	252	253	631
T	77	46	123	372	334	706	2	288	290	1119

CG chronic gastritis, PUD peptic ulcer disease, N normal gastric mucosa associated or not to gastroesophageal reflux disease (GERD), PCR polymerase chain reaction, His histology.

were confirmed by sequencing. There was no association of clarithromycin *H.pylori* resistance point mutations with patients' age or gender (data not shown).

The prevalence of *H. pylori* clarithromycin resistance found in our region was similar to that found in developed countries such as Italy and Germany [7] and in the South American developing country Paraguay [48]. These results confirm the high regional variability of *H.pylori* antibiotic resistance and spite of increasing clarithromycin resistance worldwide, in Marilia, a low resistance rate was maintained over the period of four years. Moreover, PCR/RFLP was a rapid and accurate method for the detection of clarithromycin resistance through a gene mutation directly in gastric biospsy samples and can be used together with histology to decide for prescription of clarithromycin containing regimen therapy.

H. pylori 23S rRNA domain V A2142G and A2143G point mutations are the major mutations found in *H. pylori* clinical isolates resistant to clarithromycin. We found a higher prevalence of A2143G compared to A2142G mutation in our samples which is in agreement with the majority of Brazilian studies including the States of Minas Gerais, São Paulo and Recife [20,34,36]. A2143G but not A2142G point mutation shows a synergistic effect of clarithromycin and amoxicillin, which have been used together in the first-line *H. pylori* regimen [49], reinforcing the necessity to investigate this clarithromycin 23S rDNA point mutation before treatment. One sample harbored both A2142G and A2143G mutations at domain V of the *H. pylori* 23S rDNA that was also found in three *H.pylori* isolates obtained from patients of the Brazilian State of Minas Gerais [20]. These results together with the occurrence of partial digestion of a 768 bp 23S rDNA PCR fragment (Figure 1) can be indicative of stomach colonization of multiple strains of *H.pylori* [50].

In Minas Gerais, Brazil, clarithromycin resistance has increased from 4,48% in 1996 to 19,05% in 2000 [20], probably due to the use of macrolides in the treatment of other infectious diseases. We did not find any significant difference in samples resistant to clarithromycin according to the period of the study (data not shown). These data indicate that in our region the prescription and utilization of macrolides is not performed on a high scale. More studies are necessary to confirm this hypothesis.

Clarithromycin resistance reduces the clinical efficacy of clarithromycin-based triple therapy. However, as prevalence of primary resistance of *H.pylori* to clarithromycin due to the rDNA 23S A2142G and A2143G nucleotide substitutions remains low in Marilia, the standard clarithromycin containing triple therapy is still valid as the most effective empirical first-line eradication therapy for *H. pylori* infection.

Conclusions

The developed PCR assay targeted to the 23S rDNA gene of *H. pylori* is rapid and accurate and can be used as a practical method for the detection of *H.pylori* infection directly on gastric biopsy specimens. Furthermore, the *H. pylori* 23S rDNA PCR fragment obtained can be used to detect point mutations from 1728 to 2495 bp of the *H. pylori* 23S rDNA domain V associated to clarithromycin resistance. Prevalence of primary resistance of *H.pylori* to clarithromycin due to 23S rDNA A2142G and A2143G nucleotide substitutions remains low in Marilia, thus the standard clarithromycin containing triple therapy is still valid as the most effective empirical first-line eradication therapy for *H. pylori* infection.

Abbreviations
PUD: Peptic ulcer disease; CG: Chronic gastritis; GERD: Gastroesophageal reflux disease; PCR: Polymerase chain reaction; RFLP: Restriction fragment length polymorphism.

Competing interests
The authors declare that they have no competing interest.

Authors' contributions
RBS carried out the processing of the samples, molecular studies, interpretation of data and participated to the draft of the manuscript. RABL, GACL and THH carried out the molecular studies and contributed to the acquisition and interpretation of molecular data; MAS designed the experiments, contributed to data analysis and drafted the manuscript. All authors read and approved the final manuscript.

Acknowledgments
We are grateful to Dr. Adriana Augusta Pimenta de Barros for her care to all of the patients included in the study and to Alex Gusmão da Silva for his contribution in carrying out the statistical analysis. This work was supported by the Fundação de Amparo a Pesquisa do Estado de São Paulo (FAPESP), Research Grants 03/01223-0, 08/01394-4; Fellowships RABL 2008/01395-0, GACL 2005/02482-6, THH 2003/03675-7.

Bibliography

1. Megraud F: Helicobacter pylori infection: Review and practice. *Presse Med* 2010, 39(7–8):815–822.

2. Wilhelmsen I, Berstad A: Quality of life and relapse of duodenal ulcer before and after eradication of Helicobacter pylori. *Scand J Gastroenterol* 1994, 29(10):874–879.

3. Na HS, Hong SJ, Yoon HJ, Maeng JH, Ko BM, Jung IS, Ryu CB, Kim JO, Cho JY, Lee JS, et al: Eradication rate of first-line and second-line therapy for Helicobacter pylori infection, and reinfection rate after successful eradication. *Korean J Gastroenterol* 2007, 50(3):170–175.

4. Chisholm SA, Teare EL, Davies K, Owen RJ: Surveillance of primary antibiotic resistance of Helicobacter pylori at centres in England and Wales over a six-year period (2000–2005). *Euro Surveill* 2007, 12(7):E3–4.

5. Coelho LG, Zaterka S: Second Brazilian Consensus Conference on Helicobacter pylori infection. *Arq Gastroenterol* 2005, 42(2):128–132.

6. McNamara D, O'Morain C: Consensus guidelines: agreement and debate surrounding the optimal management of Helicobacter pylori infection. *Can J Gastroenterol* 2000, 14(6):511–517.

7. Malfertheiner P, Megraud F, O'Morain C, Bazzoli F, El-Omar E, Graham D, Hunt R, Rokkas T, Vakil N, Kuipers EJ: Current concepts in the management of Helicobacter pylori infection: the Maastricht III Consensus Report. *Gut* 2007, 56(6):772–781.

8. Chey WD, Wong BC: American College of Gastroenterology guideline on the management of Helicobacter pylori infection. *Am J Gastroenterol* 2007, 102(8):1808–1825.

9. Rimbara E, Fischbach LA, Graham DY: Optimal therapy for Helicobacter pylori infections. *Nat Rev Gastroenterol Hepatol* 2011, 8(2):79–88.

10. Graham DY, Fischbach L: Helicobacter pylori infection. *N Engl J Med* 2010, 363(6):595–596. author reply 596.

11. Qasim A, O'Morain CA: Review article: treatment of Helicobacter pylori infection and factors influencing eradication. *Aliment Pharmacol Ther* 2002, 16(Suppl 1):24–30.

12. Wermeille J, Cunningham M, Dederding JP, Girard L, Baumann R, Zelger G, Buri P, Metry JM, Sitavanc R, Gallaz L, et al: Failure of Helicobacter pylori eradication: is poor compliance the main cause? *Gastroenterol Clin Biol* 2002, 26(3):216–219.

13. Egan BJ, Marzio L, O'Connor H, O'Morain C: Treatment of Helicobacter pylori infection. *Helicobacter* 2008, 13(Suppl 1):35–40.

14. Silva FM, Eisig JN, Teixeira AC, Barbuti RC, Navarro-Rodriguez T, Mattar R: Short-term triple therapy with azithromycin for Helicobacter pylori eradication: low cost, high compliance, but low efficacy. *BMC Gastroenterol* 2008, 8:20.

15. Broutet N, Tchamgoue S, Pereira E, Lamouliatte H, Salamon R, Megraud F: Risk factors for failure of Helicobacter pylori therapy–results of an individual data analysis of 2751 patients. *Aliment Pharmacol Ther* 2003, 17(1):99–109.

16. Kato M, Yamaoka Y, Kim JJ, Reddy R, Asaka M, Kashima K, Osato MS, El-Zaatari FA, Graham DY, Kwon DH: Regional differences in metronidazole resistance and increasing clarithromycin resistance among Helicobacter pylori isolates from Japan. *Antimicrob Agents Chemother* 2000, 44(8):2214–2216.

17. Lee JH, Shin JH, Roe IH, Sohn SG, Kang GH, Lee HK, Jeong BC, Lee SH: Impact of clarithromycin resistance on eradication of Helicobacter pylori in infected adults. *Antimicrob Agents Chemother* 2005, 49(4):1600–1603.

18. Giorgio F, Principi M, De Francesco V, Zullo A, Losurdo G, Di Leo A, Ierardi E: Primary clarithromycin resistance to Helicobacter pylori: Is this the main reason for triple therapy failure? *World journal of gastrointestinal pathophysiology* 2013, 4(3):43–46.

19. Mendonca S, Ecclissato C, Sartori MS, Godoy AP, Guerzoni RA, Degger M, Pedrazzoli J Jr: Prevalence of Helicobacter pylori resistance to metronidazole, clarithromycin, amoxicillin, tetracycline, and furazolidone in Brazil. *Helicobacter* 2000, 5(2):79–83.

20. Prazeres Magalhaes P, De Magalhaes Queiroz DM, Campos Barbosa DV, Aguiar Rocha G, Nogueira Mendes E, Santos A, Valle Correa PR, Camargos Rocha AM, Martins Teixeira L: Affonso de Oliveira C: Helicobacter pylori primary resistance to metronidazole and clarithromycin in Brazil. *Antimicrob Agents Chemother* 2002, 46(6):2021–2023.

21. Ribeiro ML, Vitiello L, Miranda MC, Benvengo YH, Godoy AP, Mendonca S, Pedrazzoli J Jr: Mutations in the 23S rRNA gene are associated with clarithromycin resistance in Helicobacter pylori isolates in Brazil. *Ann Clin Microbiol Antimicrob* 2003, 2:11.

22. Eisig JN, Silva FM, Barbuti RC, Navarro-Rodriguez T, Moraes-Filho JP, Pedrazzoli J Jr: Helicobacter pylori antibiotic resistance in Brazil: clarithromycin is still a good option. *Arq Gastroenterol* 2011, 48(4):261–264.

23. Garcia GT, Aranda KR, Goncalves ME, Cardoso SR, Iriya K, Silva NP, Scaletsky IC: High prevalence of clarithromycin resistance and cagA, vacA, iceA2, and babA2 genotypes of Helicobacter pylori in Brazilian children. *J Clin Microbiol* 2010, 48(11):4266–4268.

24. Megraud F: Current recommendations for Helicobacter pylori therapies in a world of evolving resistance. *Gut Microbes* 2013, 4:6.

25. Woo HY, Park DI, Park H, Kim MK, Kim DH, Kim IS, Kim YJ: Dual-priming oligonucleotide-based multiplex PCR for the detection of Helicobacter pylori and determination of clarithromycin resistance with gastric biopsy specimens. *Helicobacter* 2009, 14(1):22–28.

26. Chisholm SA, Owen RJ, Teare EL, Saverymuttu S: PCR-based diagnosis of Helicobacter pylori infection and real-time determination of clarithromycin resistance directly from human gastric biopsy samples. *J Clin Microbiol* 2001, 39(4):1217–1220.

27. Tajbakhsh S, Samarbaf-Zadeh AR, Moosavian M: Comparison of fluorescent in situ hybridization and histological method for the diagnosis of Helicobacter pylori in gastric biopsy samples. *Med Sci Monit* 2008, 14(9):BR183–187.

28. Burucoa C, Garnier M, Silvain C, Fauchere JL: Quadruplex real-time PCR assay using allele-specific scorpion primers for detection of mutations conferring clarithromycin resistance to Helicobacter pylori. *J Clin Microbiol* 2008, 46(7):2320–2326.

29. Suzuki RB, Almeida CM, Speranca MA: Absence of Helicobacter pylori high tetracycline resistant 16S rDNA AGA926-928TTC genotype in gastric biopsy specimens from dyspeptic patients of a city in the interior of Sao Paulo, Brazil. *BMC Gastroenterol* 2012, 12:49.

30. Moazed D, Noller HF: Chloramphenicol, erythromycin, carbomycin and vernamycin B protect overlapping sites in the peptidyl transferase region of 23S ribosomal RNA. *Biochimie* 1987, 69(8):879–884.

31. Taylor DE, Ge Z, Purych D, Lo T, Hiratsuka K: Cloning and sequence analysis of two copies of a 23S rRNA gene from Helicobacter pylori and association of clarithromycin resistance with 23S rRNA mutations. *Antimicrob Agents Chemother* 1997, 41(12):2621–2628.

32. Versalovic J, Shortridge D, Kibler K, Griffy MV, Beyer J, Flamm RK, Tanaka SK, Graham DY, Go MF: Mutations in 23S rRNA are associated with clarithromycin resistance in Helicobacter pylori. *Antimicrob Agents Chemother* 1996, 40(2):477–480.

33. Stone GG, Shortridge D, Flamm RK, Versalovic J, Beyer J, Idler K, Zulawinski L, Tanaka SK: Identification of a 23S rRNA gene mutation in clarithromycin-resistant Helicobacter pylori. *Helicobacter* 1996, 1(4):227–228.

34. Toracchio S, Aceto GM, Mariani-Costantini R, Battista P, Marzio L: Identification of a novel mutation affecting domain V of the 23S rRNA gene in Helicobacter pylori. *Helicobacter* 2004, 9(5):396–399.

35. Fontana C, Favaro M, Minelli S, Criscuolo AA, Pietroiusti A, Galante A, Favalli C: New site of modification of 23S rRNA associated with clarithromycin resistance of Helicobacter pylori clinical isolates. *Antimicrob Agents Chemother* 2002, 46(12):3765–3769.

36. Rimbara E, Noguchi N, Kawai T, Sasatsu M: Novel mutation in 23S rRNA that confers low-level resistance to clarithromycin in Helicobacter pylori. *Antimicrob Agents Chemother* 2008, 52(9):3465–3466.

37. Scaletsky IC, Aranda KR, Garcia GT, Goncalves ME, Cardoso SR, Iriya K, Silva NP: Application of real-time PCR stool assay for Helicobacter pylori detection and clarithromycin susceptibility testing in Brazilian children. *Helicobacter* 2011, 16(4):311–315.

38. Lins AK, Lima RA, Magalhaes M: Clarithromycin-resistant Helicobacter pylori in Recife, Brazil, directly identified from gastric biopsies by polymerase chain reaction. *Arquivos de gastroenterologia* 2010, 47(4):379–382.

39. van Doorn LJ, Glupczynski Y, Kusters JG, Megraud F, Midolo P, Maggi-Solca N, Queiroz DM, Nouhan N, Stet E, Quint WG: Accurate prediction of macrolide resistance in Helicobacter pylori by a PCR line probe assay for detection of mutations in the 23S rRNA gene: multicenter validation study. *Antimicrob Agents Chemother* 2001, 45(5):1500–1504.

40. Assumpcao MB, Martins LC, Melo Barbosa HP, Barile KA, de Almeida SS, Assumpcao PP, Corvelo TC: Helicobacter pylori in dental plaque and stomach of patients from Northern Brazil. *World J Gastroenterol* 2010, 16(24):3033–3039.

41. Rotimi O, Cairns A, Gray S, Moayyedi P, Dixon MF: Histological identification of Helicobacter pylori: comparison of staining methods. *J Clin Pathol* 2000, 53(10):756–759.

42. Altschul SF, Madden TL, Schaffer AA, Zhang J, Zhang Z, Miller W, Lipman DJ: **Gapped BLAST and PSI-BLAST: a new generation of protein database search programs.** *Nucleic Acids Res* 1997, **25**(17):3389–3402.

43. Suzuki RB, Cola RF, Cola LT, Ferrari CG, Ellinger F, Therezo AL, Silva LC, Eterovic A, Speranca MA: **Different risk factors influence peptic ulcer disease development in a Brazilian population.** *World J Gastroenterol* 2012, **18**(38):5404–5411.

44. Morris A, Ali MR, Brown P, Lane M, Patton K: **Campylobacter pylori infection in biopsy specimens of gastric antrum: laboratory diagnosis and estimation of sampling error.** *J Clin Pathol* 1989, **42**(7):727–732.

45. Sugiyama T, Sakaki N, Kozawa H, Sato R, Fujioka T, Satoh K, Sugano K, Sekine H, Takagi A, Ajioka Y, *et al*: **Sensitivity of biopsy site in evaluating regression of gastric atrophy after Helicobacter pylori eradication treatment.** *Aliment Pharmacol Ther* 2002, **16**(Suppl 2):187–190.

46. Megraud F, Lehours P: **Helicobacter pylori detection and antimicrobial susceptibility testing.** *Clin Microbiol Rev* 2007, **20**(2):280–322.

47. Godoy AP, Ribeiro ML, Benvengo YH, Vitiello L, Miranda Mde C, Mendonca S, Pedrazzoli J Jr: **Analysis of antimicrobial susceptibility and virulence factors in Helicobacter pylori clinical isolates.** *BMC Gastroenterol* 2003, **3**:20.

48. Farina N, Kasamatsu E, Samudio M, Moran M, Sanabria R, Laspina F: **Antimicrobial susceptibility of H pylori strains obtained from Paraguayan patients.** *Revista medica de Chile* 2007, **135**(8):1009–1014.

49. Sakinc T, Baars B, Wuppenhorst N, Kist M, Huebner J, Opferkuch W: **Influence of a 23S ribosomal RNA mutation in Helicobacter pylori strains on the in vitro synergistic effect of clarithromycin and amoxicillin.** *BMC research notes* 2012, **5**:603.

50. Figueiredo C, Van Doorn LJ, Nogueira C, Soares JM, Pinho C, Figueira P, Quint WG, Carneiro F: **Helicobacter pylori genotypes are associated with clinical outcome in Portuguese patients and show a high prevalence of infections with multiple strains.** *Scand J Gastroenterol* 2001, **36**(2):128–135.

4

Clinical relevance of the *cagA*, *tnpA* and *tnpB* genes in *Helicobacter pylori*

Amin Talebi Bezmin Abadi[1,2], Ashraf Mohhabati Mobarez[2], Marc JM Bonten[1], Jaap A Wagenaar[3] and Johannes G Kusters[1]*

Abstract

Background: Numerous proteins have been proposed as virulence factors for the gram negative gastric bacterium *Helicobacter pylori* but only for a few this has unequivocally been demonstrated. The aim of the current study was to evaluate the association of the putative virulence factors *tnpA* and *tnpB (no cagA)* with *H. pylori* associated gastroduodenal diseases.

Methods: A PCR based assay was used to determine the presence of the *tnpA* and *tnpB* genes, as well as of *cagA*, in 360*H. pylori* strains isolated from *H. pylori* infected patients.

Results: Of 360*H. pylori* culture positive patients (196 men, 164 women; average age 42.1 years (range 17–73), 95 had gastritis, 92 had gastric ulcers, 108 had duodenal ulcers, and 65 had gastric cancer. Using the gastritis group as a reference a significantly aberrant gene distribution was observed for the *tnpA* (Relative risk: 1.45; 95% CI 1.04-1.93), the *cagA* (Relative risk: 1.81; 95% CI 1.44-2.29), but not the *tnpB* gene in the gastric cancer group.

Conclusions: The increased incidence of the *tnpA* gene in gastric cancer patients suggests a role of the *tnpA* gene in the development of *H. pylori* induced gastric cancer.

Keywords: Helicobacter pylori, Disease association, Gastric cancer, Duodenal ulcer, Virulence factor

Background

Helicobacter pylori is the most prevalent pathogenic microorganism colonizing the gastric mucosa of humans. Infection rates range between 85-95% in developing countries and 30-50% in developed countries [1]. Colonization always results in acute gastritis and chronic gastritis when left untreated [2]. Additional complications such as gastric ulcers (GU), duodenal ulcers (DU), or gastric cancer (GC) may develop in some of these *H. pylori* infected patients [3]. The outcome of the infection is determined by both the duration of infection and environmental, host, and bacterial factors [4]. *H. pylori* strains display extensive genetic variability with considerable variation in the presence of virulence factors, which is thought to cause the many different clinical presentations of *H. pylori* infections [5-7]. The CagA protein is a commonly accepted virulence factor and the *cagA* gene is often used as a marker for the

presence of the *cag* (cytotoxin-associated gene) pathogenicity island (*cag*PAI) [4]. Patients infected with *H. pylori* strains that carry *cagA* have a higher risk for developing peptic ulcer and gastric cancer [8]. Other virulence determinants located on the *cag*PAI such as *cagE*, *cagG*, *cagH*, *cagI*, *cagL*, and *cagM* are required for *cag*PAI mediated NF-κB induction, and *cagT* and *cagY* are required for the formation of a needle-like structure that serves to inject *cagA* into the host cell [9,10]. Although these factors play a critical role in the pathogenesis of *H. pylori*, their association with specific disease outcomes is not as obvious as with *cagA*. It has been reported that in some *H. pylori* strains the *cag*PAI is split into two separate regions due to the integration of the IS*605* insertion sequence [10]. The putative IS*605* transposases (*tnpA* and *tnpB*) that can mediate this *cag*PAI disruption [10] might affect the virulence of *H. pylori* [11], but the exact biological role and clinical relevance of these two determinants is poorly studied. Iran is a developing country with a high prevalence of *H. pylori*, among both symptomatic and asymptomatic individuals, and with a prevalence as high as 95% in the northern part

* Correspondence: h.kusters@umcutrecht.nl
[1]Department of Medical Microbiology, University Medical Center Utrecht, Heidelberglaan 100, Utrecht 3584 CX, The Netherlands
Full list of author information is available at the end of the article

of the country [12,13]. This high prevalence is coupled to an even higher rate of *H. pylori* induced peptic ulcer disease and gastric cancers [14]. This makes it an ideal geographically confined region to study the effect of genetic variation of this gastric pathogen on infection associated disorders. In this study we determined associations of the presence of *tnpA* and *tnpB* and clinical manifestations of *H. pylori* infections in patients from the North of Iran.

Methods

Patients

All patients suspect of a *H. pylori* infection that visited the Tooba Medical Center, in Sari, Iran for endoscopic examination between May 2008 and October 2010 were invited to participate in this study. Patients participating in this study underwent routine gastroscopic examination. The standard number of gastric biopsy samples for patients' suspect of Helicobacter infection was obtained for routine culture and histological investigations and no extra samples were taken for this study. One of the gastric biopsy samples was sent to the pathology lab where it was tested by routine histopathological techniques and evaluated by standard criteria. Histology grading was performed by the updated Sydney criteria [15]. The other routinely obtained biopsy samples were used for microbiological culture and Rapid Urease Test (RUT), as described below. Ages below 16 years were excluded due to ethical considerations. Also antibiotic use within four months prior to endoscopy, or use of anti-secretory drugs within one month before endoscopy were used as exclusion criteria. This study was approved by the local ethics committee of Tarbiat Modares University, as no extra biopsy samples were needed for this study and that the obtained data could not be traced back to the patient level.

Microbiological analysis

One of the biopsy samples was routinely tested by the gastroenterologist by Rapid Urease Test; and if positive a second sample was obtained and placed in 200 µl sterile thioglycolate (Merck, Germany) broth and then immediately shipped to the diagnostic laboratory for routine culture. Upon arrival in the microbiology lab this sample was immediately grinded and 100 µl of the resultant homogenate was inoculated on a Colombia agar (Merck, Germany) plate supplemented with 7% defibrinated sheep blood (Jihad Daneshgahi, Tehran, Iran), 10% Fetal Calf Serum (FCS) and antibiotics (DENT, Supplement, Oxoid) [15]. Plates were incubated at 37°C, in 10% CO_2 conditions provided by incubator (Binder, USA) and high humidity until typical *H. pylori* colonies appeared or for a maximum of 7 days if no suspect colonies were observed. Colony shape, morphology in microscopic examination, routine biochemical tests such as urease, catalase and oxidase tests were performed for identification of *H. pylori* strains.

DNA extraction and PCR

Bacterial DNA was extracted from single colonies of *H. pylori* using a commercially available kit (ExiPrep™ Bacteria Genomic DNA Kit, Bioneer, Daejeon, South Korea). Genotyping was performed by PCR, using specific primers for *cagA, tnpA* and *tnpB* as previously described (Table 1). In addition a *glmM* PCR (Table 1) was carried out [16], both as an additional control for *H. pylori* identification and quality check of the isolated DNA (positive PCR control). The PCR amplified fragments were size separated on 2% agarose gel (Sinagene, Tehran, Iran) and the ethidium bromide stained DNA was visualized using UV illumination.

Statistical analysis

The chi-square and Fisher exact test was used to test for the association between patient demographics, *H. pylori* genotypes, and disease groups. A *P* value of less than 0.05 was accepted as statistically significant. Microsoft Excel 2010 was used to calculate the *P* values, odds ratio (OR) and 95% confidence interval (95% CI).

Results

376 patients suspect for *H. pylori* infection (positive RUT test) were enrolled, but *H. pylori* specific growth was not observed from the biopsy specimen in 16 of them. The remaining 360 patients that were *H. pylori* culture positive (96%) comprised 95 patients with gastritis (G), 92 with gastric ulcer (GU), 108 with duodenal ulcer, and 65 with gastric cancer (GC) (Table 2). The average age was 42.1 years (range 17 to 73 year) and there were slightly more men (n = 196) than women (n = 164). Detailed demographic data of dyspeptic patients according to age, disease symptoms, and histological findings are shown in Table 2. There were slightly more males with duodenal ulcers, and less with gastric ulcers, but there were no statistically significant associations between age, gender, histopathological findings, and *H. pylori* associated disease groups.

Table 1 Primers used in this study

Primers	5′-3′ Sequence	Reference
glmM	AAGCTTTTAGGGGTGTTAGGGGTTT	[20]
	AAGCTTACTTTCTAACACTAACGC	
tnpA	ATCAGTCCAAAAAGTTTTTTCTTTCC	[13]
	TAAGGGGGTATATTTCAACCAACCG	
tnpB	CGCTCTCCCTAAATTCAAAGAGGGC	[13]
	AGCTAGGGAAAAATCTGTCTATGCC	
cagA	ATAATGCTAAATTAGACAACTTGAGCGA	[5]
	TTAGAATAATCAACAAACATCACGCCAT	

Table 2 Detailed demographic data of dyspeptic patients according to the age and pathologic findings

Disease type	Sample size	Male (%)	Pathology findings	Age range detailed data for each disease groups				
				<30	31-40	41-50	51-60	>60
G	95	51 (53.6)	Mild (n = 14)	6	7	1	0	0
			Moderate (n = 67)	33	26	6	2	0
			Atrophic (n = 20)	8	5	6	1	0
GU	92	38 (41.3)	Mild (n = 15)	2	3	4	4	2
			Moderate (n = 84)	7	12	21	11	33
			Atrophic (n = 13)	0	2	2	6	3
DU	108	72 (66)	Mild (n = 23)	4	5	5	6	3
			Moderate (n = 57)	6	18	13	12	8
			Atrophic (n = 23)	6	7	7	6	4
GC	65	35 (53.8)	Mild (n = 7)	0	0	1	2	4
			Moderate (n = 47)	0	0	17	16	14
			Atrophic (n = 11)	0	0	6	1	4

PCR screening of *tnpA, tnpB* and *cagA*

The overall prevalence of the *tnpA, tnpB,* and *cagA* genes were 47.5%, 13.1%, and 59.2%, respectively, and the prevalence of these genes in the four disease groups is listed in Table 3. No significant associations were observed between the presence of the *tnpA, tnpB* and *cagA* genes and histological findings. Statistical analysis did however reveal a significant association between the presence of the *cagA* gene and GC [Relative risk: 1.81; 95% CI 1.44-2.29], and a weak, but significant correlation was observed between the presence of the *cagA* gene and DU [Relative risk: 1.30; 95% CI 1.01-1.69] and the *tnpA* gene with GC [Relative risk: 1.45; 95% CI 1.04-1.93] (Table 3). No significant association was observed for *tnpB* and gastroduodenal diseases.

Discussion and conclusions

To our knowledge, this is the largest study (n = 360) investigating the distribution of the *H. pylori* virulence *tnpA, tnpB* and *cagA* in dyspeptic patients. In the first study on *tnpA* and *tnpB* by Matter *et al.* [11], 63% of 215 clinical *H. pylori* isolates were *tnpA* positive and 13.5% were positive for *tnpB*, with a statistically significant association between peptic ulcer disease (PUD) and *tnpA* positive strains. This association was not apparent for *tnpB*. In the current study there was a similar

prevalence of *tnpA* and *tnpB* [171/360; 47.5% and 47/360; 13.1%, for *tnpA* and *tnpB* respectively], and a similar association between *cagA* and gastric cancer patients as observed in a preliminary study by Matter *et al.* [11]. Unfortunately in their study the associations of *tnpA* and *tnpB* with *H. pylori* associated disease types were not determined. In a more recent but smaller study Matter *et al.* investigated associations between presence of *tnpA* and *tnpB* and gastric cancer in Brazilian patients with gastric cancer (n = 34) and gastritis (n = 34) [17]. The patient population studied here is from the North of Iran (state of Mazandaran), and has been reported to not only have a very high *H. pylori* infection rate but also a very high rate patients suffering from *H. pylori* induced disease [18] This high *H. pylori* prevalence facilitates the collection of a large number of strains from a well defined, small geographical region and this facilitated a study on the putative association between the presence of tnpA/B and the clinical outcome of the *H.pylori* infection. The prevalence of *tnpA* and *tnpB* among gastric cancer and gastritis patients in the Iranian population included in the current study was 42.1% and 60.0% for *tnpA*, and 16.8% and 15.4% for *tnpB*, respectively, which, again, was comparable to the findings in the Brazilian population with gastric cancer or gastritis (29.4% and 73.5% for *tnpA*; and 2.9% and 5.9% for *tnpB*, respectively). Kersulyte *et al.*

Table 3 Prevalence of the *tnpA, tnpB,* and *cagA* genes in the four patient groups

Disease groups	tnpA			tnpB			cagA		
	Positives	Relative risk	95% CI	Positives	Relative risk	95% CI	Positives	Relative risk	95% CI
Gastritis (n = 95) (Control group)	40 (42.1%)	Reference		16 (16.8%)	Reference		45 (47.4%)	Reference	
Gastric ulcer (n = 92)	48 (52.2%)	1.23	0.97-1.61	10 (10.9%)	0.64	0.30-1.34	45 (48.9%)	1.03	0.76-1.39
Duodenal ulcer (n = 108)	44 (40.7%)	0.96	0.69-1.34	11 (10.2%)	0.59	0.29-1.22	67 (62%)	1.30	1.01-1.69
Gastric cancer (n = 65)	39 (60.0%)	1.45	1.04-1.93	10 (15.4%)	0.91	0.44-1.88	56 (86.2%)	1.81	1.44-2.29

[19] also reported a higher frequency of *tnpA* in Peruvian gastric cancer strains than in gastritis strains (9/14 (46%) versus 15/45 (33%), respectively). Although the observed associations between *tnpA* and gastric cancer are similar in the populations in Peru, Brazil and Iran [11,19], there are striking differences for associations of *cagA* with disease status between these populations. We observed a clear association between the presence of *cagA* and gastric cancer in the Iranian population, while Matter *et al.* [11] did not observe such an association in Brazil. While most studies report an association between the presence of *cagA* and gastric cancer some studies do not observe this association [20,21]. In this particular case it may be due to the low number of patients included in their study (n = 64; versus 160 in our study). After the recognition of *H. pylori* as an important gastric pathogen [21], many attempts have been made to identify *H. pylori* virulence factors predicting clinical outcome as this might assist physicians in prediction of disease progression [22]. When using the gastritis group as controls for gene distribution we observed an increased prevalence of the *tnpA* and *cagA* genes in the gastric cancer group. To our knowledge this study represents the largest cohort tested thus far for the prevalence of *tnpA* for an association with the various *H. pylori* infection associated disease groups. While it is tempting to conclude from the increased prevalence of *tnpA* and *cagA* in the gastric cancer group that these genes may serve as useful biomarkers for gastric cancer one cannot draw that conclusion from a cross-sectional study like ours. Also our study design did not include a questionnaire on the disease history of our patients and hence we are unable to correlate clinical symptoms such as bleeding, reflux, abdominal pain etc. with the presence/absence of these virulence factors. A large prospective cohort study would be required to establish reliable positive and negative predictive values of these putative biomarkers. Due to the long time between infection and cancer development such a study would require long follow-up times, and since only few infected individuals develop cancer a large study cohort would be required. In addition there are ethical issues with such a study as the hypothesis to be tested is that patients infected with *tnpA* positive *H. pylori* strains are more prone to developing gastric cancer than patients infected with *tnpA* negative strains. In order to test this hypothesis one must establish the presence of the *tnpA*$^{+/-}$ *H. pylori* strain at the start of the study while refraining from eradication of these potentially carcinogenic strains for a long period of time. In spite of the shortcomings of our cross-sectional study it provides strong indications for the clinical relevance of the *tnpA* gene of *H. pylori* strains isolated from the Iranian population where the prevalence of *H. pylori* is relatively high [13] and this high prevalence is coupled to a high incidence of *H. pylori* induced peptic ulcer disease and gastric cancers [23]. In conclusion *tnpA* but not *tnpB* is clearly associated with a more severe disease outcome of *Hc pylori* infections. As such *tnpA* could be a valuable novel biomarker but clearly further studies are required to confirm these results especially since at present no obvious biological explanation for a GC inducing function of this putative transposase can be provided.

Competing interests
The authors declare that they have no competing interests.

Authors' contributions
ATBA, JGK and AMM build the strain collection, collected the patient status data, carried out the molecular genetic studies, performed the initial statistical analyses, and drafted the manuscript. ATBA, JGK, JAW and MJB participated in the design of the study, the drafting of the mansuscirpt and assisted with the statistical analysis. All authors read and approved the final manuscript.

Author details
[1]Department of Medical Microbiology, University Medical Center Utrecht, Heidelberglaan 100, Utrecht 3584 CX, The Netherlands. [2]Department of Medical Bacteriology, School of Medical Sciences, Tarbiat Modares University, Tehran, Iran. [3]Department of Infectious Diseases and Immunology, Faculty of Veterinary Medicine, Utrecht University, Utrecht, Netherlands.

References
1. Basso D, Plebani M, Kusters JG: Pathogenesis of Helicobacter pylori infection. *Helicobacter* 2010, **15**(Suppl 1):14–20.
2. Sheu BS, *et al*: Helicobacter pylori colonization of the human gastric epithelium: a bug's first step is a novel target for us. *J Gastroenterol Hepatol* 2010, **25**(1):26–32.
3. Hussein NR: The association of dupA and Helicobacter pylori-related gastroduodenal diseases. *Eur J Clin Microbiol Infect Dis* 2010, **29**(7):817–821.
4. Kusters JG, van Vliet AH, Kuipers EJ: Pathogenesis of Helicobacter pylori infection. *Clin Microbiol Rev* 2006, **19**(3):449–490.
5. Kuipers EJ, *et al*: Review article: the development of atrophic gastritis–Helicobacter pylori and the effects of acid suppressive therapy. *Aliment Pharmacol Ther* 1995, **9**(4):331–340.
6. Taghvaei T, *et al*: Prevalence of horB gene among the Helicobacter pylori strains isolated from dyspeptic patients: first report from Iran. *Intern Emerg Med* 2012, **7**(6):505–508.
7. Talebi Bezmin Abadi A, Ghasemzadeh A, Mohabati Mobarez A: Low frequency of cagA-positive Helicobacter pylori strains isolated from Iranian patients with MALT lymphoma. *Intern Emerg Med* 2013, **8**(1):49–53.
8. Saito Y, *et al*: Conversion of Helicobacter pylori CagA from senescence inducer to oncogenic driver through polarity-dependent regulation of p21. *J Exp Med* 2010, **207**(10):2157–2174.
9. Pachathundikandi SK, Tegtmeyer N, Backert: Signal transduction of Helicobacter pylori during interaction with host cell protein receptors of epithelial and immune cells. *S Gut Microbes* 2013, **4**(6):454–474.
10. Censini S, *et al*: cag, a pathogenicity island of Helicobacter pylori, encodes type I-specific and disease-associated virulence factors. *Proc Natl Acad Sci U S A* 1996, **93**(25):14648–14653.
11. Mattar R, *et al*: Helicobacter pylori cag pathogenicity island genes: clinical relevance for peptic ulcer disease development in Brazil. *J Med Microbiol* 2007, **56**(Pt 1):9–14.
12. Malekzadeh R, Derakhshan MH, Malekzadeh Z: Gastric cancer in Iran: epidemiology and risk factors. *Arch Iran Med* 2009, **12**(6):576–583.
13. Talebi Bezmin Abadi A, *et al*: Antibiotic resistance of Helicobacter pylori in Mazandaran, North of Iran. *Helicobacter* 2010, **15**((6):505–509.
14. Salehi Z, *et al*: Helicobacter pylori cagA status and peptic ulcer disease in Iran. *Dig Dis Sci* 2009, **54**(3):608–613.
15. Dixon MF, Genta RM, Yardley JH, Correa P: Classification and grading of gastritis. The updated Sydney system. International workshop on the

histopathology of gastritis, Houston 1994. *Am J Surg Pathol* 1996, **20**(10):1161–1181.

16. Espinoza MG, *et al*: Detection of the glmM gene in Helicobacter pylori isolates with a novel primer by PCR. *J Clin Microbiol* 2011, **49**(4):1650–1652.

17. Mattar R, *et al*: Association of LEC and tnpA Helicobacter pylori genes with gastric cancer in a Brazilian population. *Infect Agent Cancer* 2010, **5**:1.

18. Abadi AT, Taghvaei T, Wolfram L, Kusters JG: Infection with Helicobacter pylori strains lacking dupA is associated with an increased risk of gastric ulcer and gastric cancer development. *Med Microbiol* 2012, **61**(Pt 1):23–30.

19. Kersulyte D, *et al*: Sequence organization and insertion specificity of the novel chimeric ISHp609 transposable element of Helicobacter pylori. *J Bacteriol* 2004, **186**(22):7521–7528.

20. Kidd M, Louw JA, Marks IN: Helicobacter pylori in Africa: observations on an 'enigma within an enigma'. *J Gastroenterol Hepatol* 1999, **14**(9):851–858.

21. Ahmad T, *et al*: Prevalence of Helicobacter pylori pathogenicity-associated cagA and vacA genotypes among Pakistani dyspeptic patients. *FEMS Immunol Med Microbiol* 2009, **55**(1):34–38.

22. Talebi Bezmin Abadi A, *et al*: Helicobacter pylori homB, but not cagA, is associated with gastric cancer in Iran. *J Clin Microbiol* 2011, **49**(9):3191–3197.

23. Talebi Bezmin Abadi A, *et al*: High correlation of babA (2)-positive strains of Helicobacter pylori with the presence of gastric cancer. *Intern Emerg Med* 2013, **8**:497–501.

5

High prevalence of Helicobacter pylori infection in Behcet's disease

Kamran B Lankarani[1*], Mohammad Reza Ravanbod[2], Elham Aflaki[3], Mohammad Ali Nazarinia[3] and Akbar Rajaee[3]

Abstract

Background: Behcet's disease (BD) is a multisystem disease of unknown etiology. There are several clues which may indicate an ethiopathogenesis role for Helicobacter pylori infection in this disease.

Methods: In a case control study in an out patient department, 48 patients with BD were compared to age, sex matched controls regarding presence of H. pylori infection by serology and urea breath test (UBT).

Results: Ongoing H. pylori infection was more prevalent among patients with BD using result of UBT with odds ratio of 3.1 (95% CI: 1.34 – 7.26, PV < 0.001).

Conclusion: H. pylori infection may have a role in the pathogenesis of BD.

Keywords: Helicobacter pylori, Behcet's disease, Pathogenesis, Urea breath test

Background

Behcet's disease is a systemic disease of unknown etiology affecting multiple organs including skin, eye, mucosa of gastrointestinal and genitourinary tract, joints, endothelial surface of arteries and veins [1].

The disease is most common along the silk route but has been reported from almost all continents [1,2].

It has clear differences with many other rheumatologic disorders which have autoimmune basis in their pathogenesis and the role of environmental factors were considered prominent in this disease [2-4].

There are several clues which may indicate an ethiopathogenesis role for Helicobacter pylori infection in this disease. This infection is most prevalent in areas where BD is common [5-7]. The geographic distribution of the most grave complication of this infection, gastric cancer have many similarities to BD [8,9].

This study was designed to find any possible relation between H. pylori infection either current or in past with BD.

Methods

Patients with a definite diagnosis of BD, based on international study group criteria [10] who were in regular follow-up for at least one year in Behcet's disease Clinic in Motahari Clinic, Shiraz University of Medical Sciences, Islamic Republic of Iran, were studied. Clinical manifestations and organ involvement along with demographic features were recorded.

For the control group, age and sex matched healthy asymptomatic people who were referred for routine check-ups as a part of their regular health surveillance were studied. Specific questions regarding presence of any gastrointestinal compliant and/or previous or current history of gastrointestinal diseases were obtained from both control and study groups and any subject with positive history were excluded. Other exclusion criteria in both cases and controls were: pregnancy, use of proton pump inhibitor or antibiotics in the past month, any co morbid condition such as renal failure, liver disease, chronic obstructive pulmonary disease, congestive heart failure, age under 18 or over 65 years.

Anti Helicobacter Pylori antibody IgG were assayed by ELISA (RADIM, Iran) in both groups. Urea breath test (UBT) was also done for all cases and controls as described elsewhere with carbon 14 after overnight fasting and tooth brushing [11]. If the result of any of these tests were positive, patients were considered infected with H. pylori.

The study design was approved by the ethics committee of the Shiraz University of Medical Sciences.

Informed consent from both groups was taken. Odds ratio, with 95% confidence interval Chi Square (Pearson) and X2 Fisher Exact tests were calculated when appropriate.

* Correspondence: lankaran@sums.ac.ir
[1]Health policy Research Center, Shiraz University of Medical Sciences, P.O. Box 71345–1414, Shiraz, Islamic Republic of Iran
Full list of author information is available at the end of the article

Table 1 Demographic features and Helicobacter pylori status of patients with BD and control group

	Mean age ± SD	Male	Serology positive	UBT positive	Cumulative number of HP infection*
Case	33.2±8.6	17	29	34	37
Controls	32.7±8.8	17	23	20	27
PV	NS	NS	NS	< 0.01	< 0.05

*Total number of HP infection when either serology and or UBT were positive.

Results

48 patients (17 males) with BD fulfilled our criteria and were studied. The same number of healthy people was enrolled in the control group.

Both groups were comparable regarding mean age and sex ratio (Table 1).

H. pylori infection as determined by positive UBT was more prevalent in patients with BD, but the results of serology were not significantly different between the two groups.

When a cumulative number of infected patients using two methods was utilized, the odds ratio for H. pylori was 2.4026 (95% CI: 0.99 – 5.828, PV: <0.05).

When the result of UBT alone was considered, the ratio was 3.1 (95% CI: 1.34 – 7.26, PV < 0.001).

The odds ratios of H. pylori infection for each major organ involvement in patients with BD are shown in Table 2, using a cumulative number of infected patients.

There was only one patient with neurobehcet in this series who was H. pylori infected, therefore the odds ratio could not be calculated for this manifestation.

Discussion

Despite description of BD for more than 2000 years, the pathogenesis of this disease is not clear [3,12,13]. Both genetic and environmental factors are considered to have ethiopathogentic role in BD [14]. It has been shown that Turkish immigrants to Germany have higher incidence of BD compared to native Germans but the incidence of BD is much lower than Turkish population living in Turkey [13,15]. The same pattern is reported for Japanese immigrants to Hawaii, mainland United States and south America [13,16].

Among the environmental factors, the role of infectious agents have been proposed [13]. Viral, bacterial, mycobacterial and even fungal agents have been studied in these patients with variable results.

Several investigators have studied the role of H. pylori infection in BD. Almost all of these studies are from Turkey [17-20]. Avci and colleagues from Turkey probably were the first group to publish on this issue [17]. In their serologic case control study, they did not find no higher prevalence of H. pylori infection in BD compared to control group but H. pylori eradication in a small group of their patients resulted in alleviation of symptoms. Ersoy and Cakmak and their colleagues in two

other different studies from Turkey could not find any relation between BD and H. pylori in endoscopic biopsies [18,19]. Another group from Turkey reported significantly higher prevalence of cytotoxin-associated gene A positivity in BD [21]. In the latter study prevalence of anti H. pylori immunoglobulin G antibody was not significantly higher in BD which is in concordance to previous studies but patients' symptoms improved after H. pylori eradication like Avci's report.

Interestingly there are only case reports on association of H. pylori infection and BD from Japan [22].

In this study from Iran, with a prevalence BD of 80 per 100,000 of inhabitants [7], we found higher prevalence of H. pylori infection in patients with BD. This relation was more prominent when result of UBT was used with OR of 3.1 (95% CI: 1.34 – 7.26, PV < 0.001). Using serology, there was no significant difference between case and control group regarding prevalence of H. pylori infection as was reported by previous researchers.

The reason that serologic evidence of H. pylori infection was not different between two groups might be related to the fact that serology can not differentiate between ongoing infection or previous exposure [23]. It seems BD has a correlation with ongoing infection, as even in previous studies who failed to show a correlation between infection and BD, there were symptomatic improvement with H. pylori eradication in those who were infected [17,21]. Although two previous studies using endoscopic biopsies were not able to show such a relation [18,19], but we should note that there are several intervening factors which may result in false negativity of endoscopic biopsies for H. pylori infection detection.

Table 2 Correlation of clinical findings in BD with HP infection

	Total number	HP infected	OR	95% CI for OR	P value
Positive pathergy test	13	10	0.99	0.22-4.49	0.987
Urogenital ulcers	23	18	1.14	0.30-4.39	0.852
Arthritis	9	8	2.76	0.31-24.89	0.366
Uveitis	12	7	0.28	0.07-1.19	0.084
DVT*	4	3	0.88	0.08-9.44	0.918
Acneiform rash	16	14	2.74	0.52-14.55	0.237
Erythema nodosum	4	3	0.88	0.08-9.44	0.918

*DVT: Deep Vein Thrombosis.

These include inadequate specimens, use of proton pump inhibitors and other acid suppressive agents, recent use of antibiotics among others [23]. In our study we strictly excluded patients who had factors which could interfere with result of UBT and this may explain the different results.

Although the odds ratio for H. pylori infection using cumulative number of infected patients by both UBT and serology was 2.4026 with a p value of less than 0.05. This may be related to relatively small size of our study group [24].

Whether any specific presentation of BD is related to H. pylori infection, has been investigated in few studies. Researchers from Turkey did not find any relation between deep vein thrombosis and H. pylori infection in BD [20]. In our own study we could not find statistically significant correlation between H. pylori infection and BD manifestations, but it seems the limited number of our cases have been contributing. Larger studies are needed to investigate such relation.

The possible mechanism of action of bacterial infections including H. pylori in the pathogensis of BD may involve molecular homology of bacterial antigens and human heat shock protein (HSP) which is now proposed as the possible antigen in BD [3,4]. This antigen is expressed outside of cellular membrane in response to shock and other stresses and physiologic stimuli. Elevated HSP and antibody against this protein have been shown in sera of patients with BD [25]. The mucosal expression of HSP was also found to be higher in BD [26]. There is homology between bacterial antigens and human HSP. Although much of this homology has been reported for Streptococcus sanguis [27], the same homology has also been reported for H. pylori [28]. This would stimulate δγ T cells. This stimulation would be further augmented with exposure to human HSP and start a cascade of proinflammatory reactions.

Conclusions

In conclusion our study from Iran using UBT could reveal a correlation between ongoing H. pylori infection and BD in contrary to all previous reports which had some limitations in their methodologies. To find a correlation between H. pylori infection and specific manifestations of BD, larger studies are needed.

Competing interests
The authors declare that they have no competing interests.

Authors' contributions
KBL developed the idea, arranged the logistic for the study, contributed in data analysis and preparation of manuscript. MRR, MAN, EA and contributed in data gathering and analysis of data and preparation of the manuscript. AR contributed to data gathering and preparation of the manuscript. All authors read and approved the final manuscript.

Acknowledgement
This work was supported by a grant from Shiraz University of Medical Sciences to the corresponding author.

Author details
[1]Health policy Research Center, Shiraz University of Medical Sciences, P.O. Box 71345-1414, Shiraz, Islamic Republic of Iran. [2]Bushehr University of Medical Sciences, Bushehr, Islamic Republic of Iran. [3]Rheumatology Research Center, Shiraz University of Medical Sciences, Shiraz, Islamic Republic of Iran.

References
1. Davatchi F, Shahram F, Chams-Davatchi C, Shams H, Nadji A, Akhlaghi M, Faezi T, Ghodsi Z, Faridar A, Ashofteh F, Sadeghi Abdollahi B: Behcet's disease: from East to West. Clin Rheumatol 2010, 29:823–833.
2. Mendes D, Correia M, Barbedo M, Vaio T, Mota M, Goncalves O, Valente J: Behcet's disease–a contemporary review. J Autoimmun 2009, 32:178–188.
3. Mendoza-Pinto C, Garcia-Carrasco M, Jimenez-Hernandez M, Jimenez Hernandez C, Riebeling-Navarro C, Nava Zavala A, Vera Recabarren M, Espinosa G, Jara Quezada J, Cervera R: Etiopathogenesis of Behcet's disease. Autoimmun Rev 2010, 9:241–245.
4. Pleyer U, Hazirolan D, Stubiger N: Comments on the pathogenesis of Behcet's disease. A key to understanding new therapies? Ophthalmologe 2012, 109(6):563–567. Epub 2012/06/16. Anmerkungen zur Pathogenese des Morbus Behcet. Ein Schlussel zum Verstandnis neuer Therapien?
5. Tan HJ, Goh KL: Changing epidemiology of Helicobacter pylori in Asia. J Dig Dis 2008, 9(4):186–189. Epub 2008/10/31.
6. Goh KL, Chan WK, Shiota S, Yamaoka Y: Epidemiology of Helicobacter pylori infection and public health implications. Helicobacter 2011, 16(Suppl 1):1–9. Epub 2011/09/16.
7. Tonkic A, Tonkic M, Lehours P, Megraud F: Epidemiology and diagnosis of Helicobacter pylori infection. Helicobacter 2012, 17(Suppl 1):1–8. Epub 2012/09/14.
8. Fock KM, Ang TL: Epidemiology of Helicobacter pylori infection and gastric cancer in Asia. J Gastroenterol Hepatol 2010, 25(3):479–486. Epub 2010/04/08.
9. Krejs GJ: Gastric cancer: epidemiology and risk factors. Dig Dis 2010, 28(4–5):600–603. Epub 2010/11/20.
10. Davatchi F: Diagnosis/Classification Criteria for Behcet's Disease. Patholog Res Int 2012, 2012:607921. Epub 2011/10/01.
11. Marshall BJ, Plankey MW, Hoffman SR, Boyd CL, Dye KR, Frierson HF Jr, Guerrant RL, McCallum RW: A 20-minute breath test for helicobacter pylori. Am J Gastroenterol 1991, 86:438–445.
12. Kaklamani VG, Vaiopoulos G, Kaklamanis PG: Behcet's Disease. Semin Arthritis Rheum 1998, 27(4):197–217. Epub 1998/03/26.
13. Galeone M, Colucci R, D'Erme AM, Moretti S, Lotti T: Potential Infectious Etiology of Behcet's Disease. Patholog Res Int 2012, 2012:595380. Epub 2012/01/19.
14. Pineton de Chambrun M, Wechsler B, Geri G, Cacoub P, Saadoun D: New insights into the pathogenesis of Behcet's disease. Autoimmun Rev 2012, 11(10):687–698. Epub 2011/12/27.
15. Zouboulis CC, Kotter I, Djawari D, Kirch W, Kohl PK, Ochsendorf FR, Keitel W, Stadler R, Wollina U, Proksch E, Sohnchen R, Weber H, Gollnick HP, Holzle E, Fritz K, Licht T, Orfanos CE: Epidemiological features of Adamantiades-Behcet's disease in Germany and in Europe. Yonsei Med J 1997, 38:411–422.
16. Hirohata T, Kuratsune M, Nomura A, Jimi S: Prevalence of Behcet's syndrome in Hawaii. With particular reference to the comparison of the Japanese in Hawaii and Japan. Hawaii Med J 1975, 34(7):244–246. Epub 1975/07/01.
17. Avci O, Ellidokuz E, Simsek I, Buyukgebiz B, Gunes AT: Helicobacter pylori and Behcet's disease. Dermatology 1999, 199(2):140–143. Epub 1999/11/13.
18. Cakmak SK, Cakmak A, Gul U, Sulaimanov M, Bingol P, Hazinedaroglu MS: Upper gastrointestinal abnormalities and Helicobacter pylori in Behcet's disease. Int J Dermatol 2009, 48(11):1174–1176. Epub 2010/01/13.
19. Ersoy O, Ersoy R, Yayar O, Demirci H, Tatlican S: H pylori infection in patients with Behcet's disease. World J Gastroenterol 2007, 13(21):2983–2985. Epub 2007/06/26.

20. Senturk O, Ozgur O, Hulagu OS, Canturk NZ, Celebi A, Karakaya AT: **Effect of Helicobacter pylori infection on deep vein thrombosis seen in patients with Behcet's disease.** *East Afr Med J* 2006, **83**(1):49–51. Epub 2006/04/29.

21. Apan TZ, Gursel R, Dolgun A: **Increased seropositivity of Helicobacter pylori cytotoxin-associated gene-A in Behcet's disease.** *Clin Rheumatol* 2007, **26**(6):885–889. Epub 2006/10/06.

22. Nojima M, Abe T, Igarashi S, Honma T, Oki M, Oikawa H, Matsumoto S, Nishimura S, Matsunaga T, Yawata A, Kimura H, Takahashi H, Imai K: **A case of gastric mucosal bridge with Behcet's disease.** *Nihon Rinsho Meneki Gakkai Kaishi* 2004, **27**:177–180.

23. Malfertheiner P, Megraud F, O'Morain CA, Atherton J, Axon AT, Bazzoli F, Gensini GF, Gisbert JP, Graham DY, Rokkas T, El-Omar EM, Kuipers EJ: **Management of Helicobacter pylori infection–the Maastricht IV/Florence Consensus Report.** *Gut* 2012, **61**:646–664.

24. Szumilas M: **Explaining odds ratios.** *J Can Acad Child Adolesc Psychiatry* 2010, **19**(3):227–229.

25. Birtas-Atesoglu E, Inanc N, Yavuz S, Ergun T, Direskeneli H: **Serum levels of free heat shock protein 70 and anti-HSP70 are elevated in Behcet's disease.** *Clin Exp Rheumatol* 2008, **26**(4 Suppl 50):S96–S98. Epub 2008/11/26.

26. Deniz E, Guc U, Buyukbabani N, Gul A: **HSP 60 expression in recurrent oral ulcerations of Behcet's disease.** *Oral Surg Oral Med Oral Pathol Oral Radiol Endod* 2010, **110**:196–200.

27. Kaneko F, Oyama N, Yanagihori H, Isogai E, Yokota K, Oguma K: **The role of streptococcal hypersensitivity in the pathogenesis of Behcet's Disease.** *Eur J Dermatol* 2008, **18**(5):489–498. Epub 2008/08/12.

28. Zhebrun AB, Mukomolov SL, Narvskaia OV: **Genotyping and molecular marking of bacteria and viruses in epidemiological surveillance of actual infections.** *Zh Mikrobiol Epidemiol Immunobiol* 2011, (4):28–36. Epub 2011/09/15.

6

The EPIYA-ABCC motif pattern in *CagA* of *Helicobacter pylori* is associated with peptic ulcer and gastric cancer in Mexican population

Fredy Omar Beltrán-Anaya[1†], Tomás Manuel Poblete[1†], Adolfo Román-Román[1], Salomón Reyes[2], José de Sampedro[3], Oscar Peralta-Zaragoza[4], Miguel Ángel Rodríguez[5], Oscar del Moral-Hernández[5], Berenice Illades-Aguiar[5] and Gloria Fernández-Tilapa[1*†]

Abstract

Background: *Helicobacter pylori* chronic infection is associated with chronic gastritis, peptic ulcer, and gastric cancer. Cytotoxin-associated gene A (*cagA*)-positive *H. pylori* strains increase the risk of gastric pathology. The carcinogenic potential of CagA is linked to its polymorphic EPIYA motif variants. The goals of this study were to investigate the frequency of *cagA*-positive *Helicobacter pylori* in Mexican patients with gastric pathologies and to assess the association of *cagA* EPIYA motif patterns with peptic ulcer and gastric cancer.

Methods: A total of 499 patients were studied; of these, 402 had chronic gastritis, 77 had peptic ulcer, and 20 had gastric cancer. *H. pylori* DNA, *cagA*, and the EPIYA motifs were detected in total DNA from gastric biopsies by PCR. The type and number of EPIYA segments were determined by the electrophoretic patterns. To confirm the PCR results, 20 amplicons of the *cagA* 3' variable region were sequenced, and analyzed *in silico*, and the amino acid sequence was predicted with MEGA software, version 5. The odds ratio (OR) was calculated to determine the associations between the EPIYA motif type and gastric pathology and between the number of EPIYA-C segments and peptic ulcers and gastric cancer.

Results: *H. pylori* DNA was found in 287 (57.5%) of the 499 patients, and 214 (74%) of these patients were *cagA*-positive. The frequency of *cagA*-positive *H. pylori* was 74.6% (164/220) in chronic gastritis patients, 73.6% (39/53) in peptic ulcer patients, and 78.6% (11/14) in gastric cancer patients. The EPIYA-ABC pattern was more frequently observed in chronic gastritis patients (79.3%, 130/164), while the EPIYA-ABCC sequence was more frequently observed in peptic ulcer (64.1%, 25/39) and gastric cancer patients (54.5%, 6/11). However, the risks of peptic ulcer (OR = 7.0, 95% CI = 3.3–15.1; p < 0.001) and gastric cancer (OR = 5.9, 95% CI = 1.5–22.1) were significantly increased in individuals who harbored the EPIYA-ABCC *cagA* gene pattern.

Conclusions: *cagA*-positive *H. pylori* is highly prevalent in southern Mexico, and all CagA variants were of the western type. The *cagA* alleles that code for EPIYA-ABCC motif patterns are associated with peptic ulcers and gastric cancer.

Keywords: *cagA* gene 3' region, CRPIA, EPIYA, CagA, *H. pylori*

* Correspondence: gferti@hotmail.com
†Equal contributors
[1]Clinical Research Laboratory, Academic Unit of Chemical-Biological Sciences, Autonomous University of Guerrero, Chilpancingo, Guerrero C.P. 39090, Mexico
Full list of author information is available at the end of the article

Background

Chronic *Helicobacter pylori* infection is etiologically related to chronic gastritis, gastric ulcers, and gastric cancer [1-4]. Cytotoxin-associated gene A (CagA)-producing strains seem to induce gastrointestinal disease more frequently than non-producing strains [5,6]. While the presence of CagA does not explain the variability in the clinical results, this oncoprotein is associated with severe gastroduodenal pathology [7-15]. *CagA*-positive strains are known to induce more intense gastric mucosal inflammation compared to *cagA*-negative strains. This pro-inflammatory potential of *cagA*-positive *H. pylori* could explain its association with severe atrophic gastritis and gastric adenocarcinoma [16,17]. The CagA oncoprotein is released within epithelial cells via a type IV secretion system [18,19]. Upon translocation, CagA localizes to the internal surface of the plasma membrane, where it is phosphorylated on C-terminal variable region tyrosine residues by multiple host Src tyrosine kinase family member proteins [20-22]. The phosphorylation motifs are defined by the Glu-Pro-Ile-Tyr-Ala (EPIYA) sequence and are classified as EPIYA-A, B, C, or D according to the amino acids that flank these motifs. Western CagA strains have the A and B segments and 1 or more C segments. CagA strains from Eastern Asia have the A, B, and D segments. This explains the size variability of CagA proteins (range, 120–145 kDa) [3,9,23]. The main phosphorylation target in CagA is the tyrosine in the EPIYA-C and EPIYA-D motifs. The phosphorylation level is proportional to the number of EPIYA-C motifs, and thus, increased motif numbers increase the pro-inflammatory and carcinogenic potential of the protein. Phosphorylated CagA forms complexes with the SHP-2 phosphatase, resulting in abnormal signaling. This leads to subsequent cellular alterations that increase the risk of cells altered by precancerous genetic changes [3,23-28]. In epithelial cells, SHP-2 binds more tightly to EPIYA-D than to EPIYA-C. However, CagA proteins with EPIYA-ABCCC have the same carcinogenic potential as those with EPIYA-D [25]. Western CagA-producing *H. pylori* strains with EPIYA-C sequences are more virulent and carcinogenic than CagA-producing strains with EPIYA-A and B motifs [15,29,30].

The prevalence of *cagA*-positive *H. pylori* is 90–95% in Asian countries and 50–60% in western countries [3,23]. *CagA* genotype distribution varies among regions and ethnic groups. For example, the Amerindian (AM) *cagA* allelic variants, which are found in the inhabitants of the Peruvian Shimaa village, encode CagA isoforms that contain altered or degenerate EPIYA-B motifs, specifically ESIYT in AM-I and GSIYD in AM-II. Additionally, the AM CagA contains attenuated conserved repeats that are responsible for phosphorylation-independent activity (CRPIA). The AM strains have attenuated proliferation and induce low-grade inflammation, resulting in low virulence and a decreased risk of severe pathology [26,31].

CagA is one of the most studied genes worldwide. In Mexico, the seroprevalence of *cagA*-positive *H. pylori* varies between 40% and 90% in patients with gastric pathology from different zones throughout the country [8,32-36]. In patients from Mexico City who presented gastroduodenal pathology, the EPIYA segments of *cagA*-positive strain were of the western type [37]. In another study conducted in children with abdominal pain and adults with duodenal ulcers, gastric ulcers, or non-ulcerous dyspepsia, the identified EPIYA patterns were ACC, ABC, ABCC, ABCCC, and ABABC [37]. The following sequences were identified in gastric cancer and chronic gastritis cases: ABC, ABCC, ABABC, AABCC, and ABCCC [38]. However, to date, no studies have been conducted to explore the association between the type and number of EPIYA segments and severe gastric pathologies in southern Mexico. The analysis of the association between the EPIYA-C motif number and peptic ulcers and gastric cancer, will help to clarify the relationship between CagA variants and gastric disease severity in *H. pylori*-infected Mexican patients. The goal of this study was to investigate the prevalence of *cagA*-positive *H. pylori* and the EPIYA motif types in the gastric mucosa of patients with chronic gastritis, peptic ulcers, and gastric cancer to determine whether the EPIYA-C motif number is associated with ulcers and gastric cancer.

In this study, we found a high prevalence of western-type *cagA*-positive *H. pylori* infection, with a predominant EPIYA-ABCC pattern in Mexican patients with peptic ulcers and gastric cancer. Interestingly, the presence of a CagA protein with 2 or more EPIYA-C motifs was associated with severe gastric pathology.

Methods

Patients

A total of 499 patients were studied. The study subjects were sequentially selected from patients who suffered from dyspepsia symptoms and had been subjected to upper gastrointestinal tract endoscopy at the Chilpancingo's General Hospital "Dr. Raymundo Abarca Alarcón" or at the State Institute of Oncology in Acapulco, Guerrero, Mexico. The subjects were recruited between April 18, 2007 and April 19, 2013. Patients in this study had not received treatment with antimicrobial agents, proton pump inhibitors, or gastric pH-neutralizing agents for a month before the endoscopic treatment. Patients who received immunosuppressive or non-steroid anti-inflammatory treatment were excluded from the study. Either the patients or their parents signed an informed consent letter. This project was approved by the Bioethics Committee of the Autonomous University of Guerrero and the participating hospitals.

Biopsy collection

Endoscopies were conducted after an overnight fast with a video processor and a video gastroscope (Fujinon, Wayne, NJ, USA). Two biopsies from the gastric antrum or body, the ulcer edge, or the tumor were collected. One biopsy was immediately fixed in 10% formalin for histological analysis, while the other was placed in a buffered solution (10 mM Tris, pH 8.0, 20 mM EDTA, pH 8.0, 0.5% SDS) for the molecular diagnosis of *H. pylori*. The latter biopsies were stored at −20°C until processing.

Histology

The formalin-fixed biopsies were embedded in paraffin, and 4-μm sections were stained with hematoxylin-eosin for histological analysis. Histopathological findings were used to determine each patient's diagnosis. Gastritis was classified according to the updated Sydney system.

H. pylori detection

Total DNA was extracted from gastric biopsies according to the phenol-chloroform-iso-amyl alcohol technique after proteinase K digestion [39]. The specific presence of the *H. pylori* 16S rRNA gene was assessed according to the methods previously described by Román-Román *et al.* [40]. For all reactions, DNA samples from the *cagA*-positive ATCC43504 and J99 *H. pylori* strains were used as positive controls. For negative controls, DNA was substituted with sterile deionized water. All reactions were performed in a Mastercycler Ep gradient thermocycler (Eppendorf, Hamburg, Germany).

CagA gene amplification

H. pylori 16S rRNA gene-positive samples were subjected to PCR to detect the *cagA* gene using the primers described previously by Figura *et al.*, [9]. These oligonucleotides amplified a 298-bp fragment within the constant region [9]. To amplify a 550- to 850-bp region within the 3′ variable region of the *cagA* gene the primers cag2 and cag4 described previously by Argent *et al.*, were using [41,42], Table 1. The reaction mix consisted of 1.7 mM MgCl2, 0.2 mM dNTPs (Invitrogen, Carlsbad, CA, USA),

5 pmol of each oligonucleotide, 1 U of Platinum® Taq DNA polymerase (Invitrogen Carlsbad, CA, USA), and 300 ng of total DNA in a total volume of 25 μl. The following amplification conditions were used: 1 cycle at 94°C for 5 min; 30 cycles at 94°C for 40 s, 56°C for 30 s, and 72°C for 50 s; and a final extension cycle at 72°C for 10 min. The PCR products were subjected to electrophoresis on a 1.5% agarose gel, followed by ethidium bromide staining and analysis under an ultraviolet (UV) light. Samples were considered CagA-positive when at least 1 of the 2 bands was observed.

Amplification of the cagA gene 3′ variable region and EPIYA motif prediction

Each *cagA*-positive sample was subjected to 4 PCR reactions to identify the EPIYA motifs. The sense oligonucleotide primer cag28F was used in all 4 reactions, while the antisense oligonucleotide primers cagA-P1C, cagAP2TA [41], CagAWest, and CagAEast [42] were used in separate reactions to amplify the EPIYA-A (~264 bp), B (~306 bp), C (~501 bp), and D (495 bp) motifs, respectively, Table 1. All PCR samples were prepared with 0.2 mM dNTPs (Invitrogen Carlsbad, CA, USA), 1.5 mM MgCl$_2$, 10 pmol of each oligonucleotide, 1 U of Platinum® Taq DNA Polymerase (Invitrogen Carlsbad, CA, USA), and 300 ng of total gastric biopsy DNA in a final volume of 25 μl. The following amplification conditions were used: 1 cycle at 94°C for 5 min; 35 cycles at 94°C for 1 min, 58°C for 30 s, and 72°C for 1 min; and a final extension cycle at 72°C for 10 min. The PCR products were separated by electrophoresis on a 1.5% agarose gel, followed by ethidium bromide staining and UV light analysis.

Sequencing and bioinformatics analysis of the cagA gene 3′ variable region

A subset of 20 samples was randomly selected for sequencing to confirm the PCR results. Cag28F and cag4 primers were used to amplify the variable region and generate ~650 to ~850-bp amplicons. The PCR reaction was conducted in a 50-μl volume with 15 pmol of each primer, 0.3 mM dNTPs, 2 mM MgCl$_2$, and 1 U of Platinum® Taq DNA

Table 1 PCR primers used in this study

Primer name and reference	Primer sequence (5'to 3')	Motif amplied	Size (bp)
cagAF D008 [9]	ACAATGCTAAATTAGACAACTTGAGCGA	Constant region of the *cag*A gene	298
cagAR R008 [9]	TTAGAATAATCAACAAACATCACGCCAT		
cag2F [30,41]	GGAACCCTAGTCGGTAATG	*cagA* 3′ variable region	550 to 850
cag4 [30,41]	ATCTTTGAGCTTGTCTATCG		
*cagA*28F [41]	TTCTCAAAGGAGCAATGGC	Forward for all EPIYA motifs	
cagA-P1C [41,42]	GTCCTGCTTTCTTTTTATTAACTTKAGC	*EPIYA-A*	*264*
cagA-P2TA [41,42]	TTTAGCAACTTGAGTATAAATGGG	*EPIYA-B*	*306*
*cagA*West [42]	TTTCAAAGGGAAAGGTCCGCC	*EPIYA-C*	*501*
*cagA*East [42]	AGAGGGAAGCCTGCTTGATT	*EPIYA-D*	*495*

Polymerase (Invitrogen Carlsbad, CA, USA) per reaction. The amplification conditions were as follows: 1 cycle at 94°C for 5 min; 30 cycles at 94°C for 40 s, 55.5°C for 30 s, and 72°C for 50 s; and a final extension cycle at 72°C for 7 min. The PCR products were purified with the Pure-Link® PCR Purification Kit (Invitrogen Carlsbad, CA, USA) according to the manufacturer's instructions. The purified products were sequenced with the BigDye terminator v1.1 sequencing kit (Applied Biosystems, Foster City, CA, USA) and analyzed with an ABI PRISM 310 Genetic Analyzer (Applied Biosystems). The nucleotide sequences were transformed into amino acid sequences with MEGA v5 software [43]. The ClustalW option within the MEGA software was used to generate a multiple amino acid sequence alignment. The partial CagA protein sequence from the *H. pylori* strain 43526 (GenBank: AF001357.1) was used as a reference.

Statistical analysis

Kruskal-Wallis, ANOVA, χ^2, and Fisher's exact test analyses were used to determine significant differences. Associations between the presence of *H. pylori*, CagA, and the EPIYA-C motif number were determined in multinomial logistic regression models at a confidence interval of 95%. A p-value < 0.05 indicated statistical significance. All analyses were conducted with the Stata v11.1 software package (StataCorp, College Station, TX, USA).

Results

Population characteristics

Of the 499 studied patients, 402 (80.6%) were diagnosed with chronic gastritis, 77 (15.4%) with peptic ulcers, and 20 (4%) with gastric cancer. The age of patients ranged from 11 to 80 years old. The cancer patients were significantly older (p < 0.001) than those in the other groups, and the female gender was predominant in all 3 groups.

Education years were significantly different among the groups (p < 0.001), Table 2.

CagA status of *Helicobacter pylori* infections

The presence of the *H. pylori* 16S rRNA gene was detected in the gastric mucosa samples from 287 (57.5%) patients. The difference in the infection frequencies according to the diagnosis was significant (p = 0.037), and a higher prevalence was observed in gastric cancer patients (70%), Figure 1A. The *H. pylori cagA* gene was found in 214 (74%) of the 287 infected patients, Figure 1B. However, no significant differences in the frequencies of *cagA*-positive *H. pylori* were found among the study groups (p = 0.930). The congruence between the two PCR assays for determining *cagA* status was 88% (Kappa correlation coefficient = 0.8857 p <0.001), data not shown

EPIYA segments and EPIYA-C motif numbers

The PCR products amplified from *cagA*-positive samples showed four electrophoretic patterns that corresponded to the following combinations of EPIYA motifs: ABC, ABCC, ABBC, and ABBCCC. The EPIYA-D motif was not detected, Figure 2.

The EPIYA-ABC segment was detected in 148 (69.2%) patients, while the ABCC motif was detected in 64 (29.9%) of the 214 *H. pylori cagA*-positive subjects. The EPIYA ABBCCC motif was only detected in one patient with chronic gastritis, while the ABBC motif was only detected in one patient with gastric cancer, Figure 1C. The EPIYA-ABC pattern was found in 130 (79.3%) of the 164 *cagA*-positive *H. pylori* patients with chronic gastritis and was more frequent in this group than in ulcer and cancer. CagA-positive *H. pylori* with two EPIYA-C motifs was more frequently detected in patients with ulcers and gastric cancer (64.1% and 54.6%, respectively), Table 3, Figure 1C. The results were confirmed by sequencing a ~650- to ~850-bp fragment

Table 2 Sociodemographic characteristics in Mexican patients with chronic gastritis, peptic ulcers, and gastric cancer

	Diagnosis			
	Chronic gastritis n = 402	Peptic ulcer n = 77	Gastric cancer n = 20	*p* value
Age (mean ± SD)	47.4 ± 16.7	52.8 ± 16.5	58.7 ± 16)	0.0009[†]
Gender n (%)				
Male	155 (38.6)	33 (42.9)	9 (45)	0.682[◊]
Female	247 (61.4)	44 (57.1)	11 (55)	
Smoking habit n (%)				
No	239 (59.5)	36 (41.8)	10 (50)	0.096[◊]
Current smoker or former smoker	163 (40.5)	41 (53.2)	10 (50)	
Alcohol consumption n (%)				
No	100 (24.9)	22 (28.6)	6 (30)	0.716[◊]
Consumes or consumed	302 (75.1)	55 (71.4)	14 (70)	
Education [median (ranges), years]	12 (6–17)	12 (6–17)	6 (0–7.5)	0.0001[■]

[†]ANOVA test; [■]Kruskal-Wallis test; [◊] χ^2 test.

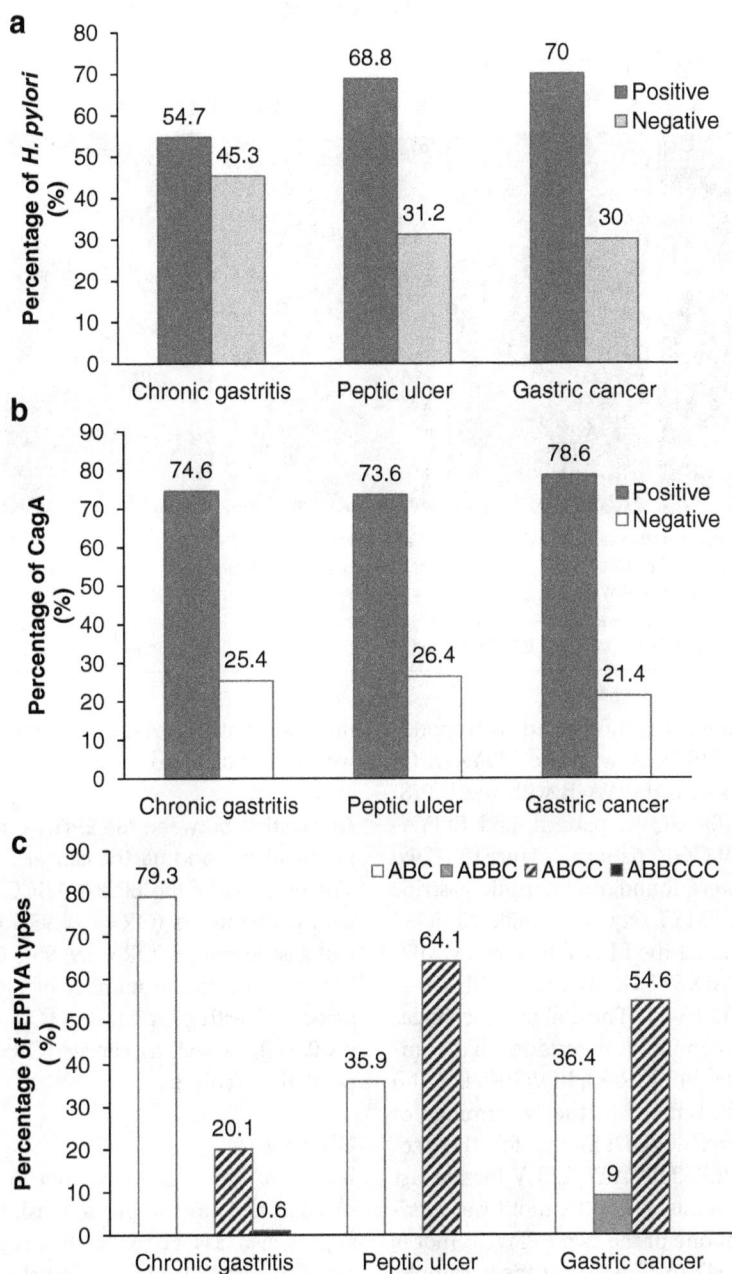

Figure 1 Prevalence of *H. pylori, cagA,* and EPIYA patterns according to histopathological diagnoses. **A**) Percentage of patients with *H. pylori* infection according to gastric disease. There were statistically significant differences in the prevalence of *H. pylori* among the study groups (p = 0.037, χ^2 test). **B**) Percentage of *cagA* among patients with *H. pylori* infection. The prevalence of *cagA*-positive *H. pylori* was very similar among the study groups (p = 0.930, χ^2 test). **C**) The prevalence of the different EPIYA patterns in the *cagA* gene is shown. The EPIYA-ABC and ABCC sequences were differentially distributed among patients with chronic gastritis, peptic ulcers, and gastric cancer (p = 0.000; Fisher's exact test).

within the 3′ variable region of the *cagA* gene in 20 randomly selected samples. The agreement between the results of PCR and sequencing was 100%.

Bioinformatic analysis of the CagA amino acid sequence

The *cagA* DNA sequences from the following amplicons were analyzed: 9 gastric cancer amplicons (MX02-C,

MX21-C, MX22-C, MX05-C, MX12-C, MX03-C, MX08-C, MX17-C, MX16-C); 9 chronic gastritis amplicons (MX66-G, MX51-G, MX52-G, MX637-G, MX006-G, MX44-G, MX43-G, MX45-G, MX392-G) and two peptic ulcer amplicons (MX204-GU, MX327-GU). An *in silico* amino acid prediction was conducted to identify the EPIYA and CagA multimerization (CM, also known as

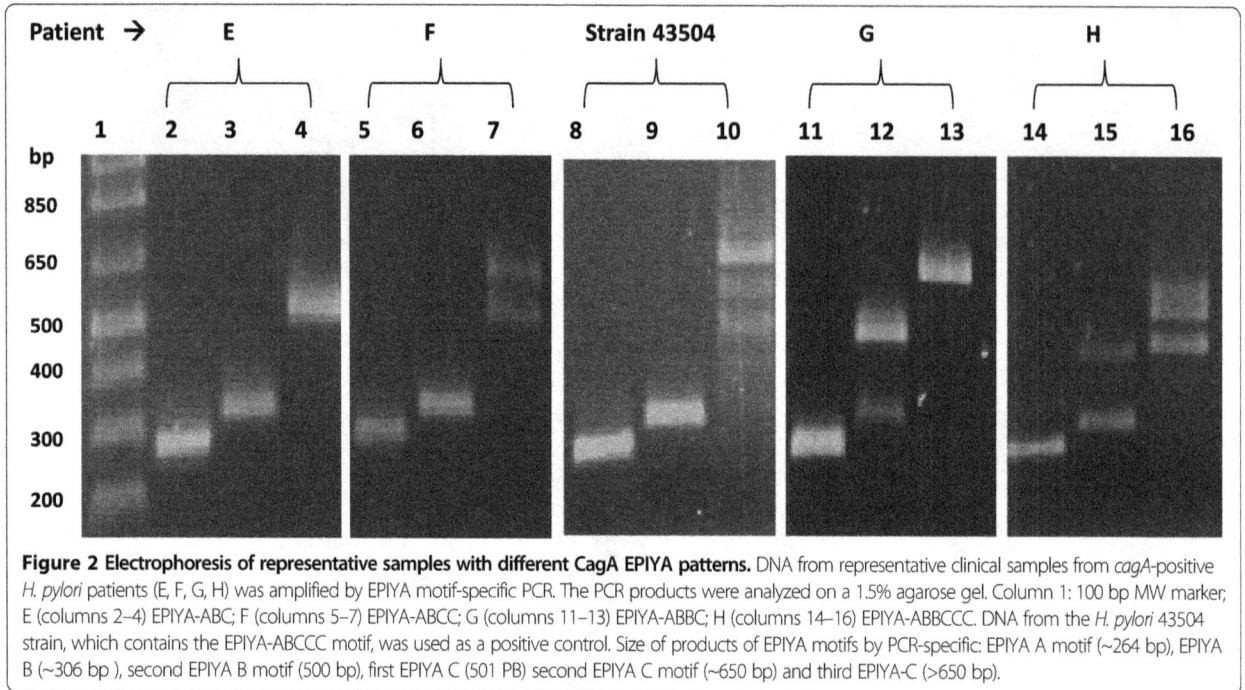

Figure 2 Electrophoresis of representative samples with different CagA EPIYA patterns. DNA from representative clinical samples from *cagA*-positive *H. pylori* patients (E, F, G, H) was amplified by EPIYA motif-specific PCR. The PCR products were analyzed on a 1.5% agarose gel. Column 1: 100 bp MW marker; E (columns 2–4) EPIYA-ABC; F (columns 5–7) EPIYA-ABCC; G (columns 11–13) EPIYA-ABBC; H (columns 14–16) EPIYA-ABBCCC. DNA from the *H. pylori* 43504 strain, which contains the EPIYA-ABCCC motif, was used as a positive control. Size of products of EPIYA motifs by PCR-specific: EPIYA A motif (~264 bp), EPIYA B (~306 bp), second EPIYA B motif (500 bp), first EPIYA C (501 PB) second EPIYA C motif (~650 bp) and third EPIYA-C (>650 bp).

CRPIA) motifs [26]. The following motifs and corresponding patterns were found: EPIYA-A with the EPIYA(K/Q) VNKKK (A/T/V/S)GQ pattern, EPIYA-B with the E(P/S) IY(A/T)(Q/K)VAKKV(N/T)(A/Q)KI pattern, and EPIYA-C with the EPIYATIDDLGGP pattern, Figure 3. Two EPIYA-B motif variants were found; one chronic gastritis sample (MX44-G) had an ESIYT sequence, while 10 (50%) of the 20 sequences contained the EPIYT pattern (MX02-C, MX22-C, MX05-C, MX637-G, MX03-C, MX08-C, MX327-GU, MX43-G, MX16-C). The following changes were found among the 16 amino acid residues that comprise the CRPIA motif: FPLK(R/K)H(D/G)KVD(D/N) LSKVG for the first CRPIA motif in the N-terminus of EPIYA-C, FPLK(R/K)H(D/G)KVDDLSKVG for the second CRPIA motif, and FPLKRHDKVDDLSKV for the last CRPIA motif in the C-terminus. A CRPIA motif was identified in the N-terminus of one of the two EPIYA-B motifs in the CagA-containing MX16-C gastric cancer sample. Within this sequence, the amino acids GKDKGPE were found in the N-terminus of the EPIYA-A motif (Figure 3). All CRPIA motifs were of the western type, Figure 3. Nucleotide and predict protein sequences of all strains were deposited in GenBank, accession numbers [GenBank: KF800898.1- GenBank:KF800917.1].

Association between *H. pylori* infection, *cagA*-positive strains, peptic ulcers, and gastric cancer

H. pylori infection was associated with peptic ulcers (OR = 1.8; 95% CI = 1.0–3.0) but not with gastric cancer (OR = 1.9; 95% CI = 0.72–5.1). On the other hand, infection with *cagA*-positive strains was not associated with either ulcers or gastric cancer, Table 3.

Association between the EPIYA-C motifs number with peptic ulcers, and gastric cancer

The presence of the EPIYA-ABCC segment was associated with peptic ulcers (OR = 7.0; 95% CI = 3.3–15.1; p < 0.001) and gastric cancer (OR = 5.9; 95% CI = 1.5–22.1; p = 0.008). The increase in the number of EPIYA-C repeats was also associated with peptic ulcers (OR = 6.8; 95% CI = 3.2–15.6; p < 0.001), as well as cancer (OR = 4.5; 95% CI = 1.3-15.9; p = 0.017), Table 3.

Discussion

Infection with a *cagA*-positive *H. pylori* strain is recognized as the most important risk factor for gastric cancer and is also associated with atrophic gastritis and duodenal ulcers [29,44]. Nonetheless, the majority of infected patients do not develop serious diseases.

In the present study, we found that 57.5% of patients with gastric pathologies were *H. pylori*-positive, and 74% of the infecting strains harbored the *cagA* gene. The global prevalence of *cagA*-positive *H. pylori*, which ranges from 43% to 90%, is in accordance with the previously reported seroprevalence in a Mexican population with gastric pathologies [8,32-36]. However, serology might overestimate the frequency of *H. pylori* and *cagA*-positive strains as it is unable to differentiate between current and past infections. The discrepancies in the prevalence of *H. pylori* can be explained by differences in the diagnostic method used, age of patients, geographic area and the environmental

Table 3 Association of H. pylori, cagA and EPIYA-C motif number with chronic gastritis, peptic ulcer and gastric cancer

Diagnosis	H. pylori			
	Negative	Positive	OR	CI 95%
G	182	220	1.0	-
PU	24	53	1.8[c]	1.0-3.0
GC	6	14	1.9	0.72-5.1
Total	**212**	**287**		
	CagA			
	Negative	Positive	OR	CI 95%
G	56	164	1.0	-
PU	14	39	0.9	0.5- 1.9
GC	3	11	1.2	0.3 – 4.6
Total	**73**	**214**		
	EPIYA motif			
	ABC	ABCC	OR	IC95%
G	130	33	1.0	-
PU	14	25	7.0[a]	3.3 – 15.1
GC	4	6	5.9[b]	1.5-22.1
Total	**148**	**64**		
	Number of EPIYA-C			
	1 C*	≥2 C[φ]	OR	IC95%
G	130	34	1.0	-
PU	14	25	6.8[a]	3.2-15.6
GC	5	6	4.5[c]	1.3-15.9
Total	**149**	**65**		

G; chronic gastritis, UP peptic ulcer, CG: gastric cancer. [a]$p < 0.001$; [b]$p <0.01$; [c]$p < 0.05$. * The EPIYA-ABBC was added; [φ] the EPIYA-ABBCCC was added
Note: Only the most frequent EPIYA motifs were considered.

health conditions in which people live. Another possible explanation is that the rate of infection is decreasing [36]. In our study, the prevalence of cagA-positive H. pylori in patients with chronic gastritis was higher (74.6%) than the rate reported in 2009 by Paniagua et al. (52.4%) via multiplex PCR [45]. In gastric cancer patients, the prevalence of cagA was higher (78.6%) than the seroprevalence reported in 2008 by Carmolinga et al. (66.2%) [8]. In this work, the frequency of H. pylori cagA-positive that we found was similar to antibodies prevalence in Mexican subjects and, unlike to other studies, the strengths of our study are in the sample size and the high sensitivity and specificity of the methods used to detect H. pylori and cagA.

Some authors have found an association between CagA and the severity of gastric pathologies [7,11-14]. It has been proposed that this relationship might be explained by the number of EPIYA-C motifs in the protein as these motifs influence the degree of virulence and oncogenic potential of cagA-positive H. pylori [7,46]. It is likely that

determining the EPIYA motifs in CagA, rather than detecting cagA per se, would be a better marker for assessing the risk of serious gastric pathology [41,47]. In our study, 100% of the EPIYA motifs identified in CagA were of the western type, and their distributions among the pathologies were significantly different ($p \le 0.001$). In 69.1% of the cases, the cagA gene contained an EPIYA-C motif in the typical ABC sequence, and this was more frequent in patients with chronic gastritis (79.3%). This result was similar to that reported by Batista et al. for Brazilian populations (70.6% in total of cases and 79.4% in patients with gastritis), [48] but higher than that found in Colombian patients by Quiroga et al. (49% in total of cases and 59.6% in patients with gastriris), [29] and by Acosta et al. (62.3% in total of cases and 52.6%, in gastritis) [49]. Interestingly, Rizzato et al. [38] detected the EPIYA-ABC pattern in 82% of Venezuelan and Mexican patients with chronic gastritis and gastric cancer, without finding frequency differences between the groups. Reyes-León et al. [37] found that the ABC sequence was more frequent (50%) in children from Mexico City with chronic abdominal pain. These findings emphasize the differences in the geographic distribution of H. pylori strains, and these differences might be related to the uneven prevalence of gastric cancer in the inhabitants of different Mexican regions.

The frequency of cases that harbored cagA-positive H. pylori with two EPIYA-C motifs was higher in gastric cancer patients (64%) and thus higher than the frequencies reported by Acosta (27.7%) and Quiroga (35.3%) in Colombia and by Batista in Brazil (34.6%) [29,48,49]. We found that the cagA allele that encoded two EPIYA-C segments was also predominant in patients with peptic ulcers (54.5%). This frequency is higher than that reported by Torres in Cuban patients (15.7%) [50]. Unexpectedly, the only motif with three EPIYA-C repeats (ABBCCC) was found in a patient with chronic gastritis. Reportedly, an increase in the number of phosphorylation sites in the C-terminus of CagA is associated with the carcinogenic potential of H. pylori [15,37,49]. Thus, it is likely that those patients with chronic gastritis infected with a H. pylori strain with cagA gene that encodes two or more EPIYA-C motifs (21%) are at higher risk of developing more serious diseases.

The amino acid sequences obtained during a bioinformatics analysis revealed that the alanine-to-threonine substitution in the EPIYA-B (EPIYT) motif occurred frequently (10 out of 20 sequences) in the studied groups. These findings are in accordance with those reported by Rizzato et al. in 2012 for Mexican and Venezuelan subjects with chronic gastritis and gastric cancer (50% of the B motifs harbored the EPIYT variant, with no significant differences between the groups) [38]. ABCC isolates bearing this modification have also been reported to cause decreased levels of cellular elongation and IL-8 secretion compared to those that bear

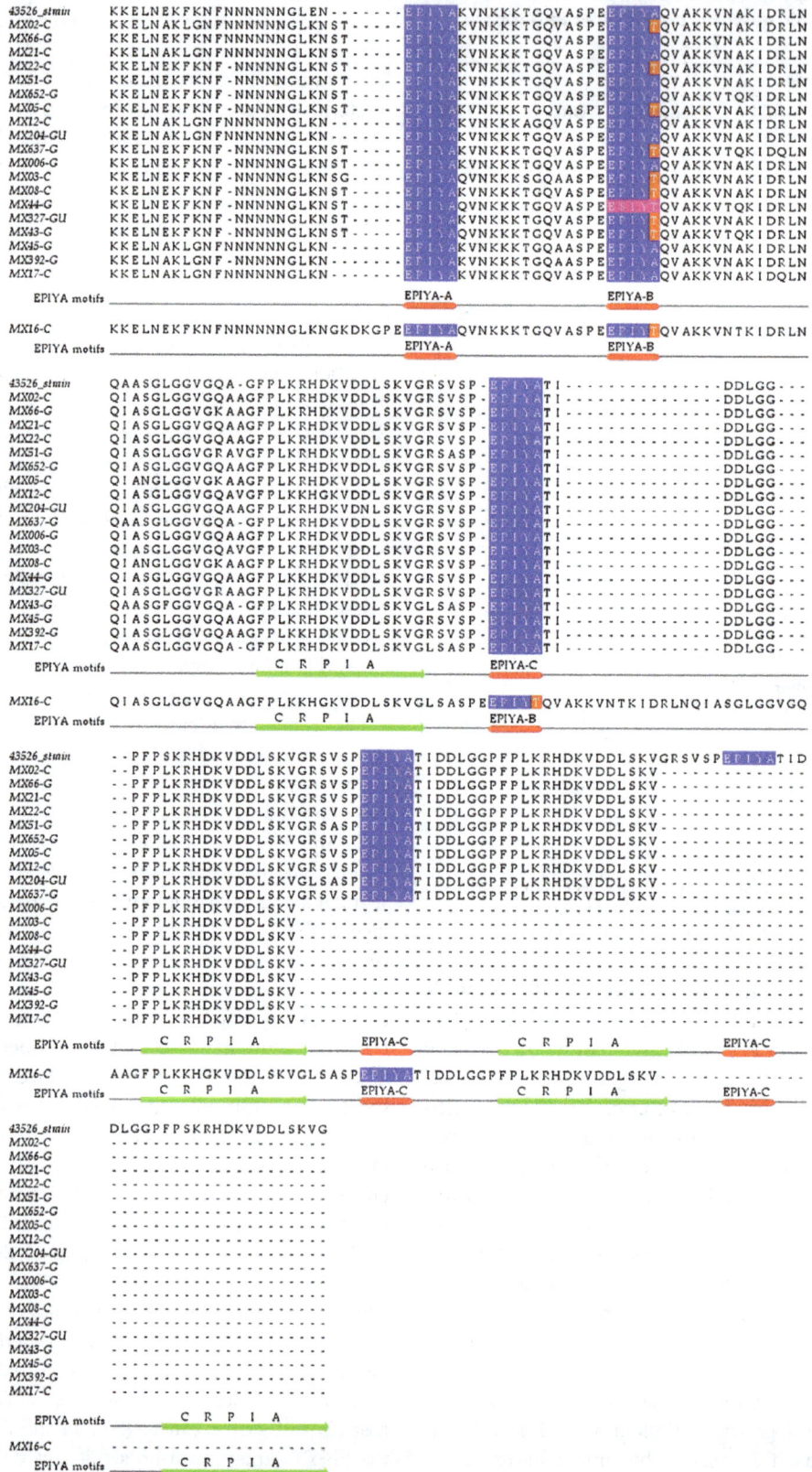

Figure 3 (See legend on next page.)

the normal ABCC pattern [37]. It is possible that, in a Mexican population, the frequency of CagA isoforms with the EPIYT amino acid sequence in EPIYA-B is associated with the prevalence of gastroduodenal diseases. However, the existing epidemiological and experimental studies are insufficient to further support this hypothesis.

The ESIYT modification in EPIYA-B was identified in one chronic gastritis sample. This sequence belonged to the AM-I CagA variant, which has been associated with low *H. pylori* virulence in comparison to the western or Asian strains [26]. However, the AM-I and II CagA variants, such as those found in indigenous Mexican groups with Amerindian ancestry, show degeneration or elimination in their CRPIA motifs [26,31,51]. Interestingly, the CagA variants with the ESIYT sequence found in the present study contained western-type CRPIA and therefore differed from the Amerindian variants [31]. A CRPIA sequence in the N-terminus of the EPIYA-B motif was also detected in a gastric cancer sample. This finding agrees with those reported by Sicinschi *et al.*, Sgouras *et al.* and Acosta *et al.*, who noted that in some CagA variants, the CRPIA segment can be found in the N-termini of the EPIYA-A and B motifs [15,49,52]. The localization of the CRPIA motif within EPIYA-B might result from recombination between *H. pylori* strains with different *cagA* allelotypes or from the insertion of DNA sequences that contribute to *H. pylori* diversification [53,54]. The CRPIA sequences stabilize the CagA protein, influence its half-life and are associated with oncoprotein activity in epithelial cells [15]. Thus, our results highlight the need to evaluate the functional importance of the EPIYT and ESIYT variants in EPIYA-B. Furthermore, it is necessary to assess the effects that the observed sequence variants and the localization of the CRPIA motifs in the ABCC pattern exert on CagA activity. It is likely that the prevalence of some of these variants could explain why the gastric cancer incidence rates of male and female Mexican patients (9.4 and 6.7/100,000, respectively) are similar to those reported in Southeastern Asian countries (10.2 and 4.7/100,000 in men and women, respectively) [55], despite the differences in the *cagA*-positive *H. pylori* prevalence (90–95% in Japan, Korea, and China; 50–60% in Mexico).

The association of *cagA* polymorphisms with severe gastric pathologies [7,29,48-50,52] or with pre-cancerous lesions is controversial [10,15,30,32], and only a few studies have been conducted in Hispanic populations with gastric ulcers [50]. This is the first study to investigate the prevalence of *cagA* variants in southern Mexico. Our results show that the presence of two or more EPIYA-C repeats within the *cagA* gene represents a higher risk of peptic ulcers and gastric cancer. It is likely that this increase in the number of EPIYA-C repeats plays an important role in the development of such diseases in individuals from this particular geographic region. A total of 51.5% of the samples with two EPIYA-C repeats came from patients with chronic gastritis. It is likely that some of these individuals have a higher risk of cancer development [29] given that the increase in the number of EPIYA-C motifs increases the CagA phosphorylation status and its interactions with cellular proteins that induce epithelial cell elongation, cell turnover, and pro-inflammatory cytokine production, thus facilitating the development of gastric cancer [29,41]. These findings might also be related to other clinical results.

The virulence factors of *H. pylori* are important risk determinants but are not sufficient to induce the full development of severe gastroduodenal disease. The host's genetic and sociocultural factors also contribute to the risk of pre-cancerous lesions and gastric cancer [56,57].

Conclusions

In conclusion, the present study shows that *cagA*-positive *H. pylori* infection is highly prevalent in patients from southern Mexico with chronic gastritis, peptic ulcers, and gastric cancer. All CagA isoforms were of the western type. The *cagA* allele that encodes the EPIYA-ABC pattern was most frequently observed in chronic gastritis samples, while the EPIYA-ABCC isoform predominated in peptic ulcer and gastric cancer samples. *CagA* variants that encode two or more EPIYA-C motifs are associated with peptic ulcer and gastric cancer. Likely, either the EPIYA-ABCC sequence or patterns with two or more EPIYA-C motifs are a risk marker for severe gastric pathologies.

Competing interests
The authors declare that they have no competing interests.

Authors' contributions
GFT and ARR designed and coordinated the research. SR and JS conducted the endoscopic study and obtained patient biopsies. FOBA and TMP conducted the research. MAR and OMH conducted the sequencing reactions. OPZ conducted the bioinformatics analysis. FOBA, BIA, and GFT analyzed the data and wrote the manuscript. All authors read and approved the final manuscript.

Acknowledgements
The authors wish to thank gastroenterologists as well as the nurses and support personnel who assisted in obtaining samples. We also want to thank Martín O. Morrugares Ixtepan, Specialist in Pathological Anatomy with subspecialty in Oncological Pathology, who was responsible for the histopathological diagnosis. Special thanks to Dr. Victor Hugo Garzon Barrientos and Dr. José Eduardo Navarro Zarza, who approved the project. This study was supported by the Autonomous University of Guerrero (2010–2012 funding period) and the Secretariat of Public Education (via PROMEP 2007 key PROMEP UAGUER-EXB-096 and PIFI-2010 support for ex-fellows). During the investigation, Tomás Manuel Poblete and Fredy Omar Beltrán were fellows of CONACYT, Mexico.

Author details
[1]Clinical Research Laboratory, Academic Unit of Chemical-Biological Sciences, Autonomous University of Guerrero, Chilpancingo, Guerrero C.P. 39090, Mexico. [2]State Institute of Oncology "Dr. Arturo Beltrán Ortega", Acapulco, Guerrero C. P. 39570, Mexico. [3]General Hospital "Dr. Raymundo Abarca Alarcón", Chilpancingo, Guerrero C.P. 39090, Mexico. [4]Department of Chronic Infections and Cancer, Infectious Diseases Research Center, National Institute of Public Health, Av. Universidad No. 655, Cerrada los Pinos y Caminera, Colonia Santa María Ahuacatitlan, Cuernavaca, Morelos C.P. 62100, Mexico. [5]Laboratory of Molecular Biomedicine, Academic Unit of Chemical-Biological Sciences, Autonomous University of Guerrero, Chilpancingo, Guerrero C.P. 39090, Mexico.

References
1. de Martel C, Forman D, Plummer M: **Gastric cancer: epidemiology and risk factors.** *Gastroenterol Clin N Am* 2013, **42**:219–40.
2. Wroblewski LE, Peek RM Jr, Wilson KT: *Helicobacter pylori* **and gastric cancer: factors that modulate disease risk.** *Clin Microbiol Rev* 2010, **23**:713–39.
3. Hatakeyama M: *Helicobacter pylori* **and gastric carcinogenesis.** *J Gastroenterol* 2009, **44**:239–48.
4. Kuipers EJ, Perez-Perez GI, Meuwissen SG, Blaser MJ: *Helicobacter pylori* **and atrophic gastritis: importance of the** *cagA* **status.** *J Natl Cancer Inst* 1995, **87**:1777–80.
5. Proenca Modena JL, Lopes Sales AI, Olszanski Acrani G, Russo R, Vilela Ribeiro MA, Fukuhara Y, da Silveira WD, Modena JL, de Oliveira RB, Brocchi M: **Association between** *Helicobacter pylori* **genotypes and gastric disorders in relation to the cag pathogenicity island.** *Diagn Microbiol Infect Dis* 2007, **59**:7–16.
6. Secka O, Antonio M, Berg DE, Tapgun M, Bottomley C, Thomas V, Walton R, Corrah T, Thomas JE, Adegbola RA: **Mixed infection with** *cagA* **positive and** *cagA* **negative strains of** *Helicobacter pylori* **lowers disease burden in The Gambia.** *PLoS One* 2011, **6**:e27954.
7. Basso D, Zambon CF, Letley DP, Stranges A, Marchet A, Rhead JL, Schiavon S, Guariso G, Ceroti M, Nitti D, Rugge M, Plebani M, Atherton JC: **Clinical relevance of** *Helicobacter pylori cagA* **and** *vacA* **gene polymorphisms.** *Gastroenterology* 2008, **135**:91–9.
8. Camorlinga-Ponce M, Flores-Luna L, Lazcano-Ponce E, Herrero R, Bernal-Sahagun F, Abdo-Francis JM, Aguirre-Garcia J, Munoz N, Torres J: **Age and severity of mucosal lesions influence the performance of serologic markers in** *Helicobacter pylori*-**associated gastroduodenal pathologies.** *Cancer Epidemiol Biomarkers Prev* 2008, **17**:2498–504.
9. Figura N, Vindigni C, Covacci A, Presenti L, Burronim D, Vernillo R, Banducci T, Roviello F, Marrelli D, Biscontri M, Kristodhullu S, Gennari C, Vaira D: **cagA positive and negative Helicobacter pylori strains are simultaneously**
present in the stomach of most patients with non-ulcer dyspepsia: relevance to histological damage. *Gut* 1998, **42**:772–8.
10. Flores-Luna L, Camorlinga-Ponce M, Hernandez-Suarez G, Kasamatsu E, Martinez ME, Murillo R, Lazcano E, Torres J: **The utility of serologic tests as biomarkers for** *Helicobacter pylori*-**associated precancerous lesions and gastric cancer varies between Latin American countries.** *Cancer Causes Control* 2013, **24**:241–8.
11. Huang JQ, Zheng GF, Sumanac K, Irvine EJ, Hunt RH: **Meta-analysis of the relationship between** *cagA* **seropositivity and gastric cancer.** *Gastroenterology* 2003, **125**:1636–44.
12. Palli D, Masala G, Del Giudice G, Plebani M, Basso D, Berti D, Numans ME, Ceroti M, Peeters PH, de Mesquita HB B, Buchner FL, Clavel-Chapelon F, Boutron-Ruault MC, Krogh V, Saieva C, Vineis P, Panico S, Tumino R, Nyrén O, Simán H, Berglund G, Hallmans G, Sanchez MJ, Larrãnaga N, Barricarte A, Navarro C, Quiros JR, Key T, Allen N, Bingham S: **CagA+** *Helicobacter pylori* **infection and gastric cancer risk in the EPIC-EURGAST study.** *Int J Cancer* 2007, **120**(4):859–67.
13. Sahara S, Sugimoto M, Vilaichone RK, Mahachai V, Miyajima H, Furuta T, Yamaoka Y: **Role of** *Helicobacter pylori cagA* **EPIYA motif and** *vacA* **genotypes for the development of gastrointestinal diseases in Southeast Asian countries: a meta-analysis.** *BMC Infect Dis* 2012, **12**:223.
14. Satomi S, Yamakawa A, Matsunaga S, Masaki R, Inagaki T, Okuda T, Suto H, Ito Y, Yamazaki Y, Kuriyama M, Keida Y, Kutsumi H, Azuma T: **Relationship between the diversity of the** *cagA* **gene of** *Helicobacter pylori* **and gastric cancer in Okinawa, Japan.** *J Gastroenterol* 2006, **41**:668–73.
15. Sicinschi LA, Correa P, Peek RM, Camargo MC, Piazuelo MB, Romero-Gallo J, Hobbs SS, Krishna U, Delgado A, Mera R, Bravo LE, Schneider BG: **CagA C-terminal variations in** *Helicobacter pylori* **strains from Colombian patients with gastric precancerous lesions.** *Clin Microbiol Infect* 2010, **16**:369–78.
16. Matteo MJ, Granados G, Perez CV, Olmos M, Sanchez C, Catalano M: *Helicobacter pylori cag* **pathogenicity island genotype diversity within the gastric niche of a single host.** *J Med Microbiol* 2007, **56**(Pt 5):664–9.
17. Nomura AM, Lee J, Stemmermann GN, Nomura RY, Perez-Perez GI, Blaser MJ: *Helicobacter pylori* **CagA seropositivity and gastric carcinoma risk in a Japanese American population.** *J Infect Dis* 2002, **186**:1138–44.
18. Backert S, Ziska E, Brinkmann V, Zimny-Arndt U, Fauconnier A, Jungblut PR, Naumann M, Meyer TF: **Translocation of the** *Helicobacter pylori* **CagA protein in gastric epithelial cells by a type IV secretion apparatus.** *Cell Microbiol* 2000, **2**:155–64.
19. Rohde M, Puls J, Buhrdorf R, Fischer W, Haas R: **A novel sheathed surface organelle of the** *Helicobacter pylori cag* **type IV secretion system.** *Mol Microbiol* 2003, **49**:219–34.
20. Mueller D, Tegtmeyer N, Brandt S, Yamaoka Y, De Poire E, Sgouras D, Wessler S, Torres J, Smolka A, Backert S: **c-Src and c-Abl kinases control hierarchic phosphorylation and function of the CagA effector protein in Western and East Asian** *Helicobacter pylori* **strains.** *J Clin Invest* 2012, **122**:1553–66.
21. Selbach M, Moese S, Hauck CR, Meyer TF, Backert S: **Src is the kinase of the** *Helicobacter pylori* **CagA protein in vitro and in vivo.** *J Biol Chem* 2002, **277**:6775–8.
22. Tegtmeyer N, Backert S: **Role of Abl and Src family kinases in actin-cytoskeletal rearrangements induced by the** *Helicobacter pylori* **CagA protein.** *Eur J Cell Biol* 2011, **90**:880–90.
23. Murata-Kamiya N: **Pathophysiological functions of the CagA oncoprotein during infection by** *Helicobacter pylori*. *Microbes Infect* 2011, **13**:799–807.
24. Backert S, Tegtmeyer N, Selbach M: **The versatility of** *Helicobacter pylori* **CagA effector protein functions: the master key hypothesis.** *Helicobacter* 2010, **15**:163–76.
25. Higashi H, Tsutsumi R, Muto S, Sugiyama T, Azuma T, Asaka M, Hatakeyama M: **SHP-2 tyrosine phosphatase as an intracellular target of** *Helicobacter pylori* **CagA protein.** *Science* 2002, **295**:683–6.
26. Suzuki M, Kiga K, Kersulyte D, Cok J, Hooper CC, Mimuro H, Sanada T, Suzuki S, Oyama M, Kozuka-Hata H, Kamiya S, Zou QM, Gilman RH, Berg DE, Sasakawa C: **Attenuated CagA oncoprotein in** *Helicobacter pylori* **from Amerindians in Peruvian Amazon.** *J Biol Chem* 2011, **286**:29964–72.
27. Suzuki M, Mimuro H, Kiga K, Fukumatsu M, Ishijima N, Morikawa H, Nagai S, Koyasu S, Gilman RH, Kersulyte D, Berg DE, Sasakawa C: *Helicobacter pylori* **CagA phosphorylation-independent function in epithelial proliferation and inflammation.** *Cell Host Microbe* 2009, **5**:23–34.
28. Yamazaki S, Yamakawa A, Ito Y, Ohtani M, Higashi H, Hatakeyama M, Azuma T: **The CagA protein of** *Helicobacter pylori* **is translocated into epithelial**

cells and binds to SHP-2 in human gastric mucosa. *J Infect Dis* 2003, 187:334–7.

29. Quiroga AJ, Huertas A, Combita AL, Bravo MM: Variation in the number of EPIYA-C repeats in CagA protein from Colombian *Helicobacter pylori* strains and its ability middle to induce hummingbird phenotype in gastric epithelial cells. *Biomedica* 2010, 30:251–8.

30. Salih BA, Bolek BK, Arikan S: DNA sequence analysis of cagA 3′ motifs of *Helicobacter pylori* strains from patients with peptic ulcer diseases. *J Med Microbiol* 2010, 59(Pt 2):144–8.

31. Camorlinga-Ponce M, Perez-Perez G, Gonzalez-Valencia G, Mendoza I, Penaloza-Espinosa R, Ramos I, Kersulyte D, Reyes-Leon A, Romo C, Granados J, Muñoz L, Berg DE, Torres J: *Helicobacter pylori* genotyping from American indigenous groups shows novel Amerindian vacA and cagA alleles and Asian. African and European admixture. *PLoS One* 2011, 6:e27212.

32. Bosques-Padilla FJ, Tijerina-Menchaca R, Perez-Perez GI, Flores-Gutierrez JP, Garza-Gonzalez E: Comparison of *Helicobacter pylori* prevalence in symptomatic patients in northeastern Mexico with the rest of the country: its association with gastrointestinal disease. *Arch Med Res* 2003, 34:60–3.

33. Lopez-Carrillo L, Camargo MC, Schneider BG, Sicinschi LA, Hernandez-Ramirez RU, Correa P, Cebrian ME: Capsaicin consumption, *Helicobacter pylori* CagA status and IL1B-31C > T genotypes: a host and environment interaction in gastric cancer. *Food Chem Toxicol* 2012, 50:2118–22.

34. Lopez-Carrillo L, Torres-Lopez J, Galvan-Portillo M, Munoz L, Lopez-Cervantes M: *Helicobacter pylori*-CagA seropositivity and nitrite and ascorbic acid food intake as predictors for gastric cancer. *Eur J Cancer* 2004, 40:1752–9.

35. Sicinschi LA, Lopez-Carrillo L, Camargo MC, Correa P, Sierra RA, Henry RR, Chen J, Zabaleta J, Piazuelo MB, Schneider BG: Gastric cancer risk in a Mexican population: role of *Helicobacter pylori* CagA positive infection and polymorphisms in interleukin-1 and −10 genes. *Int J Cancer* 2006, 118:649–57.

36. Torres J, Lopez L, Lazcano E, Camorlinga M, Flores L, Munoz O: Trends in *Helicobacter pylori* infection and gastric cancer in Mexico. *Cancer Epidemiol Biomarkers Prev* 2005, 14:1874–7.

37. Reyes-Leon A, Atherton JC, Argent RH, Puente JL, Torres J: Heterogeneity in the activity of Mexican *Helicobacter pylori* strains in gastric epithelial cells and its association with diversity in the cagA gene. *Infect Immun* 2007, 75:3445–54.

38. Rizzato C, Torres J, Plummer M, Munoz N, Franceschi S, Camorlinga-Ponce M, Fuentes-Panana EM, Canzian F, Kato I: Variations in *Helicobacter pylori* cytotoxin-associated genes and their influence in progression to gastric cancer: implications for prevention. *PLoS One* 2012, 7:e29605.

39. Green MR, Sambrook J: *Molecular cloning: a laboratory manual*. New York: Cold Spring Harbor Laboratory Press; 2012.

40. Roman-Roman A, Giono-Cerezo S, Camorlinga-Ponce M, Martinez-Carrillo DN, Loaiza-Loeza S, Fernandez-Tilapa G: vacA genotypes of *Helicobacter pylori* in the oral cavity and stomach of patients with chronic gastritis and gastric ulcer. *Enferm Infecc Microbiol Clin* 2013, 31:130–5.

41. Argent RH, Zhang Y, Atherton JC: Simple method for determination of the number of *Helicobacter pylori* CagA variable-region EPIYA tyrosine phosphorylation motifs by PCR. *J Clin Microbiol* 2005, 43:791–5.

42. Schmidt HM, Goh KL, Fock KM, Hilmi I, Dhamodaran S, Forman D, Mitchell H: Distinct cagA EPIYA motifs are associated with ethnic diversity in Malaysia and Singapore. *Helicobacter* 2009, 14:256–63.

43. Tamura K, Peterson D, Peterson N, Stecher G, Nei M, Kumar S: MEGA5: molecular evolutionary genetics analysis using maximum likelihood, evolutionary distance, and maximum parsimony methods. *Mol Biol Evol* 2011, 28:2731–9.

44. Queiroz DM, Silva CI, Goncalves MH, Braga-Neto MB, Fialho AB, Fialho AM, Rocha GA, Rocha AM, Batista SA, Guerrant RL, Lima AA, Braga LL: Higher frequency of cagA EPIYA-C phosphorylation sites in H. pylori strains from first-degree relatives of gastric cancer patients. *BMC Gastroenterol* 2012, 12:107.

45. Paniagua GL, Monroy E, Rodriguez R, Arroniz S, Rodriguez C, Cortes JL, Camacho A, Negrete E, Vaca S: Frequency of vacA, cagA and babA2 virulence markers in *Helicobacter pylori* strains isolated from Mexican patients with chronic gastritis. *Ann Clin Microbiol Antimicrob* 2009, 8:14.

46. Azuma T, Ohtani M, Yamazaki Y, Higashi H, Hatakeyama M: Meta-analysis of the relationship between CagA seropositivity and gastric cancer. *Gastroenterology* 2004, 126:1926–7. author reply 1927–1928.

47. Kumar S, Kumar A, Dixit VK: Diversity in the cag pathogenicity island of *Helicobacter pylori* isolates in populations from North and South India. *J Med Microbiol* 2010, 59(Pt 1):32–40.

48. Batista SA, Rocha GA, Rocha AM, Saraiva IE, Cabral MM, Oliveira RC, Queiroz DM: Higher number of *Helicobacter pylori* CagA EPIYA C phosphorylation sites increases the risk of gastric cancer, but not duodenal ulcer. *BMC Microbiol* 2011, 11:61.

49. Acosta N, Quiroga A, Delgado P, Bravo MM, Jaramillo C: *Helicobacter pylori* CagA protein polymorphisms and their lack of association with pathogenesis. *World J Gastroenterol* 2010, 16:3936–43.

50. Torres LE, Gonzalez L, Melian K, Alonso J, Moreno A, Hernandez M, Reyes O, Bermudez L, Campos J, Perez-Perez G, Rodríguez BL: EPIYA motif patterns among Cuban *Helicobacter pylori* CagA positive strains. *Biomedica* 2012, 32:23–31.

51. Kersulyte D, Kalia A, Gilman RH, Mendez M, Herrera P, Cabrera L, Velapatino B, Balqui J, Paredes Puente dela Vega F, Rodriguez Ulloa CA, Cok J, Hooper CC, Dailide G, Tamma S, Berg DE: *Helicobacter pylori* from Peruvian amerindians: traces of human migrations in strains from remote Amazon, and genome sequence of an Amerind strain. *PLoS One* 2010, 5:e15076.

52. Sgouras DN, Panayotopoulou EG, Papadakos K, Martinez-Gonzalez B, Roumbani A, Panayiotou J, VanVliet-Constantinidou C, Mentis AF, Roma-Giannikou E: CagA and VacA polymorphisms do not correlate with severity of histopathological lesions in *Helicobacter pylori*-infected Greek children. *J Clin Microbiol* 2009, 47:2426–34.

53. Furuta Y, Yahara K, Hatakeyama M, Kobayashi I: Evolution of cagA oncogene of *Helicobacter pylori* through recombination. *PLoS One* 2011, 6:e23499.

54. Ishikawa S, Ohta T, Hatakeyama M: Stability of *Helicobacter pylori* CagA oncoprotein in human gastric epithelial cells. *FEBS Lett* 2009, 583:2414–8.

55. Ferlay J, Shin H, Bray F, Forman D, Mathers C, Parkin D: GLOBOCAN 2008 v2.0, Cancer Incidence and Mortality Worldwide: IARC CancerBase No. 10 [Internet]. Lyon, France: International Agency for Research on Cancer; 2010. Available from: http://globocan.iarc.fr.

56. Tarkhashvili N, Chakvetadze N, Mebonia N, Chubinidze M, Bakanidze L, Shengelidze V, Mirtskhulava M, Chachava T, Katsitadze G, Gabunia U, Kordzaia D, Imnadze P, Guarner J, Sobel J: Traditional risk factors for *Helicobacter pylori* infection not found among patients undergoing diagnostic upper endoscopy-Republic of Georgia, 2007–2008. *Int J Infect Dis* 2012, 16:e697–702.

57. Wu Y, Fan Y, Jiang Y, Wang Y, Liu H, Wei M: Analysis of risk factors associated with precancerous lesion of gastric cancer in patients from eastern China: a comparative study. *J Cancer Res Ther* 2013, 9:205–9.

7

Helicobacter pylori infection is not associated with fatty liver disease including non-alcoholic fatty liver disease

Kazuya Okushin[1†], Yu Takahashi[1†], Nobutake Yamamichi[1*], Takeshi Shimamoto[2], Kenichiro Enooku[1], Hidetaka Fujinaga[1], Takeya Tsutsumi[1], Yoshizumi Shintani[1], Yoshiki Sakaguchi[1], Satoshi Ono[1], Shinya Kodashima[1], Mitsuhiro Fujishiro[1], Kyoji Moriya[1], Hiroshi Yotsuyanagi[1], Toru Mitsushima[2] and Kazuhiko Koike[1]

Abstract

Background: Fatty liver disease (FLD) including non-alcoholic fatty liver disease (NAFLD), a rapidly emerging and widely recognized liver disease today, is regarded as a hepatic manifestation of metabolic syndrome. *Helicobacter pylori*, one of the most common pathogens worldwide, has been reported to be associated with metabolic syndrome, but whether there is a direct association with FLD is as of yet unclear. The aim of this study was to clarify the association of FLD and NAFLD with causative background factors including *Helicobacter pylori* infection.

Methods: This was a cross-sectional study of Japanese adults who received medical checkups at a single medical center in 2010.Univariate and multivariate statistical analysis was performed to evaluate background factors for ultrasonography diagnosed FLD. Subjects free from alcohol influence were similarly analyzed for NAFLD.

Results: Of a total of 13,737 subjects, FLD was detected in 1,456 of 6,318 females (23.0 %) and 3,498 of 7,419 males (47.1%). Multivariable analyses revealed that body mass index (standardized coefficients of females and males (β-F/M) =143.5/102.5), serum ALT (β-F/M = 25.8/75.7), age (β-F/M = 34.3/17.2), and platelet count (β-F/M = 17.8/15.2) were positively associated with FLD in both genders. Of the 5,289 subjects free from alcohol influence, NAFLD was detected in 881 of 3,473 females (25.4%) and 921 of 1,816 males (50.7%). Body mass index (β-F/M = 113.3/55.3), serum ALT (β-F/M = 21.6/53.8), and platelet count (β-F/M = 13.8/11.8) were positively associated with NAFLD in both genders. Metabolic syndrome was positively associated with FLD and NAFLD only in males. In contrast, *Helicobacter pylori* infection status was neither associated with FLD nor NAFLD regardless of gender.

Conclusions: Body mass index, serum ALT and platelet count were significantly associated with FLD and NAFLD, whereas infection of *Helicobacter pylori* was not.

Keywords: Fatty liver disease, NAFLD, Metabolic syndrome, *Helicobacter pylori*

* Correspondence: nyamamic-tky@umin.ac.jp
†Equal contributors
[1]Department of Gastroenterology, Graduate School of Medicine, The University of Tokyo, Tokyo, Japan
Full list of author information is available at the end of the article

Background

Fatty liver disease (FLD) is the most common chronic liver disease in the world today. It is caused by multiple factors such as nutritional disorders, dyslipidemia, insulin resistance, genetic factors, etc. [1]. Especially, alcohol intake and metabolic abnormalities such as insulin resistance have been reported to be the main causes for FLD [2,3]. However, recent epidemiological studies have not been enough to elucidate complicated risk factors for FLD, despite the high prevalence and importance of the disease [4-6]. FLD is generally divided into alcoholic fatty liver disease (AFLD) and non-alcoholic fatty liver disease (NAFLD) according to amounts of alcohol intake. The boundary value of alcohol intake between AFLD and NAFLD is tentatively defined [7], but the effect of moderate alcohol intake upon FLD still leaves much room for discussion [8-10].

NAFLD is also common all over the world including Eastern countries [11], but the reported prevalence rate of NAFLD varies widely [12-17]. NAFLD is a concerning disease not only because of its high prevalence but also its potential risk of fatal diseases such as liver failure, hepatocellular carcinoma (HCC), cardiovascular disease, and so on [18,19]. NAFLD is regarded as a hepatic manifestation of metabolic syndrome (MS) [20]. Machado M et al. reported that the prevalence of NAFLD was 91% in obese patients who had undergone bariatric surgery [21]. It has also been reported that type 2 diabetes and other features of MS are strongly related to NAFLD [22,23].

The relationship between NAFLD and microbes in the gut has been occasionally reported [24,25]. As "Gut-Liver Axis" has been widely noticed [26,27], several liver diseases including NAFLD are thought to be influenced by gastro-intestinal tract environments mainly decided by existing microbes. Among enormously varied microbes, to our knowledge today, Helicobacter pylori (H. pylori) shows the greatest effect on the upper gastro-intestinal environment. It is well known that approximately 50% of the global population is estimated to be infected by H. pylori [28], and is also well established that chronic infection of H. pylori can be a cause of chronic atrophic gastritis, peptic ulcer disease and gastric cancer [29,30]. Recently, not a few reports concerning the influence of H. pylori on various extra-alimentary organs have been accumulated [31-34]. Among these putative extra-alimentary disorders caused by H. pylori, the relation to MS is still controversial [35-42]. Though there have been many reports discussing the relationship between H. pylori and MS, issues to clarify still remain.

Based on these reports, we hypothesized that H. pylori has some associations with FLD including NAFLD. There has previously been only one similar small-scale study which concluded that H. pylori infection is associated with NAFLD [43]. The aim of this study was to clarify the background factors of FLD and NAFLD, and the influence of H. pylori infection on these diseases.

Methods
Study subjects

This was a cross-sectional study of Japanese asymptomatic adults who received medical checkups at Kameda Medical Center Makuhari (Chiba-shi, Chiba, Japan) in 2010, and voluntarily consented to entry into our study. This study was approved by the ethics committees of The University of Tokyo, and written forms of informed consent were obtained from all study participants according to the Declaration of Helsinki.

If the subject had health checkups twice in 2010, the former data was used. Criteria for exclusion were age less than 20 years, insufficient data, or poor answers to the questionnaire.

Questionnaires

A detailed questionnaire including inquiries about upper gastrointestinal tract-related symptoms [44-46], medical history, family history, lifestyle factors, etc. was filled out by all the participants. This questionnaire has already been used and validated in several previous reports [31,46-49]. Answers filled out by the participants were carefully checked by the nursing staff before being recorded into our study database. The questionnaire included five yes-no questions regarding regular intake of anti-cholesterol drugs, anti-hypertensive drugs, anti-diabetic drugs and corticosteroids, and history of gastrectomy. We additionally graded alcohol intake frequency on a 5-grade scale (never, rarely, sometimes, almost daily, and daily per week). In this analysis, "never" and "rarely" are regarded as non-drinker, "sometimes" is regarded as occasional-drinker, and "almost daily" and "daily" are regarded as daily-drinker. As for the amount of alcohol intake, we defined one drink unit is equivalent to a 12-ounce beer, a 4-ounce glass of wine, or a 1-ounce shot of hard liquor. And we also categorized the subjects into four groups according to: less than two units at a time, two to three units at a time, three to four units at a time and more than four units at a time. We further categorized smoking habit into three groups, current smoking (current-smoker), past habitual smoking (former-smoker), and lifelong nonsmoking (never-smoker).

Diagnosis of fatty liver disease (FLD)

Fatty liver disease (FLD) was diagnosed by abdominal ultrasonography. Routine ultrasonography evaluation of six intra-abdominal organs (liver, gallbladder, pancreas, kidneys, spleen, and abdominal aorta) was performed by well-trained operators. Characteristic findings of fatty liver are as follows; i) an increase of liver brightness, ii) an increase of hepato-renal echo contrast, iii) deep attenuation of hepatic echo, iv) existence of intra-hepatic vascular blurring, v) existence of focal hypoechoic lesion, and vi) existence of borderline blurring between liver and gallbladder, or right kidney. Fatty liver was diagnosed when the ultrasonographic findings satisfied both i) and ii) in addition to at least one of the findings between iii) to vi) [50]. The diagnosis was double-checked by the operators and gastroenterologists.

Definition of non-alcoholic fatty liver disease (NAFLD)

NAFLD was defined according to the guideline published from AASLD (American Association for the Study of Liver Diseases), ACG (American College of Gastroenterology), and AGA (American Gastroenterological Association) in 2012 [7]. In this present study, we defined NAFLD according to the characteristic findings as follows; i) with evidence of fatty liver by ultrasonography (see above), and ii) with no causes for secondary hepatic fat accumulation including any viral hepatitis and steatogenic medication. With regard to alcohol intake, more than 21 drink units per week in males and more than 14 drink units per week in females were widely recognized as significant alcohol intake. To exclude alcohol influence strictly, we omitted all occasional-drinkers, all daily-drinkers, and Non-drinkers who occasionally drunk more than four units at one time.

Evaluation of serum anti-helicobacter pylori antibody

Serum anti-*H. pylori* antibody was measured using a commercial EIA kit (E-plate "EIKEN" *H. pylori* antibody, EIKEN Chemical Co Ltd, Tokyo, Japan) as we have previously reported [48]. According to the manufacturer's instruction, an antibody titer above 10 U/ml was considered as *H. pylori*-positive. We omitted individuals who had histories of eradications of *H. pylori* from analysis.

Definition of metabolic syndrome (MS)

The definition of MS was based on the Japanese criteria published in 2005 [51]. The diagnostic criteria is visceral obesity in combination with any two of the following three standards; i) systolic blood pressure (SBP) greater than 130 mmHg and/or diastolic blood pressure (DBP) greater than 85 mmHg, ii) triglyceride (TG) greater than 150 mg/dL and/or high-density lipoprotein (HDL) cholesterol less than 40 mg/dL, iii) fasting blood sugar (FBS) greater than 110 mg/dL. Visceral obesity was defined as a waist girth of at least 85 cm in male and at least 90 cm in female.

Statistical analyses

We analyzed data of female and male separately. We used JMP11 software (SAS Institute Japan) for statistical analyses. In univariate analyses, odds ratios and 95% confidence intervals were calculated and a p value of <0.01 was considered to indicate statistical significance. Following continuous variables were compared using the Welch's t test or Wilcoxon's rank-sum test and following categorical variables were compared using the Fisher's exact test as appropriate for fatty liver status: age (continuous data), height (continuous data), weight (continuous data), BMI (body mass index, continuous data), AST (serum aspartate aminotransferase, continuous data), ALT (serum alanine aminotransferase, continuous data), GGT (gamma-glutamyl transpeptidase, continuous data), T-Bil (total bilirubin, continuous data), ALB (serum albumin, continuous data), PLT (platelet, continuous data), TC (total cholesterol, continuous data), HDL-C (high-density lipoprotein cholesterol, continuous data), LDL-C (low-density lipoprotein cholesterol, continuous data), TG (triglyceride, continuous data), HbA1c (continuous data), FBS (fasting blood sugar, continuous data), SBP (systolic blood pressure, continuous data), DBP (diastolic blood pressure, continuous data), Waist girth (continuous data), presence of MS (metabolic syndrome, categorical data), habit of drinking (categorical data), habit of smoking (categorical data), and *H. pylori* infection status (anti-*H. pylori* antibody, categorical data). Among the continuous variables, AST, ALT, GGT and TG were compared by Wilcoxon's rank-sum test and the other continuous variables were compared by Welch's t test.

In multivariate analysis, standardized coefficient and standard error of each variable for FLD and NAFLD were calculated by the regularized logistic regression via the elastic net to avoid the correlations between each variable and a p value of <0.01 was considered to indicate statistical significance.

Results

Participants

Of the 20,773 subjects who participated in this study, we excluded 2,119 subjects due to age less than 20 years old (2), insufficient data of several examination including ultrasonography and anti-*H. pylori* antibody (1,814), or poor answers to the questionnaire (1,141). The 2,119 excluded subjects had the same background characteristics as the included 18,654 subjects (Additional file 1: Table S1). Of the 18,654 subjects who met inclusion criteria (Figure 1), we further excluded 3,809 subjects who were positive for HBsAg and/or HCVAb (261), who had a history of gastrectomy (174), and who took anti-hypertensive drugs (2,256), anti-diabetic drugs (481), anti-cholesterol drugs (1,515), or corticosteroids (186), since these factors might affect fatty liver status and/or some essential laboratory tests [52,53]. Finally, we further excluded 1,108 subjects who had a history of *H. pylori* eradication.

The primary study population of 13,737 subjects was comprised of 6,318 females and 7,419 males. Among them, fatty liver (FLD) was detected in 1,456 of 6,318

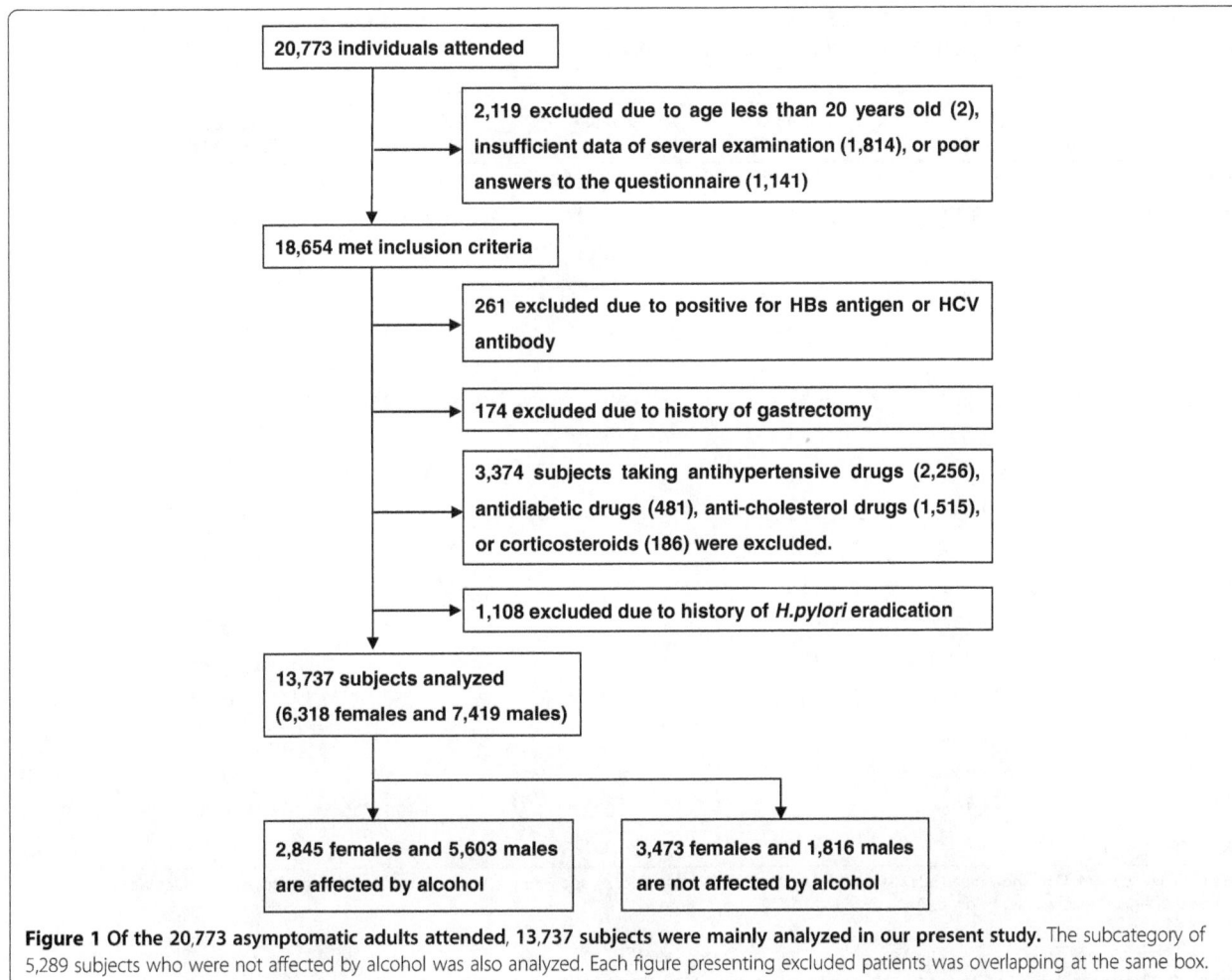

Figure 1 Of the 20,773 asymptomatic adults attended, 13,737 subjects were mainly analyzed in our present study. The subcategory of 5,289 subjects who were not affected by alcohol was also analyzed. Each figure presenting excluded patients was overlapping at the same box.

females (23.0%) and 3,498 of 7,419 males (47.1%). We also analyzed specific subjects who drank very little or no alcohol to remove the effects of alcohol intake to fatty liver status: after excluding all occasional-drinkers, all daily-drinkers, and non-drinkers who drank more than four units at a time, the residual 5,289 subjects (3,473 females and 1,816 males) were analyzed. Among them, fatty liver (i.e., NAFLD) was detected in 881 of 3,473 females (25.4%) and 921 of 1,816 males (50.7%).

Associated factors for fatty liver disease (FLD) based on the univariate analysis

We analyzed 19 continuous variables and 4 categorized variables and their association with fatty liver disease (Table 1, Table 2). Among the 23 examined factors, age, weight, BMI, AST, ALT, GGT, T-Bil, PLT, TC, HDL-C, LDL-C, TG, HbA1c, FBS, SBP, DBP, waist girth, presence of MS and drinking habit were statistically significant background factors in both genders. Height, ALB, smoking habit and *H. pylori* infection status were statistically significant background factors in one gender.

According to the results of univariate analyses and multicollinearity (0.8957 in females and 0.8723 in males between weight and BMI, 0.8521 in females and 0.7791 in males between AST and ALT), we excluded height, weight, AST and smoking habit from the next multivariate analysis. We adopted MS as a representative of waist girth, TC, HDL-C, LDL-C, TG, FBS, HbA1c, SBP and DBP. Consequently, we focused on the following nine variables for multivariate analysis: age, BMI, ALT, GGT, T-Bil, PLT, MS, drinking habit, and *H. pylori* infection status.

Associated factors for fatty liver disease (FLD) based on the multivariate analysis

As shown in Table 3, the generalized regression analysis demonstrated that BMI, ALT, age, and PLT were positively associated with FLD in both genders, and MS was positively associated only in males. Daily-drinking habit was negatively associated with FLD only in male. In contrast, GTT, T-Bil, and *H. pylori* infection status were not associated with the presence of FLD.

Table 1 Characteristics of the 13,737 subjects (6,318 females and 7,419 males) focusing on the presence of fatty liver disease (FLD) and its association with 19 continuous variables

Variables	Female			Male		
	FLD (N = 1456)	non-FLD (N = 4862)	p value	FLD (N = 3498)	non-FLD (N = 3921)	p value
Age (years old)	50.3 ± 7.9	46.9 ± 8.6	<0.0001*	48.7 ± 8.4	48.1 ± 9.5	0.0012*
Height (cm)	157.3 ± 5.6	158.2 ± 5.4	<0.0001*	170.8 ± 5.8	171.0 ± 5.9	0.0717
Weight (kg)	61.8 ± 9.6	51.4 ± 6.2	<0.0001*	72.8 ± 9.7	64.6 ± 7.8	<0.0001*
BMI (kg/m^2)	25.0 ± 3.6	20.5 ± 2.2	<0.0001*	24.9 ± 2.8	22.1 ± 2.2	<0.0001*
AST (IU/l)	21.2 ± 8.9	19.0 ± 5.4	<0.0001*	24.6 ± 10.0	21.3 ± 17.1	<0.0001*
ALT (IU/l)	23.0 ± 16.7	16.0 ± 7.6	<0.0001*	33.5 ± 22.6	21.6 ± 15.9	<0.0001*
GGT (IU/l)	28.3 ± 27.8	19.3 ± 17.3	<0.0001*	55.6 ± 58.2	38.8 ± 38.3	<0.0001*
T-Bil (mg/dl)	0.71 ± 0.27	0.76 ± 0.27	<0.0001*	0.87 ± 0.35	0.90 ± 0.37	0.0045*
ALB (g/dl)	4.26 ± 0.21	4.25 ± 0.21	0.1028	4.40 ± 0.22	4.36 ± 0.22	<0.0001*
PLT (10^4/μl)	26.1 ± 5.9	23.7 ± 5.4	<0.0001*	23.9 ± 4.9	22.9 ± 4.7	<0.0001*
TC (mg/dl)	214.0 ± 34.1	198.8 ± 33.0	<0.0001*	207.7 ± 32.5	195.4 ± 30.5	<0.0001*
HDL-C (mg/dl)	64.7 ± 14.2	75.8 ± 15.4	<0.0001*	54.1 ± 12.7	63.8 ± 15.2	<0.0001*
LDL-C (mg/dl)	135.0 ± 32.3	114.2 ± 29.9	<0.0001*	134.8 ± 30.2	119.4 ± 28.9	<0.0001*
TG (mg/dl)	107.2 ± 80.8	68.2 ± 32.0	<0.0001*	151.3 ± 97.6	98.7 ± 62.6	<0.0001*
HbA1c (%)	5.52 ± 0.56	5.30 ± 0.33	<0.0001*	5.50 ± 0.62	5.29 ± 0.37	<0.0001*
FBS (mg/dl)	94.9 ± 15.2	88.3 ± 8.5	<0.0001*	100.1 ± 16.4	94.1 ± 10.0	<0.0001*
SBP (mmHg)	118.8 ± 16.5	107.7 ± 14.5	<0.0001*	121.4 ± 15.0	115.4 ± 14.7	<0.0001*
DBP (mmHg)	73.9 ± 10.5	67.2 ± 9.6	<0.0001*	77.0 ± 10.1	73.0 ± 9.8	<0.0001*
Waist (cm)	87.2 ± 8.6	75.7 ± 6.5	<0.0001*	87.4 ± 7.1	79.8 ± 6.4	<0.0001*

FLD: fatty liver disease. Data show mean ± *SD* (standard deviation) of each variable. By applying the Welch's t test or Wilcoxon analysis, *p* values were calculated. The level of significance was set below 0.01 (*).

Table 2 Characteristics of the 13,737 subjects (6,318 females and 7,419 males) focusing on the presence of fatty liver disease (FLD) and its association with four categorized variables

Variables	Female			Male		
	FLD (N = 1456)	non-FLD (N = 4862)	p value	FLD (N = 3498)	non-FLD (N = 3921)	p value
MS			<0.0001*			<0.0001*
Non-MS	1391 (22.3 %)	4860 (77.6 %)		2945 (43.5 %)	3832 (56.5 %)	
MS	65 (97.0 %)	2 (3.0 %)		553 (86.1 %)	89 (13.9 %)	
Alcohol			<0.0001*			<0.0001*
Non-drinker	884 (25.3 %)	2604 (74.7 %)		951 (50.8 %)	923 (49.3 %)	
Occasional-drinking	368 (20.2 %)	1456 (79.8 %)		1114 (49.9 %)	1120 (50.1 %)	
Daily-drinker	204 (20.3 %)	802 (79.7 %)		1433 (43.3 %)	1878 (56.7 %)	
Smoking			0.0467			0.0045*
Current-smoker	123 (27.8 %)	319 (72.2 %)		1116 (49.3 %)	1147 (50.7 %)	
Former-smoker	174 (23.2 %)	577 (76.8 %)		1317 (47.6 %)	1450 (52.4 %)	
Never-smoker	1159 (22.6 %)	3966 (77.4 %)		1065 (44.6 %)	1324 (55.4 %)	
H. pylori Ab			<0.0001*			0.6446
Negative	1003 (21.5 %)	3665 (78.5 %)		2474 (47.0 %)	2793 (53.0 %)	
Positive	453 (27.5 %)	1197 (72.6 %)		1024 (47.6 %)	1128 (52.4 %)	

FLD: fatty liver disease, *MS*: metabolic syndrome, *Ab*: antibody. By applying the Fisher's exact test, *p* values were calculated. The level of significance was set below 0.01 (*).

Table 3 Multivariate analyses evaluating association between the presence of fatty liver disease (FLD) and 9 selected variables among the 13,737 subjects (6,318 females and 7,419 males).

Variables	Female			Male		
	Standardized coefficient	Standard error	p value	Standardized coefficient	Standard error	p value
BMI	143.5	4.8	<0.0001*	102.5	3.7	<0.0001*
ALT	25.8	5.1	<0.0001*	75.7	13.1	<0.0001*
Age	34.3	3.5	<0.0001*	17.2	2.8	<0.0001*
PLT	17.8	3.1	<0.0001*	15.2	2.6	<0.0001*
Alcohol						
Occasional-drinker	−8.1	3.7	0.0270	−5.9	2.8	0.0371
Daily-drinker	8.5	3.7	0.0209	−8.4	2.9	0.0040*
MS						
Positive	10.2	5.9	0.0804	16.4	3.2	<0.0001*
GGT	5.3	3.1	0.0919	4.0	4.1	0.3399
T-Bil	−3.1	3.3	0.3386	1.4	2.4	0.5555
H. pylori						
Positive	1.0	3.1	0.7558	−2.8	2.5	0.2642

MS: metabolic syndrome, C.I.: confidence interval, Ab: antibody, Using the logistic regression analysis, p values were calculated. The level of significance was set below 0.01 (*).

Associated factors for non-alcoholic fatty liver disease (NAFLD) based on the univariate analysis

Furthermore, we analyzed the 5,289 subjects free from alcohol influence to evaluate the relationship between NAFLD and background factors including *H. pylori* infection status. We analyzed 19 continuous variables and 3 categorized variables and their association with fatty liver disease (Tables 4 and 5). Among the 22 examined factors, weight, BMI, AST, ALT, GGT, PLT, TC, HDL-C, TG, HbA1c, FBS, SBP, DBP, waist girth, and MS were statistically significant in both genders. Age, height, T-Bil, ALB, and smoking habit were statistically significant in only one gender. However, regardless of gender, *H. pylori* infection status was not associated with the presence of NAFLD.

According to the results of univariate analyses and multicollinearity (0.9024 in female and 0.8841 in male between weight and BMI, 0.8626 in female and 0.8440 in male between AST and ALT), we excluded height, weight, AST, T-Bil, and smoking habit from the next multivariate analysis. We adopted MS as a representative of waist girth, TC, HDL-C, LDL-C, TG, FBS, HbA1c, SBP and DBP. Consequently, we chose the following seven variables for multivariate analysis: Age, BMI, ALT, GGT, PLT, MS, and *H. pylori* infection status.

Associated factors for non-alcoholic fatty liver disease (NAFLD) based on the multivariate analysis

As shown in Table 6, the generalized regression analysis displayed that BMI, ALT, and PLT were positively associated with the presence of NAFLD. Age was positively associated

with NAFLD only in females, whereas MS was positively associated only in males. Like FLD, *H. pylori* infection status did not show significant association with NAFLD, regardless of gender.

Discussion

Background factors for FLD

As for FLD, BMI, ALT, age and PLT were positively associated with the presence of FLD in both genders, which is concurrent with the recent study report from Japan [54].

Although alcohol intake has been regarded as a main cause for fatty liver for a long time [1,55-58], our result did not demonstrate a significant positive association between the frequency of alcohol intake and the presence of fatty liver. Occasional alcohol intake tended to be negatively associated with fatty liver in both genders, similarly to a recent report [8]. (Table 3). There is a possibility that the negative association of alcohol intake to FLD in daily-drinking males is attributed to the design of this study, since the evaluation of amounts of alcohol intake was not quantitatively accurate. To validate our result; the association between alcohol and fatty liver may not be as significant as previously reported, more detailed information of alcohol intake and careful setup of the study cohort will be needed in future studies.

Background factors for NAFLD

As for NAFLD, BMI, ALT, and PLT showed positive association. Unlike FLD, age was positively associated with the presence of NAFLD only in females (Table 6). Female gender, age, diabetes mellitus, hyperinsulinaemia, obesity

Table 4 Characteristics of the alcohol-free 5,289 subjects (3,473 females and 1,816 males) focusing on the presence of fatty liver (NAFLD) and its association with 19 continuous variables

Variables	Female			Male		
	NAFLD (N = 881)	non-NAFLD (N = 2592)	p value	NAFLD (N = 921)	non-NAFLD (N = 895)	p value
Age (years old)	50.8 ± 8.1	47.6 ± 8.9	<0.0001*	47.6 ± 8.6	47.4 ± 10.1	0.5126
Height (cm)	156.9 ± 5.4	157.8 ± 5.5	<0.0001*	170.7 ± 5.8	170.9 ± 6.0	0.4956
Weight (kg)	61.8 ± 9.8	51.2 ± 6.3	<0.0001*	72.8 ± 10.0	63.8 ± 8.0	<0.0001*
BMI (kg/m^2)	25.1 ± 3.7	20.5 ± 2.3	<0.0001*	25.0 ± 3.0	21.8 ± 2.3	<0.0001*
AST (IU/l)	21.4 ± 9.2	19.0 ± 5.4	<0.0001*	23.8 ± 10.6	20.0 ± 5.3	<0.0001*
ALT (IU/l)	23.5 ± 17.7	16.2 ± 7.8	<0.0001*	35.1 ± 30.7	21.3 ± 9.4	<0.0001*
GGT (IU/l)	26.4 ± 24.6	18.2 ± 14.8	<0.0001*	40.5 ± 41.0	26.6 ± 22.4	<0.0001*
T-Bil (mg/dl)	0.71 ± 0.26	0.74 ± 0.26	<0.0004*	0.85 ± 0.36	0.86 ± 0.37	0.5524
ALB (g/dl)	4.26 ± 0.22	4.24 ± 0.21	0.0148	4.41 ± 0.23	4.35 ± 0.22	<0.0001*
PLT (10^4/μl)	26.1 ± 6.0	23.7 ± 5.6	<0.0001*	24.7 ± 5.1	22.9 ± 4.9	<0.0001*
TC (mg/dl)	213.2 ± 33.4	201.2 ± 33.6	<0.0001*	207.4 ± 32.9	192.6 ± 29.9	<0.0001*
HDL-C (mg/dl)	62.9 ± 14.0	74.1 ± 15.0	<0.0001*	50.5 ± 10.7	59.5 ± 13.8	<0.0001*
LDL-C (mg/dl)	136.0 ± 31.8	118.2 ± 30.3	<0.0001*	138.6 ± 29.5	121.3 ± 27.8	<0.0001*
TG (mg/dl)	107.8 ± 71.0	69.1 ± 31.2	<0.0001*	144.1 ± 92.0	91.6 ± 47.7	<0.0001*
HbA1c (%)	5.55 ± 0.54	5.34 ± 0.35	<0.0001*	5.51 ± 0.63	5.31 ± 0.40	<0.0001*
FBS (mg/dl)	94.5 ± 14.7	88.1 ± 9.1	<0.0001*	98.4 ± 17.0	92.2 ± 8.5	<0.0001*
SBP (mmHg)	119.4 ± 16.8	107.7 ± 14.4	<0.0001*	118.6 ± 14.5	111.2 ± 13.3	<0.0001*
DBP (mmHg)	74.2 ± 10.6	66.9 ± 9.5	<0.0001*	74.9 ± 9.4	70.0 ± 8.8	<0.0001*
Waist (cm)	87.3 ± 8.7	75.7 ± 6.5	<0.0001*	87.3 ± 7.5	78.6 ± 6.6	<0.0001*

NAFLD: non-alcoholic fatty liver disease. Data show mean ± SD (standard deviation) of each variable. By applying the Welch's t test or Wilcoxon analysis, p values were calculated. The level of significance was set below 0.01 (*).

and hypertriglyceridaemia have been regarded as traditional risk factors for NAFLD [3,59-61]. Our results denoted the same tendency of these previous reports, but MS wasn't associated with the presence of NAFLD in females.

Association between H. pylori and FLD including NAFLD

Concerning *H. pylori* infection, neither FLD nor NAFLD displayed a significant association in multivariate analysis regardless of gender, though *H. pylori* infection showed significant association in univariate analysis in

Table 5 Characteristics of the alcohol-free 5,289 subjects (3,473 females and 1,816 males) focusing on the presence of fatty liver (NAFLD) and its association with three categorized variables

Variables	Female			Male		
	NAFLD (N = 881)	non-NAFLD (N = 2592)	p value	NAFLD (N = 921)	non-NAFLD (N = 895)	p value
MS			<0.0001*			<0.0001*
Non-MS	838 (24.5 %)	2590 (75.6 %)		793 (47.2 %)	886 (52.8 %)	
MS	43 (95.6 %)	2 (4.4 %)		128 (93.4 %)	9 (6.6 %)	
Smoking			0.3913			0.0033*
Current-smoker	54 (29.4 %)	130 (70.7 %)		289 (54.4 %)	242 (45.6 %)	
Former-smoker	71 (24.0 %)	225 (76.0 %)		284 (53.7 %)	245 (46.3 %)	
Never-smoker	756 (25.3 %)	2237 (74.7 %)		348 (46.0 %)	408 (54.0 %)	
H. pylori Ab			0.0145			0.8742
Negative	610 (24.2 %)	1907 (75.8 %)		669 (50.6 %)	654 (49.4 %)	
Positive	271 (28.4 %)	685 (71.7 %)		252 (51.1 %)	241 (48.9 %)	

NAFLD: non-alcoholic fatty liver disease, MS: metabolic syndrome, Ab: antibody. By applying the Fisher's exact test, p values were calculated. The level of significance was set below 0.01 (*).

Table 6 Multivariate analysis evaluating association between NAFLD and 7 selected variables among the non-drinking 5,289 subjects (3,473 females and 1,816 males)

Variables	Female			Male		
	Standardized Coefficient	Standard error	p value	Standardized Coefficient	Standard error	p value
BMI	113.3	4.9	<0.0001*	55.3	3.7	<0.0001*
ALT	21.6	6.1	0.0004*	53.8	6.5	<0.0001*
Age	25.0	3.5	<0.0001*	3.7	2.6	0.1607
PLT	13.8	3.0	<0.0001*	11.8	2.5	<0.0001*
MS						
Positive	5.9	5.0	0.2354	11.6	4.5	0.0092*
GGT	2.3	3.4	0.4975	0.24	3.9	0.9508
H. pylori						
Positive	−1.2	3.1	0.7017	−1.8	2.6	0.4764

MS: metabolic syndrome, Ab: antibody, C.I.: confidence interval. Using the logistic regression analysis, p values were calculated. The level of significance was set below 0.01 (*).

FLD in female. This suggests that upper gastro-intestinal environment caused by chronic *H. pylori* infection has no or marginal influence on the development of fatty liver. These results are consistent with some previous reports [35,36].

Limitations and future prospects
The first limitation of our study is the study design itself (i.e., cross-sectional study). A single point analysis cannot obtain accurate results, since fatty liver is thought to emerge as a consequence of several risk factors over a number of years. The second limitation is reliability of ultrasonography as a diagnostic tool for NAFLD. Diagnosis by ultrasonography has inevitable limitations due to low sensitivity for mild steatosis, inability to differentiate mild fibrosis from steatosis, and inaccurate quantification of fatty infiltration [62]. And more, interobserver and intraobserver variability in the sonographic assessment of fatty liver are well known [63]. Nevertheless, these shortcomings were thought to be minimal, because well-trained operators and gastroenterologists in a single hospital diagnosed fatty liver with prescribed findings written above in this study. In fact, we have already reported some study results based on our ultrasonography-based diagnoses [31,64]. The third limitation is the diagnostic accuracy of *H. pylori* infection based on serology. Though urea breath test (UBT) is superior to the serology test, the serology test is used due to its non-invasiveness and cost-effectiveness in our medical check up, which routinely has blood drawing. The accuracy of serology test in diagnosing *H. pylori* infection in this study was acceptable, since our recent study using the same study population showed that 97.8% (1,638 of 1,674) of the subjects with sero-positivity of *H. pylori* had chronic atrophic gastritis[49]. The fourth limi-

tation is the small number of female participants. We inferred that undetected association between MS and FLD including NAFLD might be due to the small number of female subjects who met MS criteria.

For the future prospects, we will follow this cohort to reveal the long-term effect of various associated factors upon FLD and NAFLD, such as developing NASH, liver cirrhosis, hepatocellular carcinoma, and so on.

Conclusions
Body mass index (BMI), serum ALT, and platelet count were positively associated with the presence of fatty liver disease (FLD) and non-alcoholic fatty liver disease (NAFLD) in both genders. On the other hands, *Helicobacter pylori* infection was not associated with either FLD or NAFLD.

Abbreviations
FLD: Fatty liver disease; NAFLD: Non-alcoholic fatty liver disease; AFLD: Alcoholic fatty liver disease; HCC: Hepatocellular carcinoma; *H. pylori*: Helicobacter pylori; BMI: Body mass index; AST: Aspartate aminotransferase; ALT: Alanine aminotransferase; GGT: Gamma-glutamyl transpeptidase; T-Bil: Total bilirubin; ALB: Albumin; PLT: Platelet; TC: Total cholesterol; HDL-C: High-density lipoprotein; LDL-C: Low-density lipoprotein cholesterol; TG: Triglyceride; FBS: Fasting blood sugar; SBP: Systolic blood pressure; DBP: Diastolic blood pressure; MS: Metabolic syndrome.

Competing interests
The authors declare that they have no competing interests.

Authors' contributions
KO, YT and NY contributed to the study concept and design, acquisition of data, analysis and interpretation of data, statistical analysis, and drafting of the manuscript. TS participated in support of statistical analysis. EK, HF, TT, YS, SY, SO and SK participated in critical revision of the manuscript for important intellectual content, analysis and interpretation of data. MF, KM and HY critically revised the manuscript for important intellectual content. TM and KK participated in study concept and design and study supervision.

We confirm that all authors checked and approved the final version of the manuscript.

Acknowledgements
We thank Mr. Minoru Okada and Mr. Masanori Fujiwara (Kameda Medical Center Makuhari) for maintaining the study database. We also thank Mr. Koichi Yamashita (Kameda Medical Center Makuhari) for useful advice about the diagnosis of ultrasonography-based fatty liver. This work was supported in part by Grant-in-Aid for Young Scientists (B) from the Ministry of Education, Culture, Sports, Science and Technology (MEXT); Health Sciences Research Grants of The Ministry of Health, Labour and Welfare of Japan (Research on Hepatitis); and a grant from the Smoking Research Foundation of Japan.

Author details
[1]Department of Gastroenterology, Graduate School of Medicine, The University of Tokyo, Tokyo, Japan. [2]Kameda Medical Center Makuhari (CD-2, 1–3, Nakase, Mihama-ku, Chiba-city, Japan.

Reference
1. Volzke H. Multicausality in fatty liver disease: is there a rationale to distinguish between alcoholic and non-alcoholic origin? World J Gastroenterol. 2012;18(27):3492–501.
2. Bellentani S, Saccoccio G, Costa G, Tiribelli C, Manenti F, Sodde M, et al. Drinking habits as cofactors of risk for alcohol induced liver damage. The Dionysos Study Group. Gut. 1997;41(6):845–50.
3. Bellentani S, Bedogni G, Miglioli L, Tiribelli C. The epidemiology of fatty liver. Eur J Gastroenterol Hepatol. 2004;16(11):1087–93.
4. DoS Alves De Carvalho M, Coelho Cabral P, Kruze Grande De Arruda I, Goretti Pessoa De Araujo Burgos M, Da Silva Diniz A, Barros Pernambuco JR, et al. Risk factors associated with hepatic steatosis: a study in patients in the Northeast Brazil. Nutr Hosp. 2012;27(4):1344–50.
5. Bellentani S, Saccoccio G, Masutti F, Croce LS, Brandi G, Sasso F, et al. Prevalence of and risk factors for hepatic steatosis in Northern Italy. Ann Intern Med. 2000;132(2):112–7.
6. Lau K, Lorbeer R, Haring R, Schmidt CO, Wallaschofski H, Nauck M, et al. The association between fatty liver disease and blood pressure in a population-based prospective longitudinal study. J Hypertens. 2010;28(9):1829–35.
7. Chalasani N, Younossi Z, Lavine JE, Diehl AM, Brunt EM, Cusi K, et al. The diagnosis and management of non-alcoholic fatty liver disease: practice Guideline by the American Association for the Study of Liver Diseases, American College of Gastroenterology, and the American Gastroenterological Association. Hepatol (Baltimore, Md). 2012;55(6):2005–23.
8. Sookoian S, Castano GO, Pirola CJ. Modest alcohol consumption decreases the risk of non-alcoholic fatty liver disease: a meta-analysis of 43 175 individuals. Gut. 2014;63(3):530–2.
9. Hamaguchi M, Kojima T, Ohbora A, Takeda N, Fukui M, Kato T. Protective effect of alcohol consumption for fatty liver but not metabolic syndrome. World J Gastroenterol. 2012;18(2):156–67.
10. Liangpunsakul S, Chalasani N. What should we recommend to our patients with NAFLD regarding alcohol use? Am J Gastroenterol. 2012;107(7):976–8.
11. Kojima S, Watanabe N, Numata M, Ogawa T, Matsuzaki S. Increase in the prevalence of fatty liver in Japan over the past 12 years: analysis of clinical background. J Gastroenterol. 2003;38(10):954–61.
12. Ryan CK, Johnson LA, Germin BI, Marcos A. One hundred consecutive hepatic biopsies in the workup of living donors for right lobe liver transplantation. Liver Transpl. 2002;8(12):1114–22.
13. Nadalin S, Malago M, Valentin-Gamazo C, Testa G, Baba HA, Liu C, et al. Preoperative donor liver biopsy for adult living liver transplantation: risks and benefits. Liver Transpl. 2005;11(8):980–6.
14. Tran TT, Changsri C, Shackleton CR, Poordad FF, Nissen NN, Colquhoun S, et al. Living donor liver transplantation: histological abnormalities found on liver biopsies of apparently healthy potential donors. J Gastroenterol Hepatol. 2006;21(2):381–3.
15. Lee JY, Kim KM, Lee SG, Yu E, Lim YS, Lee HC, et al. Prevalence and risk factors of non-alcoholic fatty liver disease in potential living liver donors in Korea: a review of 589 consecutive liver biopsies in a single center. J Hepatol. 2007;47(2):239–44.
16. Minervini MI, Ruppert K, Fontes P, Volpes R, Vizzini G, de Vera ME, et al. Liver biopsy findings from healthy potential living liver donors: reasons for disqualification, silent diseases and correlation with liver injury tests. J Hepatol. 2009;50(3):501–10.
17. Vernon G, Baranova A, Younossi ZM. Systematic review: the epidemiology and natural history of non-alcoholic fatty liver disease and non-alcoholic steatohepatitis in adults. Aliment Pharmacol Ther. 2011;34(3):274–85.
18. Baffy G, Brunt EM, Caldwell SH. Hepatocellular carcinoma in non-alcoholic fatty liver disease: an emerging menace. In: Journal of hepatology. Volume 56. England: Published by Elsevier B.V; 2012. p. 1384–91.
19. Rubinstein E, Lavine JE, Schwimmer JB. Hepatic, cardiovascular, and endocrine outcomes of the histological subphenotypes of nonalcoholic fatty liver disease. Semin Liver Dis. 2008;28(4):380–5.
20. de Alwis NM, Day CP. Non-alcoholic fatty liver disease: the mist gradually clears. J Hepatol. 2008;48 Suppl 1:S104–12.
21. Machado M, Marques-Vidal P, Cortez-Pinto H. Hepatic histology in obese patients undergoing bariatric surgery. J Hepatol. 2006;45(4):600–6.
22. Targher G, Bertolini L, Padovani R, Rodella S, Tessari R, Zenari L, et al. Prevalence of nonalcoholic fatty liver disease and its association with cardiovascular disease among type 2 diabetic patients. Diabetes Care. 2007;30(5):1212–8.
23. Marchesini G, Bugianesi E, Forlani G, Cerrelli F, Lenzi M, Manini R, et al. Nonalcoholic fatty liver, steatohepatitis, and the metabolic syndrome. Hepatology. 2003;37(4):917–23.
24. Frasinariu OE, Ceccarelli S, Alisi A, Moraru E, Nobili V. Gut-liver axis and fibrosis in nonalcoholic fatty liver disease: an input for novel therapies. Dig Liver Dis. 2013;45(7):543–51.
25. Henao-Mejia J, Elinav E, Jin C, Hao L, Mehal WZ, Strowig T, et al. Inflammasome-mediated dysbiosis regulates progression of NAFLD and obesity. Nature. 2012;482(7384):179–85.
26. Solga SF, Diehl AM. Gut flora-based therapy in liver disease? The liver cares about the gut. Hepatology (Baltimore, Md). 2004;39(5):1197–200.
27. Chassaing B, Etienne-Mesmin L, Gewirtz AT. Microbiota-liver axis in hepatic disease. Hepatology (Baltimore, Md). 2014;59(1):328–39.
28. Cover TL, Blaser MJ. Helicobacter pylori in health and disease. Gastroenterology. 2009;136(6):1863–73.
29. Malfertheiner P, Megraud F, O'Morain CA, Atherton J, Axon AT, Bazzoli F, et al. Management of Helicobacter pylori infection–the Maastricht IV/ Florence Consensus Report. Gut. 2012;61(5):646–64.
30. Matsuhisa T, Aftab H. Observation of gastric mucosa in Bangladesh, the country with the lowest incidence of gastric cancer, and Japan, the country with the highest incidence. Helicobacter. 2012;17(5):396–401.
31. Takahashi Y, Yamamichi N, Shimamoto T, Mochizuki S, Fujishiro M, Takeuchi C, et al. Helicobacter pylori infection is positively associated with gallstones: a large-scale cross-sectional study in Japan. J Gastroenterol. 2014;49(5):882–9.
32. Patel P, Mendall MA, Carrington D, Strachan DP, Leatham E, Molineaux N, et al. Association of Helicobacter pylori and Chlamydia pneumoniae infections with coronary heart disease and cardiovascular risk factors. BMJ. 1995;311(7007):711–4.
33. Federman DG, Kirsner RS, Moriarty JP, Concato J. The effect of antibiotic therapy for patients infected with Helicobacter pylori who have chronic urticaria. J Am Acad Dermatol. 2003;49(5):861–4.
34. Maurer KJ, Ihrig MM, Rogers AB, Ng V, Bouchard G, Leonard MR, et al. Identification of cholelithogenic enterohepatic helicobacter species and their role in murine cholesterol gallstone formation. Gastroenterology. 2005;128(4):1023–33.
35. Naja F, Nasreddine L, Hwalla N, Moghames P, Shoaib H, Fatfat M, et al. Association of H. pylori infection with insulin resistance and metabolic syndrome among Lebanese adults. Helicobacter. 2012;17(6):444–51.
36. Cho I, Blaser MJ, Francois F, Mathew JP, Ye XY, Goldberg JD, Bini EJ: Helicobacter pylori and overweight status in the United States: data from the Third National Health and Nutrition Examination Survey. In: Am J Epidemiol. Volume 162, edn. United States; 2005: 579–584.
37. Longo-Mbenza B, Nkondi Nsenga J, Vangu Ngoma D. Prevention of the metabolic syndrome insulin resistance and the atherosclerotic diseases in Africans infected by Helicobacter pylori infection and treated by antibiotics. Int J Cardiol. 2007;121(3):229–38.
38. Polyzos SA, Kountouras J, Zavos C, Deretzi G. Helicobacter pylori Infection and insulin resistance. Helicobacter. 2013;18(2):165–6.

39. Stergiopoulos C, Kountouras J, Daskalopoulou-Vlachoyianni E, Polyzos SA, Zavos C, Vlachoyiannis E, et al. Helicobacter pylori may play a role in both obstructive sleep apnea and metabolic syndrome. Sleep Med. 2012;13 (2):212–3.

40. Shin DW, Kwon HT, Kang JM, Park JH, Choi HC, Park MS, et al. Association between metabolic syndrome and Helicobacter pylori infection diagnosed by histologic status and serological status. J Clin Gastroenterol. 2012;46 (10):840–5.

41. Pietroiusti A, Diomedi M, Silvestrini M, Cupini LM, Luzzi I, Gomez-Miguel MJ, et al. Cytotoxin-associated gene-A–positive Helicobacter pylori strains are associated with atherosclerotic stroke. Circulation. 2002;106(5):580–4.

42. Gunji T, Matsuhashi N, Sato H, Fujibayashi K, Okumura M, Sasabe N, et al. Helicobacter pylori infection is significantly associated with metabolic syndrome in the Japanese population. Am J Gastroenterol. 2008;103(12):3005–10.

43. Polyzos SA, Kountouras J, Papatheodorou A, Patsiaoura K, Katsiki E, Zafeiriadou E, et al. Helicobacter pylori infection in patients with nonalcoholic fatty liver disease. Metabolism. 2013;62(1):121–6.

44. Danjo A, Yamaguchi K, Fujimoto K, Saitoh T, Inamori M, Ando T, et al. Comparison of endoscopic findings with symptom assessment systems (FSSG and QUEST) for gastroesophageal reflux disease in Japanese centres. J Gastroenterol Hepatol. 2009;24(4):633–8.

45. Kusano M, Shimoyama Y, Sugimoto S, Kawamura O, Maeda M, Minashi K, et al. Development and evaluation of FSSG: frequency scale for the symptoms of GERD. J Gastroenterol. 2004;39(9):888–91.

46. Yamamichi N, Mochizuki S, Asada-Hirayama I, Mikami-Matsuda R, Shimamoto T, Konno-Shimizu M, et al. Lifestyle factors affecting gastroesophageal reflux disease symptoms: a cross-sectional study of healthy 19864 adults using FSSG scores. BMC Med. 2012;10:45.

47. Shimamoto T, Yamamichi N, Kodashima S, Takahashi Y, Fujishiro M, Oka M, et al. No association of coffee consumption with gastric ulcer, duodenal ulcer, reflux esophagitis, and non-erosive reflux disease: a cross-sectional study of 8,013 healthy subjects in Japan. PLoS One. 2013;8(6):e65996.

48. Minatsuki C, Yamamichi N, Shimamoto T, Kakimoto H, Takahashi Y, Fujishiro M, et al. Background factors of reflux esophagitis and non-erosive reflux disease: a cross-sectional study of 10,837 subjects in Japan. PLoS One. 2013;8(7):e69891.

49. Yamamichi N, Hirano C, Shimamoto T, Minatsuki C, Takahashi Y, Nakayama C, et al. Associated factors of atrophic gastritis diagnosed by double-contrast upper gastrointestinal barium x-ray radiography: a cross-sectional study analyzing 6,901 healthy subjects in Japan. PLoS One. 2014;9(10):e111359.

50. Hamaguchi M, Kojima T, Itoh Y, Harano Y, Fujii K, Nakajima T, et al. The severity of ultrasonographic findings in nonalcoholic fatty liver disease reflects the metabolic syndrome and visceral fat accumulation. Am J Gastroenterol. 2007;102(12):2708–15.

51. [Definition and the diagnostic standard for metabolic syndrome–Committee to Evaluate Diagnostic Standards for Metabolic Syndrome]. Nihon Naika Gakkai zasshi The Journal of the Japanese Society of Internal Medicine 2005, 94(4):794–809.

52. Karcz WK, Krawczykowski D, Kuesters S, Marjanovic G, Kulemann B, Grobe H, et al. Influence of Sleeve Gastrectomy on NASH and Type 2 Diabetes Mellitus. J Obes. 2011;2011:765473.

53. Dowman JK, Tomlinson JW, Newsome PN. Systematic review: the diagnosis and staging of non-alcoholic fatty liver disease and non-alcoholic steatohepatitis. Aliment Pharmacol Ther. 2011;33(5):525–40.

54. Inabe F, Takahashi E, Moriyama K, Negami M, Otsuka H. Risk assessment chart for predicting fatty liver in Japanese subjects. Tokai J Exp Clin Med. 2012;37(4):94–101.

55. Becker U, Deis A, Sorensen TI, Gronbaek M, Borch-Johnsen K, Muller CF, et al. Prediction of risk of liver disease by alcohol intake, sex, and age: a prospective population study. Hepatology. 1996;23(5):1025–9.

56. Ludwig J, McGill DB, Lindor KD. Review: nonalcoholic steatohepatitis. J Gastroenterol Hepatol. 1997;12(5):398–403.

57. Lucey MR, Mathurin P, Morgan TR. Alcoholic hepatitis. N Engl J Med. 2009;360(26):2758–69.

58. Altamirano J, Bataller R. Alcoholic liver disease: pathogenesis and new targets for therapy. Nat Rev Gastroenterol Hepatol. 2011;8(9):491–501.

59. Mulhall BP, Ong JP, Younossi ZM. Non-alcoholic fatty liver disease: an overview. J Gastroenterol Hepatol. 2002;17(11):1136–43.

60. Sheth SG, Gordon FD, Chopra S. Nonalcoholic steatohepatitis. Ann Intern Med. 1997;126(2):137–45.

61. Bugianesi E, Leone N, Vanni E, Marchesini G, Brunello F, Carucci P, et al. Expanding the natural history of nonalcoholic steatohepatitis: from cryptogenic cirrhosis to hepatocellular carcinoma. Gastroenterology. 2002;123(1):134–40.

62. Festi D, Schiumerini R, Marzi L, Di Biase AR, Mandolesi D, Montrone L, et al. Review article: the diagnosis of non-alcoholic fatty liver disease – availability and accuracy of non-invasive methods. Aliment Pharmacol Ther. 2013;37(4):392–400.

63. Strauss S, Gavish E, Gottlieb P, Katsnelson L. Interobserver and intraobserver variability in the sonographic assessment of fatty liver. AJR Am J Roentgenol. 2007;189(6):W320–3.

64. Yamaji Y, Okamoto M, Yoshida H, Kawabe T, Wada R, Mitsushima T, et al. Cholelithiasis is a risk factor for colorectal adenoma. Am J Gastroenterol. 2008;103(11):2847–52.

8

Comparison of 10-day sequential therapy with 7-day standard triple therapy for *Helicobacter pylori* eradication in inactive peptic ulcer disease and the efficiency of sequential therapy in inactive peptic ulcer disease and non-ulcer dyspepsia

Chung-Chuan Chan[1,5†], Nai-Hsuan Chien[3,4†], Chia-Long Lee[3,5*], Yi-Chen Yang[2], Chih-Sheng Hung[3], Tien-Chien Tu[3,5] and Chi-Hwa Wu[3]

Abstract

Background: Eradication rates of standard triple therapy for *Helicobacter pylori* infections have decreased in recent years due to a worldwide increase in bacterial resistance. Sequential therapy has the advantage of a two-phase treatment regimen and achieves a superior result for *H. pylori* eradication in peptic ulcer disease. However, no study has yet compared the efficacy of sequential therapy for *H. pylori* eradication exclusively in inactive duodenal ulcer (iDU) or non-ulcer dyspepsia (NUD).

Method: We retrospectively recruited 408 patients with endoscopic proven iDU (170 patients) or NUD (238 patients) infected with *H. pylori*. Patients with iDU were assigned into two groups: iDU triple therapy group, 44 patients treated with 40 mg pantoprazole, 1000 mg amoxicillin and 500 mg clarithromycin, twice daily for 7 days; iDU sequential therapy group, 126 patients treated with 40 mg pantoprazole and 1000 mg amoxicillin, twice daily for the first 5 days, followed by 40 mg pantoprazole, 500 mg clarithromycin and 500 mg tinidazole, twice daily for the next 5 days. All patients with NUD were treated with sequential therapy and assigned as the NUD sequential group. Post-treatment *H. pylori* status was confirmed by a ^{13}C-urea breath test.

(Continued on next page)

* Correspondence: cghleecl@hotmail.com
†Equal contributors
3Division of Gastroenterology, Department of Internal Medicine, Cathay General Hospital, 280, Section 4, Jen-Ai Road, Taipei 10650, Taiwan
5Department of Internal Medicine, School of Medicine, College of Medicine, Taipei Medical University, Taipei, Taiwan
Full list of author information is available at the end of the article

(Continued from previous page)

Result: The eradication rates of intention-to-treat (ITT) and per-protocol (PP) analysis were 77.3 % (95 % CI 64.9–89.7 %) and 85.0 % (95 % CI 73.9–96.1 %) in the iDU triple therapy group and 87.3 % (95 % CI 81.5–93.1 %) and 92.4 % (95 % CI 87.6–97.2 %) in the iDU sequential therapy group. The overall eradication efficacy was superior in the sequential group than in the triple group, both with ITT analysis (83.5 % vs. 77.3 %, P = 0.29) and PP analysis (88.1 % vs. 85.0 %, P = 0.57). Eradication rates for ITT and PP analysis were 81.5 % (95 % CI 76.6–86.4 %) and 85.8 % (95 % CI 83.5–88.2 %) in the NUD sequential therapy group. Eradication rate was statistically better in the iDU sequential therapy group than the NUD sequential therapy group according to per protocol analysis (P = 0.04). Eradication rate was not significantly different between the iDU sequential- and iDU triple therapy groups according to protocol analysis (P = 0.14).

Conclusion: The sequential regimen has a better eradiation rate in the iDU group than in the NUD group. There is no statistically difference between 10-day sequential therapy and 7-day standard triple in iDU group.

Keywords: Helicobacter pylori, Inactive Duodenal ulcer, Non-ulcer dyspepsia, Sequential therapy, Triple therapy

Background

Helicobacter pylori (*H. pylori*) has been proved to be a major cause of chronic gastritis, and peptic ulcer disease [1, 2]. Furthermore, *H. pylori* infection is also a crucial cause of gastric cancer [3, 4] and is associated with an increased risk of gastric mucosa-associated lymphoid tissue (MALT) lymphoma [5]. WHO has categorized *H. pylori* as a class I carcinogenic agent in humans; therefore, its eradication has been an important step in the treatment of peptic ulcer disease and prevention of gastric malignancy [6–8].

Treatment of *H. pylori* has been evolving rapidly over the past two decades and several regimens have been proposed to maintain or even increase eradication rates. When first introduced, the now standard triple therapy using proton pump inhibitors, amoxicillin, and clarithromycin, was popular and recommended as first-line therapy for *H. pylori* in Asia and other regions of the world [7–9]. The eradication rates of this regimen, however, have declined below 80 % as observed in many of the latest studies because of increasing drug resistance, mostly to clarithromycin [10–12]. Several approaches have been proposed to overcome the low eradication rates. Sequential therapy was first proposed by Zullo *et al*, in Italy [13]. This two-phase treatment regimen, which involves a proton pump inhibitor plus amoxicillin for the first 5 days followed by a proton pump inhibitor plus clarithromycin and tinidazole or metronidazole for a further 5 days, achieved better results than standard triple therapy [14–16].

Many studies have proved that successful eradication of *H. pylori* substantially reduces the recurrent rate of duodenal ulcers [17, 18] and its recommendation has a worldwide consensus [7–9]. However, no study has yet demonstrated the efficacy of sequential therapy for *H. pylori* eradication exclusively in an inactive duodenal ulcer (iDU). On the other hand, a significant portion of non-ulcer dyspepsia (NUD) patients are infected with *H. pylori* [19] and its eradication improved dyspeptic symptoms. [20] An early study, which compared triple therapy with ranitidine bismuth citrate based quadruple therapy in treatments between peptic ulcer disease (PUD) and NUD patients, revealed better eradication results in PUD [21]. With a similar regimen in another study, there was no convincing evidence to imply that NUD patients responded to *H. pylori* eradication treatments differently from those with PUD [22].

The aim of our study was to compare the efficacy of currently used two-phase sequential therapy with standard triple therapy for *H. pylori* eradication in patients with iDU and the efficiency of sequential therapy in iDU and NUD in the Taiwanese population.

Methods

Study population and intervention

We enrolled consecutive patients with endoscopically proven iDU or NUD who were infected with *H. pylori*, which is defined as a positive rapid urease test (CLOtest; Kimbery-Clark, Roswell, GA 30076 USA) from the gastroenterology clinic in one medical center in Taipei, Taiwan. All patients were >18 years of age and had never received treatment for *H. pylori*. Additional exclusion criteria included: (i) consumption of antibiotics, nonsteroid anti-inflammatory drugs, proton pump inhibitors (PPI), H2-receptor antagonists, or bismuth salt during the previous four weeks; (ii) allergy or contraindications to antibiotics or PPI; (iii) previous gastric surgery; (iv) severe concomitant cardiopulmonary disease or serious hepatic/renal dysfunction or malignancy; and (v) pregnancy or lactation.

Patients received esophagogastroduodenoscopy (EGD; Olympus, GIF-XP 260) before enrolment to determine iDU or NUD. The study was approved by the Institutional Review Board of the Cathy General Hospital. The trial registration number is CGH-P104077, and the registration date is September 30,2015. Informed consent was obtained from all patients before EGD.

Patient selection and *H. pylori* detection

An inactive duodenal ulcer was defined as an endoscopic inspection of a white scar longer than 3 mm with converging folds, located over the duodenal bulb region. Patients with findings of coexisting active ulcers were excluded. Non-ulcer dyspepsia patients were defined as having clinical symptoms of persistent pain or discomfort focused over the epigastric region for at least one month and no abnormality could be detected during endoscopic inspection or during a normal abdominal ultrasound examination. One biopsy specimen was obtained from at least 2 cm away from the pylorus along the greater curvature side of the antrum for a rapid urea test. *H. pylori* infection was diagnosed if the rapid urea test was positive.

Therapy protocol

Patients with iDU were assigned into 2 groups according to a physician's discretion: the iDU triple therapy group (hereafter, the iDU triple group) contained 44 patients who received a triple therapy regimen: 40 mg pantoprazole, 1000 mg amoxicillin, and 500 mg clarithromycin, twice daily for 7 days. The iDU sequential therapy group (hereafter, the iDU sequential group) contained 126 patients and they received a sequential therapy regimen: 40 mg pantoprazole and 1000 mg amoxicillin, twice daily for the first 5 days, followed by 40 mg pantoprazole, 500 mg clarithromycin and 500 mg tinidazole, twice daily for the next 5 days. All 238 patients with NUD were treated with a sequential therapy regimen and assigned to the NUD sequential group.

Post treatment measurement

Results of *H. pylori* status after eradication therapy were determined using a ^{13}C-urea breath test (^{13}C-UBT). When patients had persistent epigastric symptoms, follow-up endoscopy was performed to make sure there were no newly developed lesions. Assessment of *H. pylori* status again used a rapid urease test (CLO). The ^{13}C-UBTs were performed at least 2 months apart and from the date at the end of therapy. The UBT was performed after an overnight fast. A baseline breath sample was obtained and then 75 mg of ^{13}C urea with 1.5 g of citric acid was administered as an aqueous solution. The second breath sample was collected 30 min after the intake of test solution. The result was defined positive if the difference between the baseline sample and the 30-min sample exceeded 4.5 per mil of $^{13}CO_2$. The sensitivity and specificity values of the UBT were reported as 94.7 % and 95.7 %, respectively [23]. Therapy compliance and drug adverse effects were assessed by personal interview after the end of treatment.

Statistical analysis

We used intention-to-treat (ITT) and per-protocol (PP) analysis in assessment of the eradication efficacy. Enrolled eligible patients who started medication were all included in the ITT analysis regardless of the correct protocol or compliance. Patients who did not take at least 80 % of the medication or who had incomplete treatment were excluded from PP analysis.

We compared continuous variables with the Student's test and presented an arithmetic mean and standard deviations. Qualitative variables were analyzed with the chi-square test and presented as percentage and 95 % confidence intervals (95 % CI). All statistical tests were two-sided and all P values <0.05 were considered statistically significant. The analyses were performed using SPSS for Microsoft Window (version 18; SPSS Inc., Chicago, IL, USA).

Results

Patients

From September 2007 to June 2010, we recruited 408 patients with endoscopic proven iDU or NUD and who were infected with *H. pylori*. Figure 1 shows the flow diagram of patients during the protocol. A total of 170 patients were diagnosed as iDU patients and 238 patients were diagnosed as NUD patients. Of the 170 iDU patients, 126 were assigned to the iDU sequential group and the remaining 44 patients were assigned to the iDU triple group. All 238 NUD patients were assigned to the NUD sequential group. Patients of these 3 groups all went through the complete protocol and 7 patients (5.6 %), 4 patients (9.1 %), and 12 patients (5.0 %) of the iDU sequential group, iDU triple group, and NUD sequential group, respectively, did not take the complete regimen of medication. Comparison of clinical characteristics and eradication rates between the iDU sequential group *vs.* the iDU triple group and the iDU sequential group *vs.* the NUD sequential group were performed with both ITT and PP analysis.

Eradication rates of *H. pylori*

Demographic characteristics of the sequential and triple groups are summarized in Table 1. A total of 364 patients (126 of iDU patients and 238 of NUD patients) received the sequential regimen; mean age was 51.0 ± 11.2 y and females were dominant. Forty-four patients received conventional triple therapy; mean age was 52.6 ± 9.5 y and females were dominant. The eradication efficacy was better in the sequential group than in the triple group, both with ITT analysis (83.5 % *vs.* 77.3 %) and PP analysis (88.1 % *vs.* 85.0 %). Neither analysis, however, demonstrated a significant difference in the 2 therapy regimens.

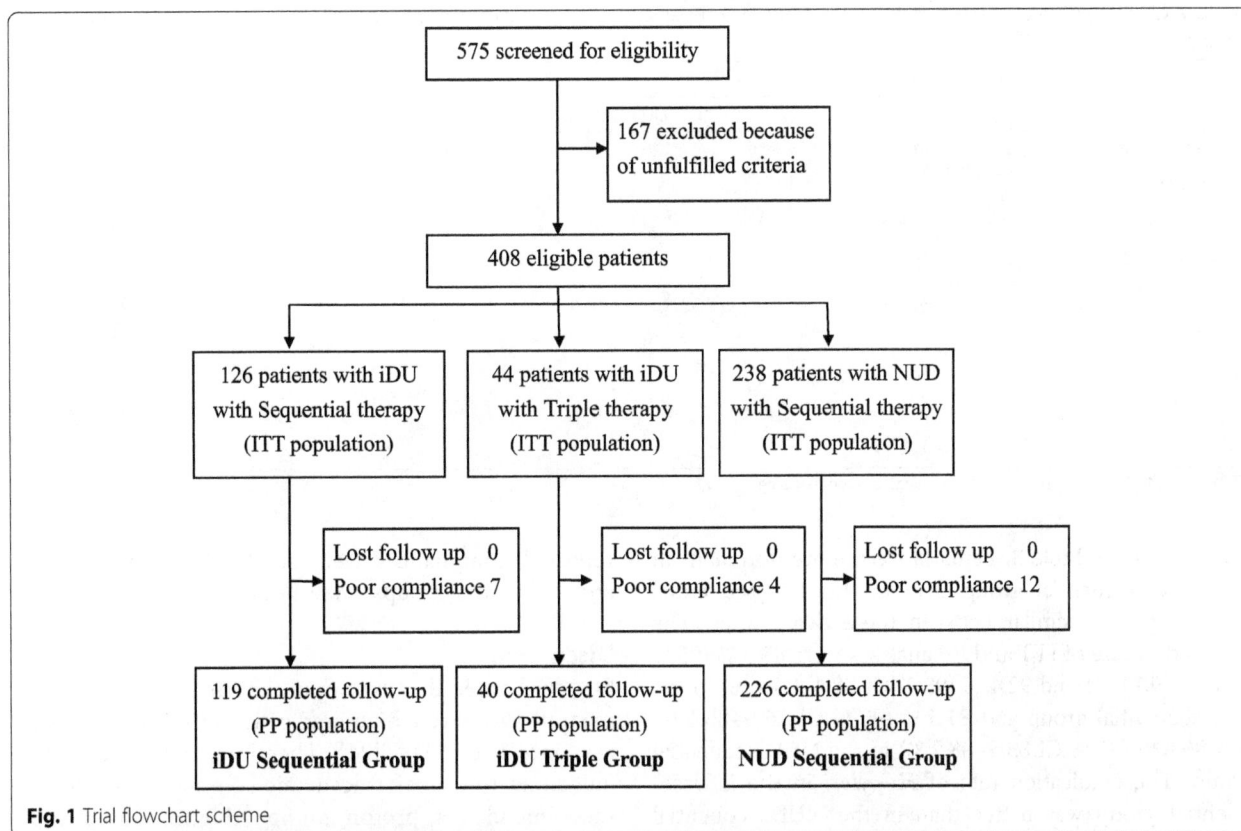

Fig. 1 Trial flowchart scheme

Demographic characteristics and eradication rate of the iDU sequential group *vs.* the iDU triple group are summarized in Table 2. Females were more dominant in the iDU triple group than in the iDU sequential group. Age was similar between these two groups. The eradication rate of ITT and PP analyses were 77.3 % (95 % CI 64.9–89.7 %) and 85.0 % (95 % CI 73.9–96.1 %) in the iDU triple group and 87.3 % (95 % CI 81.5–93.1 %) and 92.4 % (95 % CI 87.6–97.2 %) in the iDU sequential group. The eradication rate of *H. pylori* in the iDU sequential group was better than in the iDU triple group both with ITT and PP analyses. However, the differences were not significant and P values were 0.22 and 0.14, respectively.

Demographic characteristics and eradication rate of the iDU sequential group *vs.* the NUD sequential group are

Table 1 Baseline demographic and clinical characteristics of the patients

	ITT		PP	
	Triple therapy	Sequential therapy	Triple therapy	Sequential therapy
Number of patients	44	364	40	345
Age (Mean ± SD)	52.6 ± 9.5	51.0 ± 11.2	53.7 ± 9.0	51.1 ± 11.2
Gender (%)				
Male	9 (20.5 %)	135 (37.1 %)	7 (17.5 %)	127 (36.8 %)
Female	35 (79.5 %)	229 (62.9 %)	33 (82.5 %)	218 (63.2 %)
Endoscopic finding				
iDU	44 (100 %)	126 (34.6 %)		
NUD		238 (65.4 %)		
Eradication success	34	304	34	304
Eradication rate	77.3 %	83.5 %	85.0 %	88.1 %
95 % CI	64.9–89.7 %	79.9–87.3 %	73.9–96.1 %	84.7–91.5 %
P-value	0.29		0.57	

ITT intention to treat, *PP* per protocol

Table 2 Characteristics of subjects in ITT and PP and a comparison of the eradication rate between iDU triple and iDU sequential groups

	ITT		PP	
	iDU triple	iDU sequential	iDU triple	iDU sequential
Number of patients	44	126	40	119
Gender (%)				
Male	9 (20.5 %)	57 (45.2 %)	7 (17.5 %)	52 (43.7 %)
Female	35 (79.5 %)	69 (54.8 %)	33 (82.5 %)	67 (56.3 %)
Age (Mean ± SD)	52.6 ± 9.5	52.4 ± 12.3	53.7 ± 9.0	52.4 ± 12.3
Eradication success	34	110	34	110
Eradication rate	77.3 %	87.3 %	85.0 %	92.4 %
95 % CI	64.9–89.7 %	81.5–93.1 %	73.9–96.1 %	87.6–97.2 %
P-value	0.22		0.14	

ITT intention to treat, *PP* per protocol, *iDU* inactive duodenal ulcer

summarized in Table 3. Females were more dominant in the NUD sequential group than in the iDU sequential group. Age was similar between these two groups. The eradication rate of ITT and PP analyses were 87.3 % (95 % CI 81.5–93.1 %) and 92.4 % (95 % CI 88.4–96.4 %) in the iDU sequential group and 81.5 % (95 % CI 76.6–86.4 %) and 85.8 % (95 % CI 83.5–88.2 %) in the NUD sequential group. The eradication rate of *H. pylori* in the iDU sequential group was better than in the NUD sequential group both for ITT and PP analyses. Difference was significant in PP analysis but not so marked in ITT analysis; P values were 0.04 and 0.11 respectively.

Adverse events and compliance

Table 4 shows the adverse events and their incidences in conventional triple and sequential therapy groups. The overall adverse event rate was higher in the sequential group than in the triple group (36.3 % *vs.* 22.7 %, $P = 0.08$). The highest incidence of adverse events was mouth bitterness in both groups. Patients

reported compliances were similar in both the triple and sequential groups (90.9 % *vs.* 94.8 %, $P = 0.29$).

Discussion

Standard triple therapy, when first proposed, was demonstrated to have a high eradication efficacy with a success rate over 85 % [24]. Therefore, most therapeutic guidelines from major academic committees worldwide recommended a proton pump inhibitor based triple therapy plus clarithromycin and amoxicillin or metronidazole as the first-line regimen for eradication of *H. pylori* [7–9]. Unfortunately, the eradication rate of this gold standard therapy declined rapidly during the following 10 years toward unacceptable levels [25]. The frustrating outcome of the poor eradication rate led to several new strategies aimed to raise eradication efficacy. Innovative therapeutic approaches included extending therapy duration, the altering of conventionally used antibiotics to novel ones, and the addition of multi-drug regimens.

Table 3 Characteristics of subjects in ITT and PP and a comparison of the eradication rate between iDU sequential and NUD sequential groups

	ITT		PP	
	iDU Sequential	NUD Sequential	iD U Sequential	NUD Sequential
Number of patients	126	238	119	226
Gender (%)				
Male	57 (45.2 %)	78 (32.8 %)	52 (43.7 %)	75 (33.2 %)
Female	69 (54.8 %)	160 (67.2 %)	67 (56.3 %)	151 (66.8 %)
Age (Mean ± SD)	52.4 ± 12.3	50.3 ± 10.7	52.4 ± 12.3	50.4 ± 10.6
Eradication success	110	194	110	194
Eradication rate	87.3 %	81.5 %	92.4 %	85.80 %
95 % CI	81.5–93.1 %	76.6–86.4 %	88.4–96.4 %	83.5–88.2 %
P-value	0.11		0.04	

ITT intention to treat, *PP* per protocol, *iDU* inactive duodenal ulcer, *NUD* non-ulcer dyspepsia

Table 4 Adverse events in sequential therapy

Adverse event	Triple (N = 44)	iDU Sequential (N = 126)	NUD Sequential (N = 238)	Total Sequential (N = 364)
Taste disturbance	6.8 %	7.10 %	7.60 %	7.40 %
Diarrhea	0.0 %	2.40 %	0.40 %	1.10 %
Abdominal discomfort	0.0 %	3.20 %	0.40 %	1.40 %
Skin rash	0.0 %	1.60 %	0.80 %	1.10 %
Nausea	2.3 %	0.00 %	0.80 %	0.50 %
Poor appetite	0.0 %	0.00 %	0.40 %	0.30 %
Dizziness	0.0 %	2.40 %	0.40 %	1.10 %
Mouth bitterness	11.4 %	28.60 %	11.30 %	17.30 %
Loose stool	2.3 %	3.20 %	7.10 %	5.80 %
Cramp	0.0 %	0.80 %	0.00 %	0.30 %
Total	22.7 %	49.20 %	29.40 %	36.30 %
P value (triple vs total sequential)		0.08		

iDU inactive duodenal ulcer, *NUD* non-ulcer dyspepsia

A two-phase sequential regimen, by adding a fourth drug, has been shown to have promising eradication results in many studies worldwide. However, most of these trials were conducted in patients diagnosed with *H. pylori* infection and without separately analyzed eradication rates in either ulcer related or non-ulcer related groups. Our current work was a trial to compare the eradication efficacy of sequential therapy and conventional triple therapy exclusively in inactive duodenal ulcer and non-ulcer dyspepsia patients. The results demonstrated that a 10-day sequential regimen was superior to conventional triple therapy for eradication of *H. pylori* in treatment naïve patients. Overall, the eradication rate of sequential therapy was 88.1 % with PP analysis and 83.5 % with ITT analysis, which were higher than those of triple therapy (85.0 % with PP analysis and 77.3 % with ITT analysis). The result is similar to that shown in other studies in Western and Asian countries [26–31]. However, in our trial, the eradication rate of sequential therapy did not reach the good category according to the Graham's report card for grading *H. pylori* therapy [32] (90–95 % intention-to-treat) as with most other studies [15, 33, 34] and did not demonstrate a significant difference compared to triple therapy. One randomized controlled trial in southern Taiwan reported a high eradication rate (92.9 % with PP and 93.2 % with ITT analysis) of sequential therapy [35]. Patients they enrolled had either gastric ulcers or duodenal ulcers (94.3 % of total patients). We suggest the reason why our results did not yield a higher eradication efficacy may be due to the type of gastroduodenal diseases in our patients. Our patient pool only consisted of either inactive duodenal ulcer or non-ulcer dyspepsia patients.

Previous studies found that the eradication rate of standard triple therapy in non-ulcer dyspepsia tends to be lower than that in peptic-ulcer patients [21, 36]. Contrary results are observed in sequential therapy and the success rates are not significantly affected by pathological findings (peptic-ulcer *vs.* non-ulcer dyspepsia) [37, 38]. Our study's result was different, in that the eradication rate of sequential therapy (Table 3) was better in duodenal ulcer scar patients than in non-ulcer dyspepsia with ITT analysis (87.3 % *vs.* 81.5 %) and with PP analysis (92.4 % *vs.* 85.8 %), which reached a significant difference. Two large studies (DU-MACH [39] and GU-MACH [40]) have therefore looked at the impact of inflammation on H. pylori eradication. Polymorph infiltration in the antrum of patients with inflammation of grades 2/3 was associated with a significantly higher eradication rate when compared with inflammation of grades 0/1. Previous ulcer diseases may induce inflammation processes that cause degradation of the mucus and epithelial layers and altered epithelial permeability. That may allow better penetration of antibiotics from the gastric lumen and better systemic delivery of drugs. Besides, the subtype of H. Pylori that cause ulcer may be more aggressive which has a better response to the antibiotics. Therefore, we speculate that the low eradication rate of sequential therapy in non-ulcer dyspepsia patients tarnished the overall eradication rate of sequential therapy in our 364 patients with either duodenal ulcer scar or non-ulcer dyspepsia. Although eradication of *Helicobacter Pylori* is both suggested in patient with duodenal ulcer scar or non-ulcer dyspepsia, the difference in eradication rate could provide us a better outcome predication to discuss with the patient.

Although the difference was not statistically significant, subgroup analysis revealed a superior eradication rate of sequential therapy in duodenal ulcer scar patients (Table 2; ITT, 87.3 % *vs.* 77.3 %; PP, 92.4 % *vs.* 85.0 %).

Sequential therapy also achieved the acceptable effectiveness category (86–89 %, ITT) and was better than triple therapy (unacceptable category: <80 %, ITT) according to Graham's category [32]. Since many studies have proved that successful eradication of *H. pylori* substantially reduces the recurrent rate of duodenal ulcers, it is recommended by a worldwide consensus. We believe that a 10-day sequential regimen could be a valid alternative therapy in initial treatment for the eradication of *H. pylori* in duodenal ulcer scar patients.

Our data showed that the overall adverse event rate was higher in the sequential group than that in the triple group (Table 4; 36.3 % *vs.* 22.7 %). The highest incidence of adverse events was mouth bitterness in both groups. The sequential group had an even higher frequency of mouth bitterness. Nonetheless, patient-reported compliance was similar in both the triple and sequential therapy groups (90.9 % *vs.* 94.8 %).

We also performed the multivariate analysis to investigate the independent factors predicting eradication failure in this study. Table 5 showed the eradication efficiency has no relationship with age and gender. Besides, the successful eradication group has a significantly higher adverse reaction rate then the failure group. It seemed that the eradication rate was associated independently with the different protocol and presence of ulcer scar.

Furthermore, Table 6 shows the cost of each individual regimen. Clarithromycin was the most expensive drug and cost $32.30 in the standard triple therapy regimen, out of a total cost of $51.00. The sequential therapy regimen cost only $47.6. Due to the comparative expense of standard therapy, replacement of it with the less costly sequential regimen would greatly reduce total treatment

Table 5 Multivariate analysis to investigate the independent factors

	Total (N = 408)	Eradication failure (N = 70)	Eradication success (N = 338)	p-value
Age (Mean ± SD)	51.2 ± 11.1	50.7 ± 10.5	51.3 ± 11.1	0.67
Gender (%)				
Male	144	22 (31.4 %)	122 (36.1 %)	0.46
Female	264	48 (68.6 %)	216 (63.9 %)	
Adverse event (%)				
Yes	140	16 (22.9 %)	124 (36.7 %)	0.03
No	268	54 (77.1 %)	214 (63.3 %)	

There is no statistically difference between eradication rate, gender, and age. The success group have more adverse event.

iDU	Total failure in iDU (N = 26)	Failure in Triple (N = 10)	Failure in Sequential (N = 16)	p-value
Age (Mean ± SD)	51.7 ± 9.7	48.5 ± 7.9	53.7 ± 10.4	0.19
Gender (%)				
Male	9	3 (30.0 %)	6 (37.5 %)	0.7
Female	17	7 (70.0 %)	10 (62.5 %)	
Adverse event (%)				
Yes	10	2 (20.0 %)	8 (50.0 %)	0.13
No	16	8 (80.0 %)	8 (50.0 %)	

In iDU group, there is no statistically difference between failure rate, age, gender, and adverse, event.

Sequential	Total failure in Sequential (N = 60)	Failure in iDU (N = 16)	Failure in NUD (N = 44)	p-value
Age (Mean ± SD)	51.0 ± 10.9	53.7 ± 10.4	50.0 ± 11.0	0.26
Gender (%)				
Male	19	6 (37.5 %)	13 (29.5 %)	0.56
Female	41	10 (62.5 %)	31 (70.5 %)	
Adverse event (%)				
Yes	14	8 (50.0 %)	6 (13.6 %)	0.003
No	46	8 (50.0 %)	38 (86.4 %)	

In sequential group, there is no statistically difference between failure rate, age, and gender. However, the adverse rate is statistically higher in iDU group.

Table 6 The therapy dose and cost for triple and sequential therapy

Group	Regimen	Dose		Cost
Triple therapy	Pantoprazole	40 mg	BID × 7	$14.60
	Amoxicillin	1 gm	BID × 7	$4.10
	Clarithromycin	500 mg	BID × 7	$32.30
				Total $51.00
Sequential therapy	Pantoprazole	40 mg	BID × 5	$10.40
	Amoxicillin	1 gm	BID × 5	$3.00
	Pantoprazole	40 mg	BID × 5	$10.40
	Clarithromycin	500 mg	BID × 5	$23.10
	Tinidazole	500 mg	BID × 5	$0.70
				Total $47.60

costs. This economical consideration also favors the use of the latter treatment regimen.

The present study had a couple of limitations. Firstly, that patients were not randomized to receive either standard triple therapy or 10-day sequential therapy. Patients with iDU were assigned into 2 groups according to a physician's discretion, which may have introduced selection bias. Therefore, the number in the iDU triple group was too small. However, all patients were prospectively followed up with a standard protocol and were well informed about adverse problems and compliance. Secondly, bacterial culture was not performed in our protocol, and therefore the effect of antibiotic resistance was not able to be assessed. However, the resistance rates of Amoxicillin, Clarithromycin, Metronidazole, and Tetracycline in Cathy General Hospital are 13.9, 27.8, 19.4, and 0 % respectively.

Conclusion

Despite no statistically significant difference in ITT patients, 10-day sequential therapy for the eradication of *H. pylori* was superior in iDU patients than NUD patients and it reached a significant eradication effectiveness in PP patients. The sequential regimen has a better eradication rate in the iDU group than in the NUD group.

Abbreviations

H. pylori: Helicobacter pylori; iDU: inactive duodenal ulcer; NUD: non-ulcer dyspepsia; ITT: intention-to-treat; PP: per-protocol; PUD: peptic ulcer disease; EGD: esophagogastroduodenoscopy; C-UBT: ^{13}C-urea breath test; CLOtest: rapid urease test.

Competing interests

The authors declare that they have no competing interests.

Authors' contributions

CCC and CNH contributed equally to this work. CCC drafted the manuscript. CNH proposed the study protocol. YYC performed data analysis. HCS, TTC, and WCH recruited all clinical cases. LCL audited all the study details and results. All authors read and approved the final manuscript.

Acknowledgment

The author declares that this research did not receive any grant from funding agency in the public, commercial, or not-for-profit sectors.

Author details

[1]Division of Gastroenterology, Department of Internal Medicine, Hsinchu Cathay General Hospital, Hsinchu, Taiwan. [2]Committee of Medical Research and Education, Hsinchu Cathay General Hospital, Hsinchu, Taiwan. [3]Division of Gastroenterology, Department of Internal Medicine, Cathay General Hospital, 280, Section 4, Jen-Ai Road, Taipei 10650, Taiwan. [4]School of Medicine, Fu Jen Catholic University, New Taipei, Taiwan. [5]Department of Internal Medicine, School of Medicine, College of Medicine, Taipei Medical University, Taipei, Taiwan.

References

1. Suerbaum S, Michetti P. *Helicobacter pylori* infection. N Engl J Med. 2002;347: 1175–86.
2. Hsu PI, Lai KH, Lo GH, Tseng HH, Lo CC, Chen HC, et al. Risk factors for ulcer development in patients with non-ulcer dyspepsia: a prospective two year follow up study of 209 patients. Gut. 2002;51:15–20.
3. Helicobacter and Cancer Collaborative Group. Gastric cancer and *Helicobacter pylori*: a combined analysis of 12 case control studies nested within prospective cohorts. Gut. 2001;49:347–53.
4. Uemura N, Okamoto S, Yamamoto S, Matsumura N, Yamaguchi S, Yamakido M, et al. *Helicobacter* infection and the development of gastric cancer. N Engl J Med. 2001;345:784–9.
5. Parsonnet J, Hansen S, Rodriguez L, Gelb AB, Warnke RA, Jellum E, et al. *Helicobacter pylori* infection and gastric lymphoma. N Engl J Med. 1994;330: 1267–71.
6. Fuccio L, Zagari RM, Eusebi LH, Laterza L, Cennamo V, Ceroni L, et al. Meta-analysis: can *Helicobacter pylori* eradication treatment reduce the risk for gastric cancer? Ann Intern Med. 2009;151:121–8.
7. Fock KM, Katelaris P, Sugano K, Ang TL, Hunt R, Talley NJ, et al. Second Asia-Pacific Consensus Guidelines for *Helicobacter pylori* infection. J Gastroenterol Hepatol. 2009;24:1587–600.
8. Chey WD, Wong BC. Practice Parameters Committee of the American College of Gastroenterology. American College of Gastroenterology guideline on the management of Helicobacter pylori infection. Am J Gastroenterol. 2007;102:1808–25.
9. Malfertheiner P, Megraud F, O'Morain CA, Atherton J, Axon ATR, Bazzoli F, et al. The European Helicobacter Study Group (EHSG). Management of *Helicobacter pylori* infection – the Maastricht IV/ Florence consensus report. Gut. 2012;61:646–64.
10. Graham DY, Fischbach LA. *Helicobacter pylori* treatment in the era of increasing antibiotic resistance. Gut. 2010;59:1143–53.
11. Rimbara E, Fischbach LA, Graham DY. Optimal therapy for *Helicobacter pylori* infection. Nat Rev Gastroenterol Hepatol. 2011;8:79–88.
12. Megraud F, Coenen S, Versporten A, Kist M, Lopez-Brea M, Hirschl AM, et al. *Helicobacter pylori* resistance to antibiotics in Europe and its relationship to antibiotic consumption. Gut. 2013;62:34–42.
13. Zullo A, Vaira D, Vakil N, Hassan C, Gatta L, Ricci C, et al. High eradication rates of *Helicobacter pylori* with a new sequential treatment. Aliment Pharmacol Ther. 2003;17:719–26.
14. Vaira D, Zullo A, Vakil N, Gatta L, Ricci C, Perna F, et al. Sequential therapy *versus* standard triple-drug therapy for Helicobacter pylori eradication: a randomized trial. Ann Intern Med. 2007;146:556–63.
15. Jafri NS, Hornung CA, Howden CW. Meta-analysis: sequential therapy appears superior to standard therapy for helicobacter pylori infection in patients naïve to treatment. Ann Intern Med. 2008;148:923–31.
16. Gatta L, Vakil N, Leandro G, Di Mario F, Vaira D. Sequential therapy or triple therapy for *Helicobacter pylori* infection: systematic review and meta-analysis of randomized controlled trials in adults and children. Am J Gastroenterol. 2009; 104:3069–79.
17. Neil GA, Suchower LJ, Johnson E, Ronca PD, Skoglund ML. *Helicobacter pylori* eradication as a surrogate marker for the reduction of duodenal ulcer recurrence. Aliment Pharmacol Ther. 1998;12:619–33.
18. Kim JS, Kim SG, Choi IJ, Park MJ, Kim BG, Jung HC, et al. Effect of *Helicobacter pylori* eradication on duodenal ulcer scar in patient with no clinical history of duodenal ulcer. Aliment Pharmacol Ther. 2002;16:275–80.

19. Bruley des Varannes S, Flejou JF, Colin R, Zaïm M, Meunier A, Bidaut-Mazel C. There are some benefits for eradicating *Helicobacter pylori* in patients with non-ulcer dyspepsia. Aliment Pharmacol Ther. 2001;15:1177–85.

20. Jaakkimainen RL, Boyle E, Tudiver F. Is Helicobacter pylori associated with non-ulcer dyspepsia and will eradication improve symptoms? A meta-analysis. BMJ. 1999;319:1040–4.

21. Gisbert JP, Marcos S, Gisbert JL, Pajares M. *Helicobacter pylori* eradication therapy is more effect in peptic ulcer than in non-ulcer dyspepsia. Eur J Gastroenterol Hepatol. 2001;13:1303–7.

22. Huang JQ, Zheng GF, Hunt RH, Wong WM, Lam SK, Karlberg J, et al. Do patients with non-ulcer dyspepsia respond differently to *Helicobacter pylori* eradication treatments from those with peptic ulcer disease? A systematic review. World J Gastroenterol. 2005;11:2726–32.

23. Vaira D, Vakil N. Blood, urine, stool, breath, money, and *Helicobacter pylori*. Gut. 2001;48:287–9.

24. Bazzoli F, Pozzato P, Zagari M, Fossi S, Ricciardiello L, Nicolini G, et al. Efficacy of lansopraole in eradicating *Helicobacter pylori*: a meta-analysis. Helicobacter. 1998;3:195–201.

25. Laheij RJ, Rossum LG, Jansen JB, Straatman H, Verbeek AL. Evaluation of treatment regimens to cure *Helicobacter pylori* infection- a meta-analysis. Aliment Pharmacol Ther. 1999;13:857–64.

26. Sirimontaporn N, Thong-Ngam D, Tumwasorn S, Mahachai V. Ten-day sequential therapy of *Helicobacter pylori* infection in Thailand. Am J Gastroenterol. 2010;105:1071–5.

27. Park HG, Jung MK, Jung JT, Kwon JG, Kim EY, Seo HE, et al. Randomised clinical trial: a comparative study of 10-day sequential therapy with 7-day standard triple therapy for *Helicobacter pylori* infection in naïve patients. Aliment Pharmacol Ther. 2012;35:56–65.

28. Chung JW, Jung YK, Kim YI, Kwon KA, Kim JI, Lee JJ, et al. Ten-day sequential *versus* triple therapy for *Helicobacter pylori* eradications: a prospective, open-label, randomized trial. J Gastroenterol Hepatol. 2012;27: 1675–80.

29. Liou JM, Chen CC, Chen MJ, Chen CC, Chan CY, Fang YJ, et al. Sequential *versus* triple therapy for the first-line treatment of *Helicobacter pylori*: a multicentre, open-label, randomised trial. Lancet. 2013;381:205–13.

30. Zhou L, Zhang J, Chen M, Hou X, Li Z, Song Z, et al. A comparative study of sequential therapy and standard triple therapy for *Helicobacter pylori* infection: a randomized multicenter trial. Am J Gastroenterol. 2014;109:535–41.

31. Gatta L, Vakil N, Vaira D, Scarpignato C. Global eradication rates for *Helicobacter pylori* infection: systematic review and meta-analysis of sequential therapy. BMJ. 2013;347:f4587.

32. Graham DY, Lu H, Yamaoka Y. A report card to grade *Helicobacter pylori* therapy. Helicobacter. 2007;12:275–8.

33. Tong JL, Ran ZH, Shen J, Xiao SD. Sequential therapy *vs.* standard triple therapies for *Helicobacter pylori* infection: a meta-analysis. J Clin Pharm Ther. 2009;34:41–53.

34. Gisber JP, Calvet X, O'Connor A, Mégraud F, O'Morain CA. Sequential therapy for *Helicobacter pylori* eradication : a critical review. J Clin Gastroenterol. 2010;44:313–25.

35. Tsay FW, Tseng HH, Hsu PI, Wang KM, Lee CC, Chang SN, et al. Sequential therapy achieves a higher eradication rate than standard triple therapy in Taiwan. J Gastroenterol Hepatol. 2012;27:498–503.

36. de Boer WA, Tytgat GN. Should anti-Helicobacter therapy be different in patients with dyspepsia compared with patients with peptic ulcer diathesis? Eur J Gastroenterol Hepatol. 2001;13:1281–4.

37. De Francesco V, Zullo A, Hassan C, Faleo D, Ierardi E, Panella C, et al. Two new treatment regiments for *Helicobacter pylori* does not allow reaching therapeutic outcome of sequential scheme: a prospective randomized study. Dig Liver Dis. 2001;33:676–9.

38. Zullo A, De Francesco V, Hassan C, Morini S, Vaira D. The sequential therapy regimen for *Helicobacter pylori* eradication: a pooled-data analysis. Gut. 2007; 56:1353–7.

39. Zanten SJ, Bradette M, Farley A, Leddin D, Lind T, Unge P, et al. The DU-MACH study: eradication of *Helicobacter pylori* and ulcer healing in patients with acute duodenal ulcer using omeprazole based triple therapy. Aliment Pharmacol Ther. 1999;13:289–95.

40. Malfertheiner P, Bayerdörffer E, Diete U, Gil J, Lind T, Misiuna P. The GU-MACH study: the effect of 1-week omeprazole triple therapy on *Helicobacter pylori* infection in patients with gastric ulcer. Aliment Pharmacol Ther. 1999;13(6): 703–12.

9

Pharmacological regimens for eradication of Helicobacter pylori

Yiqiao Xin[1]*[iD], Jan Manson[2], Lindsay Govan[1], Robin Harbour[2], Jenny Bennison[3], Eleanor Watson[4] and Olivia Wu[1]

Abstract

Background: Approximately half of the world's population is infected with Helicobacter pylori (H.pylori), a bacterium shown to be linked with a series of gastrointestinal diseases. A growing number of systematic reviews (SRs) have been published comparing the effectiveness of different treatments for H.pylori infection but have not reached a consistent conclusion. The objective of this study is to provide an overview of SRs of pharmacological therapies for the eradication of H.pylori.

Methods: Major electronic databases were searched to identify relevant SRs published between 2002 and February 2016. Studies were considered eligible if they included RCTs comparing different pharmacological regimens for treating patients diagnosed as H.pylori infected and pooled the eradication rates in a meta-analysis. A modified version of the 'A Measurement Tool to Assess Systematic Reviews' (AMSTAR) was used to assess the methodological quality. A Bayesian random effects network meta-analysis (NMA) was conducted to compare the different proton pump inhibitors (PPI) within triple therapy.

Results: 30 SRs with pairwise meta-analysis were included. In triple therapy, the NMA ranked the esomeprazole to be the most effective PPI, followed by rabeprazole, while no difference was observed among the three old generations of PPI for the eradication of H.pylori. When comparing triple and bismuth-based therapy, the relative effectiveness appeared to be dependent on the choice of antibiotics within the triple therapy; moxifloxacin or levofloxacin-based triple therapy were both associated with greater effectiveness than bismuth-based therapy as a second-line treatment, while bismuth-based therapy achieved similar or greater eradication rate compared to clarithromycin-based therapy. Inconsistent findings were reported regarding the use of levofloxacin/moxifloxacin in the first-line treatment; this could be due to the varied resistant rate to different antibiotics across regions and populations. Critical appraisal showed a low-moderate level of overall methodological quality of included studies.

Conclusions: Our analysis suggests that the new generation of PPIs and use of moxifloxacin or levofloxacin within triple therapy as second-line treatment were associated with greater effectiveness. Given the varied antibiotic resistant rate across regions, the appropriateness of pooling results together in meta-analysis should be carefully considered and the recommendation of the choice of antibiotics should be localized.

Keywords: Helicobacter pylori, Eradication, Systematic review, Network meta-analysis

* Correspondence: yiqiao.xin@glasgow.ac.uk
[1]Health Economics and Health Technology Assessment (HEHTA), Institute of Health and Wellbeing, University of Glasgow, Glasgow, UK
Full list of author information is available at the end of the article

Background

Helicobacter pylori (H.pylori) is one of the most common human infections with a worldwide prevalence of approximately 50 %. In the United States (US) and Europe, the prevalence of H.pylori is estimated to be 20 % to 50 %, varying in different socioeconomic, age and ethnic groups and geography [1, 2]. In developing countries, the prevalence has been reported to be as high as 70 % [3]. H.pylori is usually latent and asymptomatic; however, increasing evidence has demonstrated the link between H.pylori infection and the pathogenesis of a series of upper gastrointestinal diseases: functional dyspepsia, chronic gastritis, peptic ulcer disease, gastric cancer and gastric mucosa-associated lymphoid-tissue lymphoma [4–9].

Eradication of H.pylori has been shown to be associated with increased rate of peptic ulcer healing and reduced risk of gastric cancer [10, 11]. Standard triple therapy, which includes a proton pump inhibitor (PPI), clarithromycin, and amoxicillin or metronidazole, is recommended as first-line eradication therapy for H.pylori infection in clinical guidelines worldwide [12–15]. A treatment alternative also widely recommended is bismuth-based quadruple therapy, which contains a PPI or H_2 receptor antagonist (H_2RA), bismuth, metronidazole, and tetracycline. Other treatment options include varying individual drugs within the triple therapy and quadruple therapy based regimens. More recently, sequential therapy of these multiple treatment options also has been introduced. In the US, the American College of Gastroenterology guideline (2007) recommends clarithromycin-based triple therapy for first-line eradication in patients who have not previously been treated with clarithromycin and are not allergic to penicillin. For patients who are allergic to penicillin or have previously received a macrolide antibiotic, a bismuth quadruple therapy is preferred [14].

Although these recommendations specified the type of antibiotics in the regimen, the choice of PPIs was not specified. Based on the available evidence at the time when the guidelines were produced, the relative effectiveness of PPIs was assumed to be comparable. Furthermore, in recent years, a decline in the effectiveness of the treatment regimens has been observed due to increasing clarithromycin resistance; this may have an impact on the relative effectiveness of these treatment strategies [16]. A 12-year retrospective study published in 2008 showed that the eradication rate of standard therapy decreased from 90.6 % in 1997 to 74.8 % [17].

In the past decade, several systematic reviews have evaluated the effectiveness of individual specific pharmacological regimens for H.pylori eradication. These reviews compared the eradication rate by different PPIs and antibiotics, triple versus quadruple therapy, or PPI versus H_2RA, but the conclusions of these reviews were not always consistent.

The Scottish Intercollegiate Guidelines Network (SIGN) published their recommendations on H.pylori eradication in the dyspepsia guideline in 2003 and is due to update their guidance [18]. This study aims to systematically evaluate the current evidence (since 2003) on the effectiveness of H.pylori eradication therapies for the patients diagnosed as H.pylori infection through an overview of systematic reviews.

Methods

An overview of systematic reviews was carried out according to the general principles of systematic reviewing methodology [19]. A Bayesian network meta-analysis (NMA) was conducted to compare the eradication rates by using different PPIs within triple therapy.

Eligibility criteria

All systematic reviews comparing different drug therapies for the eradication of H.pylori infection that fulfilled the following criteria were included:

- Patient — studies of adult patients who were naïve to treatment (first-line therapy) or have previous treatment failures (second-line therapy).
- Intervention/Comparator — studies comparing any pharmacological regimens.
- Outcome measure — studies reporting pooled eradication rates measured by urea breathe testing or gastric mucosal biopsy four weeks after completion of treatment, as the primary outcome. Secondary outcome measures may include adverse events rates and rates of discontinuation of therapy due to severe adverse events.
- Design — systematic reviews and meta-analyses of data from randomized controlled trials (RCTs).

Exclusion criteria

Studies were excluded if they focused on comparing the variation of dose or duration of the same drug combination; if no meta-analysis was conducted; meta-analysis included observational studies; or the included RCTs in the meta-analysis were not clearly specified. Conference abstracts were excluded due to lack of details for data extraction and quality assessment. Studies on furazolidone were excluded because it is no longer available in the US and the United Kingdom (UK) due to severe side effects. No language exclusions were applied. As this work was initiated by the SIGN guideline update, studies published prior to 2002 were excluded.

Search strategy

Four major electronic databases were searched: MEDLINE, EMBASE, the Cochrane Library and the Database of abstracts of review of effects. Relevant keywords were used to develop appropriate search strategies; these are shown in the Additional file 1. The primary search was carried out in November 2012 and updated in March 2016.

Study selection

Two reviewers (JM and YX) independently reviewed the titles and abstracts of all retrieved studies for identification of potentially relevant systematic reviews. After the initial screening, the full texts of studies deemed relevant were obtained and reviewed in detail. The discrepancy was addressed by discussion or a third reviewer (OW). Reference list of included studies was also checked to identify any potentially relevant studies that may not have been identified by the electronic searching.

Data extraction

For each included systematic review, the following data were extracted by two reviewers independently: first author, publication year and country; objective; search database and selection criteria; number of included studies in the review and meta-analysis; number of patients in the meta-analysis; patient characteristics; intervention and comparison; outcomes including eradication rate, adverse events rate, therapy discontinuation rate. In addition, as the resistant rate to antibiotics differs across regions, the country of the RCTs included in the meta-analysis was also extracted when the focus of the comparison was involved with antibiotics. To conduct the NMA, we also extracted data from the individual RCTs in the included systematic reviews, including: interventions in comparison, the total number of people in each arm and the number of people of which H.pylori had been eradicated.

Quality assessment

To assess methodological quality of the included systematic reviews, a modified version of the 'A Measurement Tool to Assess Systematic Reviews' (AMSTAR) checklist [20] was used by two reviewers (JM and YX) independently to examine the following 11 aspects: (1) clearly defined research question; (2) study selection and data extraction carried out by two independent reviewers; (3) comprehensive literature search; (4) clear selection criteria; (5) list of included and excluded studies; (6) study characteristics appropriately extracted; (7) quality assessment documented; (8) results of quality assessment appropriately considered in reaching conclusions; (9) results combined appropriately; (10) publication bias assessed; (11) conflicts of interest declared. Studies were graded as "high quality (++)", "acceptable (+)" or "low quality (0)", based on the overall risk of bias and the likelihood that results may be changed by further research.

Network meta-analysis (NMA)

A Bayesian random effect NMA was conducted to compare and rank all the PPIs within the triple therapy based on the eradication rates. When more than two interventions are being evaluated, conventional pairwise meta-analysis is limited in that it requires direct head-to-head evidence between interventions. In contrast, NMA allows the estimation of relative effects between multiple alternative interventions by incorporating both direct and indirect evidence [21, 22]. The NMA model used in this study is shown in Additional file 2. The odds ratios (ORs) for all pairwise comparisons of each treatment were calculated and presented in an interval plot. The median of the posterior distribution along with 95 % credible intervals (95%CrI) was reported. In addition, the PPIs were ranked based on their probability to be considered the best for the outcome of eradication rate of H.pylori.

Two sets of vague priors, uniform and inverse Gamma, were used for the Bayesian model, which were burned-in for 27,000 and 8,000 Markov Chain Monte Carlo iterations respectively until the convergence was met based on the Gelman-Rubin-Brooke statistic (within $1+/- 0.05$). A further approximately 40,000 iterations were run until the MC error became lower than 5 % standard error and the results became stable. The median of the posterior distribution and credible intervals for ORs was reported. The analysis was performed using WinBUGS 1.4.3 [23].

Results

Results of search and selection

The search identified 1690 studies, of which 30 studies were included in this overview of systematic reviews. The flowchart of the screening process is shown in Fig. 1. The excluded studies at full-text screening stage are listed in Additional file 3: Table S1 with reasons for exclusion.

Systematic reviews included in analysis

All the included studies were published between 2002 and 2015 in English, with the exception of three studies, which were published in Chinese [24–26]. Six studies exclusively evaluated second-line treatment for patients with at least one prior course of treatment failure [27–32]; 12 studies focused on treatment naive patients [25, 26, 33–42]; the remaining systematic reviews included RCTs for both first-line and second-line treatment. 13 studies evaluated treatments in patients with comorbid gastric diseases including peptic ulcer disease, duodenal ulcer, functional dyspepsia, chronic gastritis or other

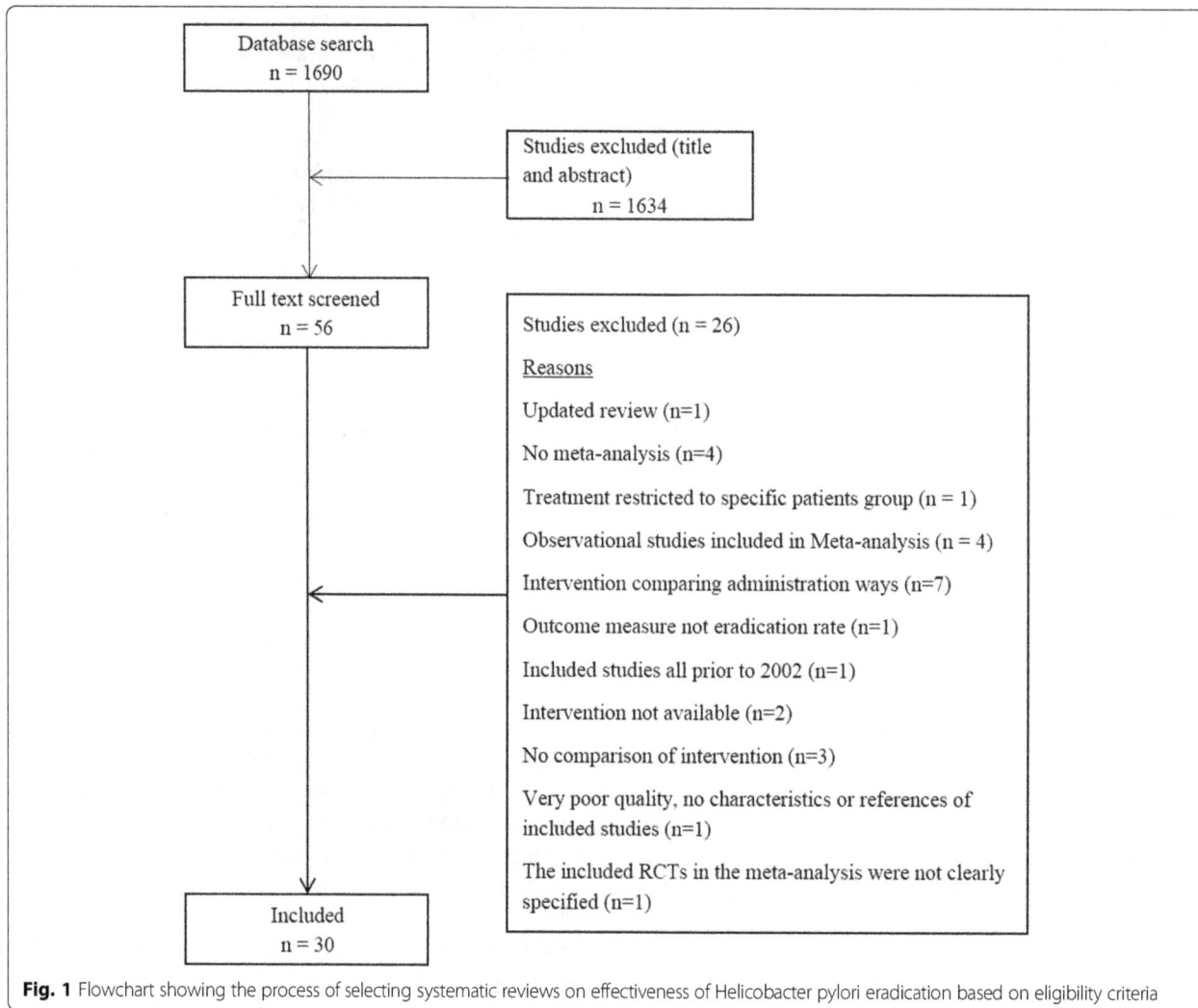

Fig. 1 Flowchart showing the process of selecting systematic reviews on effectiveness of Helicobacter pylori eradication based on eligibility criteria

non-ulcer diseases [24, 27, 37–40, 43–49] (the remaining studies did not provide such data). In addition to the eradication rate, 15 systematic reviews also compared adverse events rates [25, 28–38, 41, 47, 50] and six compared the discontinuity rate (compliance rate) [25, 29–31, 37, 50]. The pooled eradication rates of different regimens in all of the included systematic reviews ranged between 47 % (data from three RCTs relating to standard triple therapy [30]) and 94 % (data from one RCT relating to esomeprazole-based triple therapy [46]) by intention to treat (ITT) analysis.

Based on the treatment regimens under comparison, the included studies were classified into the following five categories:

- Triple therapy with different PPIs
- Triple therapy with different antibiotics
- Triple therapy versus bismuth-based therapy
- PPI versus H_2RA in triple therapy
- Other drug therapies

Triple therapy with different PPIs

Seven studies evaluated the impact of different PPIs within a triple therapy regimen on H.pylori eradication rate (Table 1) [24, 42–46, 51]. These included both new (esomeprazole, rabeprazole) and older generations of PPIs (omeprazole, pantoprazole, lansoprazole); overall, the results were mixed, but a time trend was observed that studies published from 2006 onwards [24, 42, 46] suggested consistently that new generation of PPIs achieved greater eradication rate than the older generations. Amongst the new PPIs, the reported eradication rates ranged from 77 % (data from nine RCTs relating to rabeprazole-based triple therapy [43]) to 94 % (data from one RCT relating to esomeprazole-based triple therapy [46]); for the older generation PPIs, the reported eradication rates ranged from 75 % (data from four RCTs relating to omeprazole-based triple therapy [51]) to 88 % (data from two RCTs relating to omeprazole-based triple therapy [51]). Five studies compared esomeprazole with older generation PPIs in the triple therapy, of which,

Table 1 Characteristics of systematic reviews comparing triple therapy with different PPIs (n = 7)

Author, year, country	Last search date	Disease	Intervention[c]	Comparator[c]	No. of studies in MA	No. of patients in MA	Eradication rates	Eradication rates odds ratio (95 % CI) by ITT	Quality assessment[b]
Gisbert et al. 2003-r Spain [43]	Sep 2002	HP infection; PUD/NUD/not reported	Rabeprazole	Omeprazole/Lansoprazole	12	2226	79 % vs. 77 %	1.15 (0.93–1.42)	+
			Rabeprazole	Omeprazole	9	1475	77 % vs. 77 %	1.03 (0.81–1.32)	
			Rabeprazole	Lansoprazole	7	1095	82 % vs. 79 %	1.20 (0.87–1.64)	
Vergara et al. 2003 Spain [51]	Sep 2002	HP infection	Omeprazole	Lansoprazole	4	1085	74.7 % vs. 76 %;	0.91 (0.69–1.21)[a]	+
			Omeprazole	Rabeprazole	4	825	77.9 % vs. 81.2 %	0.81 (0.58–1.15)[a]	
			Omeprazole	Esomeprazole	2	833	87.7 % vs. 89 %	0.89 (0.58–1.35)[a]	
			Lansoprazole	Rabeprazole	3	550	81 % vs. 85.7 %	0.77 (0.48–1.22)[a]	
Gisbert et al. 2004 Spain [44]	Jun 2003	HP infection; PUD +/-NUD	Esomeprazole	Omeprazole	4	1292	85 % vs. 82 %	1.19 (0.81–1.74)	+
Gisbert et al. 2004 Spain [45]	Sep 2002	HP infection; PUD +/-NUD	Pantoprazole	Omeprazole/Lansoprazole	7	1137	83 % vs. 81 %	1.00 (0.61–1.64)	+
			Pantoprazole	Omeprazole	1	974	83 % vs. 82 %	0.91 (0.49–1.69)	
			Pantoprazole	Lansoprazole	2	258	78 % vs. 75 %	1.22 (0.68–2.17)	
Wang et al. 2006 China [24]	Jul 2006	HP infection; DU, NUD, PUD	Esomeprazole	Omeprazole	11	2048	85.6 % vs. 81.6 %	1.30 (1.02–1.65)	0
Wang X et al. 2006 China [46]	2000–2005 (published date)	HP infection; PUD/NUD	Esomeprazole	Omeprazole/Pantoprazole	11	2146	86 % vs. 81 %	1.39 (1.09–1.75)	0
			Esomeprazole	Omeprazole	10	1946	85 % vs. 82 %	1.29 (1.01–1.65)	
			Esomeprazole	Pantoprazole	1	200	94 % vs. 82 %	3.44 (1.30–9.07)	
McNicholl et al. 2012 Spain [42]	Oct 2011	HP infection; naïve to therapy	Rabeprazole	Omeprazole/Lansoprazole/pantoprazole	21	2945	80.5 % vs. 76.2 %	1.21 (1.02–1.42)	0
			Esomeprazole	Omeprazole/Lansoprazole/pantoprazole	12	2598	82.3 % vs. 77.6 %	1.32 (1.01–1.73)	
			Rabeprazole	Esomeprazole	5	1574	76.7 % vs. 78.7 %	0.90 (0.70–1.17)	

HP H.pylori, PPI proton pump inhibitor, PUD peptic ulcer disease, NUD non-ulcer dyspepsia, MA meta-analysis, ITT intention to treat, CI confidence interval

[a] Peto OR is reported here

[b] Quality assessment: high quality (++): majority of criteria met, little or no risk of bias and results unlikely to be changed by further research. Acceptable (+): most criteria met, some flaws in the study with an associated risk of bias and conclusions may change in the light of further studies. Low quality (0): either most criteria not met or significant flaws relating to key aspects of study design, and conclusions likely to change in the light of further studies

[c] The antibiotics are the same type and same dose for each arm of the RCTs

three reported a statistically significant benefit of esomeprazole in H.pylori eradication with OR of approximately 1.3 [24, 42, 46]. A similar effect was reported in one of the three studies comparing the effectiveness of the rabeprazole with the older generation PPIs (OR 1.21; 95%CI 1.02–1.42) [42]. Only one study compared the effectiveness of esomeprazole with rabeprazole and found no difference in eradication rate (OR 0.90; 95%CI 0.70–1.17) [42]. Similarly, no difference was observed when comparing within older generation PPIs [45, 51].

A diagram of the PPI network is given in Fig. 2. Overall, 57 trials were included in the NMA analysis. None of the trials compared rabeprazole with pantoprazole, or lansoprazole with esomeprazole. In contrast, esomeprazole was compared with omeprazole in 15 trials. In our analysis omeprazole was used as the reference treatment since direct trials existed comparing omeprazole and each of the other PPIs and it was the most commonly used PPI in the triple therapy for H.pylori eradication. Esomeprazole was ranked first in the probability best test, with OR to be 1.29 (95 % credible interval 1.08–1.56) when compared with omeprazole, followed by rabeprazole (Table 2). The three old generations of PPIs showed similar effectiveness. The OR and interval plot for each pair of the mixed comparisons of different PPIs is shown in Fig. 3.

Triple therapy with different antibiotics

Seven studies evaluated the impact of different antibiotics within a triple therapy for the first-line treatment [25, 26, 33–37] and one study evaluated the antibiotics for both first-line and second-line treatment [47] (Table 3). Clarithromycin was used as a comparator in all the studies while the intervention antibiotics included

levofloxacin [25, 26, 35–37], azithromycin [33] and moxifloxacin [34]. Five studies compared levofloxacin-based triple therapy with standard triple therapy for first-line treatment [25, 26, 35–37], among which two studies reported improved eradication rates with levofloxacin [25, 26] while the other three studies showed no difference between the two regimens [35–37]. Similarly, for moxifloxacin, two systematic reviews reached conflict conclusions when comparing it with standard triple therapy for first-line treatment [34, 47]. The two systematic reviews included three same RCTs while one of them included an additional RCT from China [34]. With the inclusion of this RCT, the pooled result showed moxifloxacin was associated with greater eradication rate for the naïve patient (OR 1.13; 95%CI 1.01–1.27) [34] while no difference was shown in another study (OR 1.80; 95%CI 0.71–4.55) [47]. The use of moxifloxacin as second-line treatment was evaluated in one study which showed that the moxifloxacin-based triple therapy achieved greater eradication rate than the clarithromycin-based therapy (OR 1.78; 95%CI 1.16–2.73) [47]. In addition to levofloxacin and moxifloxacin, one study evaluated azithromycin-based triple therapy versus standard triple therapy as first-line treatment and did not find a difference [33].

In addition to the eradication rates, adverse events rates were also compared in seven studies, such as nausea, metallic taste and other gastrointestinal tract discomforts [25, 33–37, 47]. Compared to clarithromycin, the risk of adverse events was approximately halved with azithromycin (OR 0.58; 95%CI 0.41–0.82) [33]. Two studies compared the adverse events between moxifloxacin and clarithromycin containing triple therapy; one showed lower adverse events rate associated with moxifloxacin (OR 0.45; 95%CI 0.26–0.77) [47] while the other

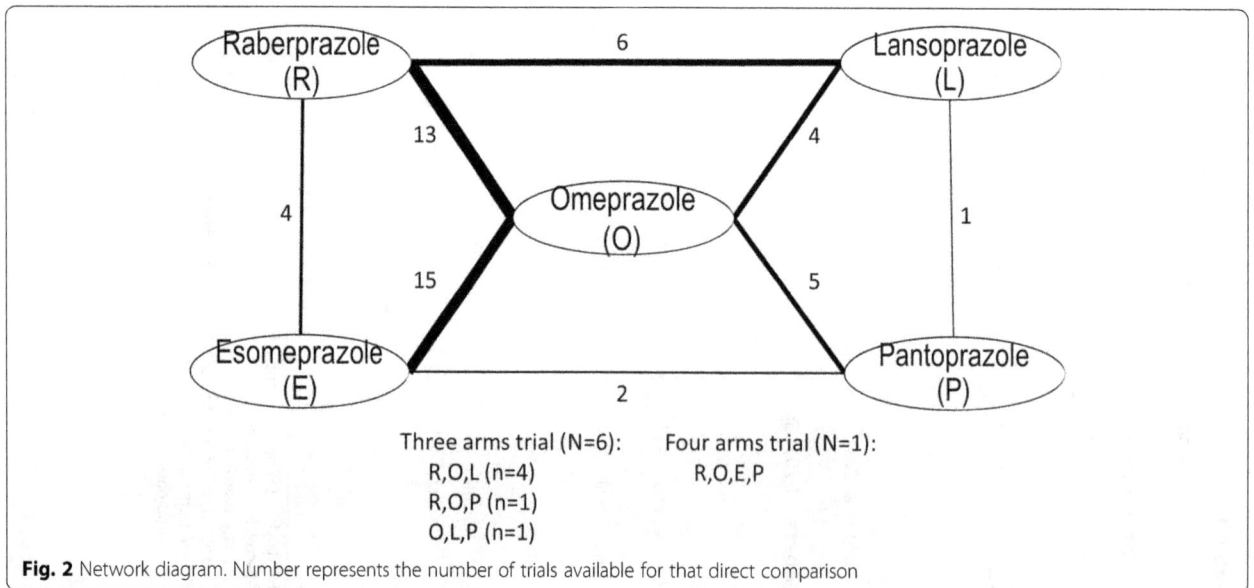

Fig. 2 Network diagram. Number represents the number of trials available for that direct comparison

Table 2 Rank order of effectiveness of PPIs for H.pylori eradication

Rank	Generation of PPI	PPI	Probability best (standard deviation)	OR (95 % credible Interval) Comparator: Omeprazole
1	New	Esomeprazole	0.820 (0.384)	1.29 (1.08 – 1.56)
2	New	Rabeprazole	0.170 (0.375)	1.77 (0.99 – 1.39)
3	Old	Pantoprazole	0.008 (0.087)	0.94 (0.72 – 1.22)
4	Old	Lansoprazole	0.003 (0.050)	0.93 (0.74 – 1.16)
5	Old	Omeprazole	0.0003 (0.018)	1

did not show any difference [34]. For levofloxacin, one study showed there were reduced adverse events rate (OR 0.57; 95%CI 0.44–0.74) [25] while three studies reported no difference when comparing to the standard therapy [35–37].

Triple therapy versus bismuth-based therapy

Nine studies compared the effectiveness, adverse events rate and therapy discontinuation rates between triple therapy and bismuth-based therapy [27–32, 38, 39, 50]. The study characteristics are presented in Table 4. For the bismuth-based therapies, seven studies evaluated bismuth-based quadruple therapy [29–32, 38, 39, 50], one evaluated ranitidine bismuth citrate (RBC) [27] and another one evaluated both quadruple therapy and RBC [28]. Overall, the quadruple therapy was associated with similar or greater eradication rate than standard triple therapy; however when levofloxacin or

moxifloxacin was contained in the triple therapy, the reverse was observed.

Two of the nine studies focused on treatment naive patients, and no difference in eradication rates was found between triple and quadruple therapy. The primary antibiotics used in both studies was clarithromycin [38, 39]. The remaining seven studies compared second-line therapy for patients with previous treatment failures [27–32, 50]. The primary antibiotics used in triple therapy varied: two studies evaluated clarithromycin [27, 50], one study with moxifloxacin [31], three studies with levofloxacin [28, 29, 32], and one study compared all of the three [30]. Clarithromycin-containing triple therapy was associated with lower eradication rates than bismuth-based therapy in two studies [27, 30] while one study showed no difference [50]. In contrast, moxifloxacin-containing triple therapy was suggested to achieve greater effectiveness than bismuth-based therapy [30, 31]. Similar

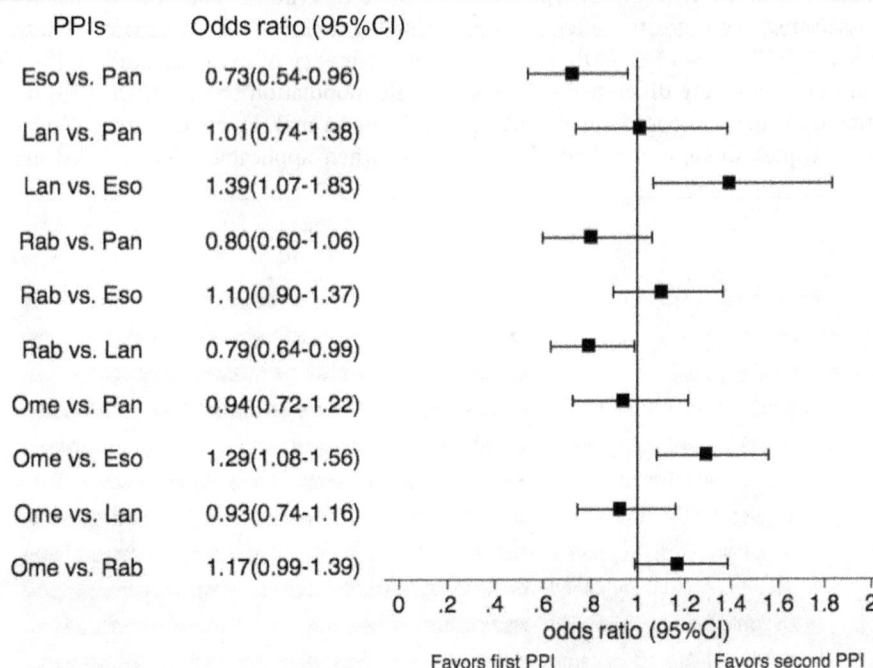

PPIs	Odds ratio (95%CI)
Eso vs. Pan	0.73(0.54-0.96)
Lan vs. Pan	1.01(0.74-1.38)
Lan vs. Eso	1.39(1.07-1.83)
Rab vs. Pan	0.80(0.60-1.06)
Rab vs. Eso	1.10(0.90-1.37)
Rab vs. Lan	0.79(0.64-0.99)
Ome vs. Pan	0.94(0.72-1.22)
Ome vs. Eso	1.29(1.08-1.56)
Ome vs. Lan	0.93(0.74-1.16)
Ome vs. Rab	1.17(0.99-1.39)

odds ratio (95%CI)

Favors first PPI   Favors second PPI

Abbreviations: PPI = proton pump inhibitor; eso = esomeprazole; lan = lansoprazole; ome = omeprazole; pan = pantoprazole; rab = rabeprazole

Fig. 3 Odds ratios and interval plot of mixed treatment comparisons between PPIs for H.pylori eradication

to moxifloxacin, triple therapy with levofloxacin appeared to be more effective than bismuth-based therapy, however statistically significant finding was only reported in one of the four studies (OR 1.18; 95%CI 1.08–1.29) [29].

The adverse events around the bismuth-based therapy included diarrhea, abdominal pain, dark stools, dizziness, headache, nausea, metallic taste and nausea [52]. Seven studies reported adverse events of the compared regimens [28–32, 38, 50]. The pooled adverse event rates of clarithromycin-based triple therapy ranged from 35.4 % [50] to 37 % [38], 10.1 % [31] to 16.75 % [30] for levofloxacin or moxifloxacin-based triple therapy, and 27.8 % [31] to 44 % [28] for bismuth-based therapy. Five studies showed a lower risk of adverse events of levofloxacin/moxifloxacin compared with the bismuth-based regimen with ORs ranging from 0.27 to 0.51 [28–32], and one study favoured bismuth when comparing with clarithromycin triple therapy [50]. One study classified adverse events by severity and reported much lower risk favouring levofloxacin compared with bismuth therapy when including only severe adverse events (OR 0.20; 95%CI 0.06–0.67) [28]. Furthermore, the discontinuation rate of triple therapy using moxifloxacin and levofloxacin was statistically significantly lower than bismuth-based therapy in three of the four studies [29–31].

PPI versus H$_2$RA in triple therapy

Three studies compared the effectiveness of PPI versus H$_2$RA within a triple therapy (Table 5) [40, 41, 53]. One systematic review based on 20 RCTs with 2374 patients showed PPI was associated with greater effectiveness than H$_2$RA (OR 1.31; 95%CI 1.09–1.58) [40]. Another study of 12 RCTs did not show any difference between the two, but its subgroup analysis based on six RCTs suggested PPI-based triple therapy reached higher

eradication rates than H$_2$RA when clarithromycin was not contained [53]. A recent systematic review of three RCTs compared lafutidine versus lansoprazole-containing triple therapy and reported no difference between the two regimens [41].

Other drug therapies

One study evaluated the impact of adding metronidazole or tinidazole (concomitant quadruple therapy) on standard triple therapy and reported greater eradication rates with concomitant therapy (OR 2.36; 95%CI 1.67–3.34) [48]. One study based on 14 RCTs assessed the combination of tetracycline and amoxicillin in triple therapy/quadruple therapy and found no difference in eradication rate when compared to other regimens when the two drugs were not combined [49]. One Japanese study evaluated the effectiveness of supplementation with rebamipide and found it was associated with greater eradication rate compared to rebamipide not-containing regimens (OR 1.59; 95%CI 1.14–2.22) [54]. The characteristics of these studies are presented in Table 6.

Quality assessment

The overall quality of the included systematic reviews was graded as low to moderate with a higher risk of bias (Fig. 4). This was primarily due to insufficient reporting and poor methodological approaches. The majority of the reviews met five to eight criteria out of the 11 total AMSTAR criteria. The criteria that were frequently not fulfilled included: (1) transparent study selection process and reference of excluded studies; (2) adequate reporting of the population characteristics; (3) using quality appropriately in making conclusions; (4) assessing publication bias when applicable. The detailed assessment for each

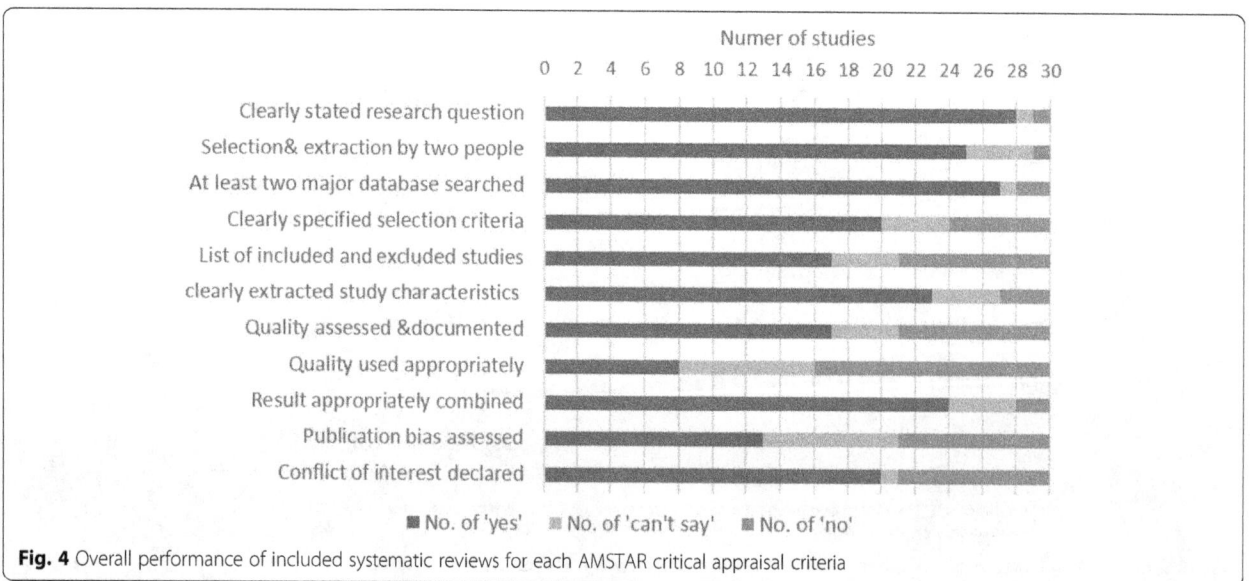

Fig. 4 Overall performance of included systematic reviews for each AMSTAR critical appraisal criteria

Table 3 Characteristics of systematic reviews comparing triple therapy with different antibiotics (n = 8)

Author, Year, country	Last search date	Disease	Countries of included RCTs[c]	Intervention	Comparator	No. of studies in MA	No. of patients in MA	Eradication rates by ITT	Eradication rates odds ratio (95 % CI) by ITT	Quality assessment[b]
Zhang et al. 2008 China [25]	May 2008	HP infection; naïve to treatment; PUD/NUD	China (8), Italy (3)	**Levofloxacin-containing triple:** levofloxacin+ +same PPI(Ome/panto/esome) + another one antibiotic (furazolidone/amoxicillin/azithromycin/metronidazole/tinidazole)	**Standard triple:** clarithromycin+	11	1926	Not reported	1.56 (1.25–1.94)	0
Dong et al. 2009 China [33]	May 2009	HP infection; naïve to treatment	China (4), Italy (5), Korea, Russia, France, Croatia, US	**Azithromycin-containing triple:** azithromycin+ + one antibiotic (levofloxacin/amoxicillin/metronidazole)+ +same PPI (ome/esome/lanso/panto)	**Azithromycin NOT-containing triple:** + two antibiotics (amoxicillin/clarithromycin/metronidazole/tinidazole)+	14	1431	72.0 % vs. 69.8 %	1.17 (0.64–2.14)	+
Yuan et al. 2009 China [34]	Dec 2008	HP infection; naïve to treatment	Italy, Croatia, Turkey, China	**Moxifloxacin-containing triple:** moxifloxacin+ + same PPI (esome/lanso/ome) + another same regimen (amoxicillin/tinidazole/metronidazole/bismuth-)	**Clarithromycin-containing triple:** clarithromycin+	4	772	84.1 % vs. 73.6 %	1.13 (1.01–1.27)[a]	+
Zhang et al. 2013 China [47]	March 2012	HP infection; PUD/NUD/others; either naïve or with previous treatment failures	Korea (2), Croatia (2), China, Italy, Turkey	**Moxifloxacin-containing triple OR Quadruple:** moxifloxacin + amoxicillin/metronidazole/tinidazole +/– RBC+ + same PPI (esome/ome/rabe/lanso)	**Standard triple or quadruple:** (+/–)Bismuth/RBC + metronidazole/tinidazole/clarithromycin/amoxicillin+	7	1263	79.0 % vs. 68.3 %	1.82 (1.17–2.81)	+
			Croatia, Turkey, Italy	**First-line** **Moxifloxacin-containing triple OR Quadruple:** moxifloxacin + amoxicillin/metronidazole/tinidazole (+/–) RBC+ + same PPI (esome/lanso)	**First-line** **Standard triple or quadruple:** (+/–) Bismuth/RBC + metronidazole/tinidazole/clarithromycin/amoxicillin +	3	717	Not reported	1.80 (0.71–4.55)	
			Croatia, Korea (2), China	**Second-line** **Moxifloxacin-containing triple:** moxifloxacin + metronidazole/amoxicillin+ + same PPI (esome/ome/rabe)	**Second-line** **Standard triple or quadruple:** (+/–) Bismuth + metronidazole/tinidazole/clarithromycin+	4	546	73.3 % vs. 60.2 %	1.78 (1.16–2.73)	
			Croatia, Korea (2), Turkey, Italy, China	**Moxifloxacin + amoxicillin** (+/–) RBC+	**Standard triple or quadruple:** (+/–) Bismuth/RBC + metronidazole/tinidazole/	6	810	Not reported	1.50 (0.95–2.38)	

Table 3 Characteristics of systematic reviews comparing triple therapy with different antibiotics (n = 8) (*Continued*)

Study	Date	Population	Countries	Intervention	Comparison	No. RCTs	No. patients	Eradication rate	RR (CI)	Quality
			Croatia (2), Italy	**Moxifloxacin + metronidazole/tinidazole+** + same PPI(esome/ome/rabe/lanso)	**Standard triple or quadruple:** (+/−) Bismuth/RBC + metronidazole/tinidazole/ clarithromycin/amoxicillin + clarithromycin/amoxicillin + + same PPI (esome/ome/rabe/lanso)	3	453	Not reported	3.00 (1.84–4.89)	++
Ye et al. 2014 China [35]	August 2013	HP infection; naïve to treatment	Germany, Egypt, Taiwan (2), China (2), Spain (2), Italy (2)	**Levofloxacin-containing triple:** levofloxacin+ +same PPI(Ome/lanso/esome) + another one antibiotic (amoxicillin/metronidazole)	**Standard triple:** clarithromycin+	10	2676	81.5 % vs. 77.2 %	1.28 (0.88–1.85)	++
Peedikayil et al. 2014 Saudi Arabia [36]	March 2013	HP infection; naïve to treatment	Egypt and Saudi Arabia, Taiwan (2), South Korea, China, Italy (2)	**Levofloxacin-containing triple:** levofloxacin+ +same PPI(Ome/lanso/esome) + another one antibiotic (amoxicillin/+metronidazole/clarithromycin/azithromycin)	**Standard triple:** clarithromycin+	7	1782	79.1 % vs. 81.4 %	0.97 (0.93–1.02)[a]	+
Xiao et al. 2014 China [37]	March 2013	HP infection; naïve to treatment, PUD/NUD/not reported	Italy (2), China (3), Spain (2), Egypt and Saudi Arabia, Korea	**Levofloxacin-containing triple:** levofloxacin+ +same PPI(Ome/lanso/esome) + another one antibiotic (amoxicillin/+metronidazole/clarithromycin/azithromycin)	**Standard triple:** clarithromycin+	9	2512	80.2 % vs. 77.4 %	1.03 (0.94–1.13)[a]	++
Gou et al. 2014 China [26]	December 2013	HP infection; naïve to treatment	All from China	**Levofloxacin-containing triple:** levofloxacin+ No details reported	**Standard triple:** clarithromycin+	21	2697	82.3 % vs.73.8 %	1.12 (1.08–1.16)[a]	0

HP H.pylori, *PPI* proton pump inhibitor, *esome* esomeprazole, *lanso* lansoprazole, *ome* omeprazole, *panto* pantoprazole, *rabe* rabeprazole, *PUD* peptic ulcer disease, *NUD* non-ulcer dyspepsia, *MA* meta-analysis, *ITT* intention to treat, *CI* confidence interval, *RCT* randomized controlled trials, *RBC* ranitidine bismuth citrate

[a] Relative risk is reported here

[b] Quality assessment: high quality (++): majority of criteria met, little or no risk of bias and results unlikely to be changed by further research. Acceptable (+): most criteria met, some flaws in the study with an associated risk of bias and conclusions may change in the light of further studies. Low quality (0): either most criteria not met or significant flaws relating to key aspects of study design, and conclusions likely to change in the light of further studies

[c] Countries of included RCTs: the number in the bracket represents the number of trials from the same country if more than one trial exists

Table 4 Characteristics of systematic reviews comparing triple therapy versus bismuth-based therapy ($n = 9$)

Author, Year, country	Last search date	Disease	Countries of included RCTs[f]	Triple therapy	Bismuth-based Quadruple therapy	No. of studies in MA	No. of patients in MA	Eradication rates by ITT	Eradication rates odds ratio (95 % CI) by ITT[d]	Quality assessment[e]
Gene et al. 2003 Spain [38]	Aug 2002	HP infection; naïve to therapy; PUD/ NUD	Spain (2), US/ Canada, unknown	PPI (ome/panto) + clarithromycin + amoxicillin	Bismuth + PPI(ome/panto) + tetracycline + metronidazole	4	981	78 % vs. 81 %	0.83 (0.61–1.14)[a]	0
Gisbert et al. 2005 Spain [27]	Sep 2004	HP infection; NUD+/–PUD; previous treatment failures	Croatia, Spain (6), Belgium, Italy (4), Greece, China	PPI (ome/lanso/panto) + clarithromycin + amoxicillin/nitroimidazole	RBC + clarithromycin + amoxicillin	14	2205	78 % vs. 79 %	**Bismuth vs. triple** 1.11 (0.88–1.40)	+
			Croatia, Italy (6), Spain, Norway, Unknown (2), The Netherlands, China	PPI (ome/lanso/panto/ rabe) + clarithromycin + amoxicillin/nitroimidazole	RBC + clarithromycin + nitroimidazole	13	1777	80 % vs. 87 %	**Bismuth vs. triple** 1.65 (1.15–2.37)	
			Taiwan, China, UK	PPI (ome) + clarithromycin + amoxicillin/ nitroimidazole	RBC + nitroimidazole + amoxicillin	3	451	75 % vs. 73 %	**Bismuth vs. triple** 0.92 (0.60–1.41)	
Gisbert et al. 2006 Spain [28]	Jul 2005	HP infection; Previous treatment failures	Italy (5), China, Spain, unknown	**Levofloxacin-containing:** levofloxacin + PPI(panto/ rabe/esome/ome) + amoxicillin/rifabutin	Bismuth + PPI(panto/rabe/ ome) + tetracycline + metronidazole; or RBC+ tetracycline + metronidazole	8	996	81 % vs. 70 %	1.80 (0.9–3.5)	0
			Not reported	**Levofloxacin + amoxicillin** + PPI(panto/ rabe/esome/ome)	Bismuth + PPI(panto/rabe/ ome) + tetracycline + metronidazole; or RBC+ tetracycline + metronidazole	not specified	Not specified	Not reported	1.7 (0.71–4.0)	
Saad et al. 2006 US [29]	Apr 2005	HP infection; failed prior course(s) of standard triple therapy	Italy (5), China	**Levofloxacin-containing:** levofloxacin+ amoxicillin + + same PPI (ome/esome/rabe/panto)	Bismuth – + metronidazole + tetracycline+	6	854	87 % vs. 60 %	1.18 (1.08–1.29)[b]	0
Li et al. 2010 China [30]	1981-Mar 2009 (Published date)	HP infection; previous treatment failures	Germany (2), Ireland	**Clarithromycin-containing:** clarithromycin+ amoxicillin+ + same PPI (ome/not specified)	Bismuth+ metronidazole + tetracycline+	3	411	46.5 % vs. 61.9 %	0.53 (0.35–0.80)	0
			Korea (2), Croatia	**Moxifloxacin-containing:** moxifloxacin + amoxicillin/ metronidazole+ +PPI(esome/ome)	Bismuth + metronidazole + tetracycline+	3	437	Not reported	1.78 (0.98–3.22)	0

Table 4 Characteristics of systematic reviews comparing triple therapy versus bismuth-based therapy (n = 9) (Continued)

Study	Published date	Indication	Countries[f]	Regimens	RCTs	n	Eradication	OR (CI)[d]	Quality[e]
			Taiwan, Korea, China (5), Italy (2)	**Levofloxacin-containing:** levofloxacin + amoxicillin/rifabutin+ + same PPI(esome/panto/lanso/rabe)	9	928	Not reported	1.43 (0.82–2.51)	0
Luther et al. 2010 US [50]	1990–2008 (Published date)	HP infection	Spain (2), Greece, Australia/New Zealand, India, US/Canada, Korea, Turkey, UK	**Clarithromycin-containing:** clarithromycin + amoxicillin + +PPI (ome/panto/lanso/not specified)	9	1679	77.0 % vs. 78.3 %	**Bismuth vs. triple** 1.00 (0.94–1.07)[b]	
Wu et al. 2011 China [31]	Dec 2010	HP infection; previous treatment failures	China (4), Korea (2), Croatia	**Moxifloxacin-containing:** Moxifloxacin + + amoxicillin/metronidazole+ + PPI (esome/ome/rabe)	7	787	74.9 % vs. 61.4 %	1.89 (1.38–2.58)	++
Di Caro et al. 2012 UK [32]	Oct 2010	HP infection; previous treatment failures	Italy (4), Spain (2), China (4), Korea (2), Taiwan, Unknown	**Levofloxacin + amoxicillin-containing:** levofloxacin + amoxicillin + PPI(panto/rabe/esome/ome/lanso)	14	1331	76.5 % vs. 67.4 %	1.59 (0.98–2.58)	0
Venerito et al. 2013 Germany [39]	Nov 2011	HP infection; naïve to therapy; PUD/NUD/others	Spain (2), Australia/New Zealand, Greece, US/Canada, India, Korea, Turkey (2), UK, China, multi European countries	**Clarithromycin-containing:** clarithromycin + amoxicillin + +PPI(ome/panto/lanso/not specified)	12	2467	68.9 % vs. 77.6 %	**Bismuth vs. triple** 0.06 (−0.01–0.13)[c]	+

Bismuth + metronidazole/ + tetracycline+ (row 1); Bismuth + metronidazole + tetracycline + (row 2); Bismuth + metronidazole/ furazolidone + tetracycline/amoxicillin/ clarithromycin+ (row 3); Bismuth quadruple therapy (not specified) (row 4); Bismuth + tetracycline + metronidazole+ (row 5)

HP H.pylori, PPI proton pump inhibitor, esome esomeprazole, lanso lansoprazole, ome omeprazole, panto pantoprazole, rabe rabeprazole, PUD peptic ulcer disease, NUD non-ulcer dyspepsia, MA meta-analysis, ITT intention to treat, CI confidence interval, RCT randomized controlled trials, RBC ranitidine bismuth citrate

[a] Peto OR is reported here

[b] Relative risk is reported here

[c] Risk difference is reported here

[d] OR > 1 indicates that triple therapy is associated with greater effectiveness than bismuth-based therapy and vice versa. When "Bismuth vs. triple" is specified in the form, OR > 1 indicates bismuth-based therapy is associated with greater effectiveness than triple therapy and vice versa

[e] Quality assessment: high quality (++): majority of criteria met, little or no risk of bias and results unlikely to be changed by further research. Acceptable (+): most criteria met, some flaws in the study with an associated risk of bias and conclusions may change in the light of further studies. Low quality (0): either most criteria not met or significant flaws relating to key aspects of study design, and conclusions likely to change in the light of further studies

[f] Countries of included RCTs: the number in the bracket represents the number of trials from the same country if more than one trials exist

Table 5 Characteristics of systematic reviews comparing PPI and H$_2$ receptor antagonists (H$_2$RAs) ($n = 3$)

Author, year, country	Last search date	Disease	H$_2$RAs	PPI	No. of studies in MA	No. of patients in MA	Eradication rates by ITT	Eradication rates odds ratio (95 % CI) by ITT	Quality assessment[a]
Gisbert et al. 2003 Spain [40]	Jan 2002	HP infection; naïve to treatment; PUD/NUD	H$_2$RAs (ranitidine/famotidine/nizatidine)+ + two same antibiotics (amoxicillin/clarithromycin/metronidazole/tinidazole) +/− bismuth-	PPI (ome/lanso)+	20	2374	69 % vs. 74 %	**Triple vs. H$_2$RAs** 1.31 (1.09-1.58)	+
Graham et al. 2003 US [53]	1990–2001 (Published date)	HP infection; either naïve or with previous treatment failures	H$_2$RAs(nizatidine/famotidine/ranitidine) + + two same antibiotics (clarithromycin/amoxicillin/metronidazole/tinidazole)	PPI (lanso/ome) +	12	1441	78 % vs. 81 %	0.83 (0.63–1.09)	0
			H$_2$RAs(not specified)+ + one same antibiotics (not specified)	**Clarithromycin-containing triple:** Clarithromycin + PPI(not specified)+	6	Not reported	79 % vs. 69 %	1.14 (0.76–1.71)	
			H$_2$RAs(not specified)+ +two same antibiotics (not specified)	**Clarithromycin NOT-containing triple:** PPI(not specified)+	6	Not reported	78 % vs. 85 %	0.64 (0.45–0.92)	
Ren et al. 2010 China [41]	Apr 2010	HP infection; naïve to treatment	**Lafutidine-containing:** H$_2$RAs(lafutidine)+ + two same antibiotics (clarithromycin + amoxicillin)	**Lanso-containing triple:** PPI(lanso) +	3	238	78 % vs. 77.5 %	1.03 (0.64–1.66)	++

HP H.pylori, *H2RAs* H2 receptor antagonists, *PPI* proton pump inhibitor, *esome* esomeprazole, *lanso* lansoprazole, *ome* omeprazole, *panto* pantoprazole, *rabe* rabeprazole, *PUD* peptic ulcer disease, *NUD* non-ulcer dyspepsia, *MA* meta-analysis, *ITT* intention to treat, *CI* confidence interval, *RCT* randomized controlled trials

[a] Quality assessment: high quality (++): majority of criteria met, little or no risk of bias and results unlikely to be changed by further research. Acceptable (+): most criteria met, some flaws in the study with an associated risk of bias and conclusions may change in the light of further studies. Low quality (0): either most criteria not met or significant flaws relating to key aspects of study design, and conclusions likely to change in the light of further studies

Table 6 Characteristics of systematic reviews comparing other regimens (n = 3)

Author, year, country	Last search date	Disease	Countries of included RCTs[b]	Intervention	Comparison	No. of studies in MA	No. of patients in MA	Eradication rates by ITT	Eradication rates odds ratio (95 % CI) by ITT	Quality assessment[a]
Gisbert and Calvet 2012 Spain [48]	December 2011	HP infection PUD/NUD/ others	Germany, UK, Japan, Italy, Japan, Korea (2)	Concomitant therapy: **metronidazole** + standard triple therapy Note: Standard triple therapy: (PPI(ome/rabe/lanso) + amoxicillin + clarithromycin)	Standard triple therapy	7	984	90 % vs. 78 %	2.36 (1.67–3.34)	0
Lv et al. 2015 China [49]	April 2014	HP infection; PUD/NUD/ others; naive to treatment or had previous treatment	China (4), Taiwan (3), Korea, Turkey	**Quadruple** regimens containing **both amoxicillin and tetracycline**	Other quadruple regimens where amoxicillin and tetracycline were not contained together	9	1453	78.1 % vs. 80.5 %	0.90 (0.46–1.78)	+
			US, Italy, Turkey, Taiwan, China	**Triple** therapy containing both **amoxicillin and tetracycline**	Other regimens where amoxicillin and tetracycline were not contained together	5	840	68.8 % vs. 66.7 %	1.21 (0.64–2.28)	
Nishizawa et al. 2014 Japan [54]	July 2014	HP infection	Japan (5), Korea	**Rebamipide containing regimen:** rebamipide+ +PPI(lanso/ome) + antibiotics (amoxicillin/ metronidazole)	**Rebamipide NOT-containing regimen:** none or mucosal protective agents other than rebamipide (teprenone/plaunotol)+	6	611	63.5 % vs. 52.7 %	1.59 (1.14–2.22)	+

HP H.pylori, *PPI* proton pump inhibitor, *esome* esomeprazole, *lanso* lansoprazole, *ome* omeprazole, *panto* pantoprazole, *rabe* rabeprazole, *PUD* peptic ulcer disease, *NUD* non-ulcer dyspepsia, *MA* meta-analysis, *ITT* intention to treat, *CI* confidence interval, *RCT* randomized controlled trials

[a] Quality assessment: high quality (++): majority of criteria met, little or no risk of bias and results unlikely to be changed by further research. Acceptable (+): most criteria met, some flaws in the study with an associated risk of bias and conclusions may change in the light of further studies. Low quality (0): either most criteria not met or significant flaws relating to key aspects of study design, and conclusions likely to change in the light of further studies

[b] Countries of included RCTs: the number in the bracket represents the number of trials from the same country if more than one trials exist

of the included studies is presented in Additional file 4: Table S2.

Discussion
Summary of findings
This overview of systematic reviews evaluated the effectiveness of pharmacological regimens for the eradication of H.pylori by searching and analysing the existing systematic reviews from 2002 to present. In triple therapy, regarding the use of different PPIs, we found that the results of studies were inconsistent; however more recently published studies tend to suggest new generation PPIs were associated with greater eradication rates than the old generation. The NMA suggested that esomeprazole was the most effective PPI with the highest probability to be the best among the five PPIs after incorporating evidence of both direct and indirect comparisons. Regarding the use of antibiotics, conflicting results exist between the studies to some extent; however this could be due to the varied resistant rate to different antibiotics across regions. This leads to the limited transferability of RCT results across countries and population and thus, there exist issues of fundamental heterogeneity when pooling results together in the meta-analysis. Concerning the comparison between triple therapy and bismuth-based therapy, there was no difference between the two regimens overall, but the antibiotics within the triple therapy may have an impact on the overall effectiveness of the drug regimen. Moxifloxacin or levofloxacin based triple therapy were associated with greater eradication rates, lower risk of adverse events and lower discontinuation rate than bismuth-based therapy for second-line treatment. With regard to the comparison between triple therapies and H_2 receptor antagonist and others, no definite conclusion could be reached due to limited available evidence.

The evidence on the effectiveness of PPI has evolved over time. Contrary to existing guidance, recent studies have shown that the new generation PPIs have achieved statistically significant greater effectiveness rate than the old generations. There is a clear time trend when evaluating the systematic reviews – systematic reviews published before 2006 reported no difference, while 2006 onwards, the statistical significant difference was shown in the pooled results. This can be explained by more recent RCTs and a more complete evidence base included in the recent systematic reviews (Additional file 5: Table S3). When comparing between triple therapy and bismuth-based therapy, the results were mixed. However, there seems to be a trend according to the choice of antibiotics in triple therapy – triple therapy achieved greater eradication rates than bismuth-based therapy when moxifloxacin or levofloxacin was used as a substitute of clarithromycin for second-line treatment.

Although generally the results of comparing triple therapy and bismuth-based therapy failed to show statistical significance, it is possible this is a sample size issue. Our results support the current guidance on the recommendations of moxifloxacin or levofloxacin as the second-line treatment for previous treatment failures of H.pylori. However, its role as a first-line therapy was found to be controversial. Two studies showed the use of levofloxacin or moxifloxacin for treating naïve patients was associated with improved eradication rate [25, 26], while three studies found no difference [35–37]. This was further investigated by two subgroup analyses from two included studies which both suggested that levofloxacin achieved statistically greater eradication rates in European countries where the resistant rates were much lower than the global average [35, 37]. Therefore, the discrepancy of the results could be attributed to the varied resistant rates to different antibiotics across regions or populations. This could also possibly explain that the two meta-analyses which pooled RCTs mostly from China showed the improved effectiveness of levofloxacin as first-line treatment [25, 26] – the resistant rate to clarithromycin could be possibly much higher than that to levofloxacin in the regions where the included RCTs were conducted.

Comparison with current guidelines
Based on current guidelines from the American College of Gastroenterology, Canadian Helicobacter Study Group and National Institute for Health and Care Excellence (NICE), a triple regimen consisting of a PPI, clarithromycin with either metronidazole or amoxicillin is recommended as first-line treatment [13–15]. In addition, both of the American and Canadian guidelines recommend the combination of PPI, bismuth, tetracycline and metronidazole as an alternative for first-line therapy [13, 14]. The alternative of bismuth quadruple therapy is raised due to the increasing clarithromycin resistance rate which has lowered the efficacy of triple therapy to 70–85 %. The American guideline also recommends to consider levofloxacin-based triple therapy when bismuth or clarithromycin-based therapies are not an option in some circumstances [14]. In 2009, the Asia–Pacific H.pylori Consensus Conference agreed that the first-line treatment should consist of either clarithromycin-based triple or bismuth quadruple therapy, and further proposed four options for second-line treatment: (i) standard triple therapy that has not been previously used; (ii) bismuth-based quadruple therapy; (iii) levofloxacin-based triple therapy; and (iv) rifabutin-based triple therapy [55].

The European Helicobacter Study Group published their latest guideline in 2012 – the Maastricht IV report [12] recommending specific H.pylori eradication strategies according to different clarithromycin resistance rates. The threshold for classifying clarithromycin resistance to the high/low area is set as 15 % −20 %. In regions with low clarithromycin resistance rates, clarithromycin-based triple therapy remains the first-line treatment, with the alternative of bismuth quadruple therapy. Where there is higher clarithromycin resistance, the bismuth-based therapy is recommended as the first-line treatment. In both circumstances, levofloxacin is recommended for second-line therapy rather than first-line for the reason of 'rapid acquisition of resistance'.

The World Gastroenterology Organization published their H.pylori guideline for developing countries in 2011, which is consistent with the above guidelines. However, it states that, due to its low cost, furazolidone may be served as an alternative option by developing countries, such as Brazil and China, despite being withdrawn in the US and the European Union due to the severe adverse events [56].

It is worth noting that the type of PPI is not specified in any of the current guidelines, which may be due to the limited availability of reliable evidence from studies when those guidelines were published. However, our review showed that the esomeprazole could achieve greater eradication rate than the older generation of PPIs. Despite the relatively high cost of newer generation of PPI, this difference in effectiveness between the generations of PPIs should be taken into account in the recommendations. Our finding supported the recommendation of bismuth-based therapy as a first-line alternative to standard triple therapy in a high clarithromycin resistant area. For the second-line treatment, our findings are consistent with the current guidelines; both moxifloxacin/levofloxacin containing triple therapy and bismuth-based therapy can achieve higher eradication rates than clarithromycin-containing triple therapy. Moreover, the former appeared to be superior to the latter in terms of eradication rates and adverse events rates.

Limitations

There are a few limitations of this study. As this is an overview of systematic reviews, our results are dependent on what has been reported in the included systematic reviews and on the methodological rigour applied in their development. For instance, similar search strategy across systematic reviews has turned out to include difference RCTs. The low-moderate overall quality of included studies may affect the impact of this overview of systematic reviews on clinical decision making. However, it is difficult to judge whether the low internal validity of the individual systematic reviews resulted from insufficient reporting or certain methodological flaws. In addition, there were some heterogeneity issues in this overview. The systematic reviews have included a mixture of population characteristics, countries of origin and comorbidities, infection epidemiology and antibiotics resistance type and thus the eradication rates varied with those factors. This may not be appropriately considered and addressed in some of the included meta-analysis, leading to the inconsistent results in our findings.

Conclusions

This overview of systematic reviews suggests that the new generation of PPIs and use of moxifloxacin or levofloxacin in triple therapy or bismuth-based therapy as second-line treatment were associated with greater effectiveness, while the comparative effectiveness of antibiotics is complex which probably depends on the resistant rate to different antibiotics in different regions. This should be explored in future research for updating the guidelines. In addition, considering the substantiated difference in the cost of treatment, estimating the cost-effectiveness of these treatments is of value to clinical decision making, especially in the area with high H.pylori prevalence. Given the variation in infection epidemiology and increasing antibiotics resistance, from a clinical perspective, the recommendations should be localized based on the specific prevalence of H.pylori infection and antibiotics resistance rate in the local region and population.

Additional files

Additional file 1: Search strategy.

Additional file 2: WinBUGS code for the network meta-analysis model.

Additional file 3: Table S1. Excluded studies based on full-text review.

Additional file 4: Table S2. Quality assessment of included studies based on revised AMSTAR checklist.

Additional file 5: Table S3. Individual study check table.

Abbreviations
AMSTAR, A measurement tool to assess systematic reviews; CI, Confidence interval; CrI, Credible interval; H.pylori, Helicobacter pylori; H$_2$RA, H$_2$ receptor antagonist; ITT, Intention to treat; NICE, National Institute for Health and Care Excellence; NMA, Network meta-analysis; OR, Odds ratio; PPI, Proton pump inhibitor; RBC, Ranitidine bismuth citrate; RCT, Randomized controlled trial; SIGN, Scottish Intercollegiate Guidelines Network; UK, United Kingdom; US, United States

Acknowledgement
Not applicable.

Funding
No funding source.

Authors' contributions
OW designed the study. JM conducted the electronic database search. JM and YX performed the selection of eligible studies. YX, JM and OW performed data extraction and critical appraisal. YX and LG carried out the network meta-analysis. YX and OW drafted the manuscript with comments

by JM, RH, JB and EW. All authors approved the final version of the article, including the authorship list.

Authors' information
Not applicable.

Competing interests
The authors declare that they have no competing interests.

Consent for publication
Not applicable.

Endnotes
Not applicable.

Author details
[1]Health Economics and Health Technology Assessment (HEHTA), Institute of Health and Wellbeing, University of Glasgow, Glasgow, UK. [2]Knowledge and Information, Healthcare Improvement Scotland, Glasgow, UK. [3]Scottish Intercollegiate Guideline Network (SIGN), NHS Education for Scotland, Royal College of General Practitioners (Scotland), Mill Lane Surgery, Edinburgh, UK. [4]Department of gastroenterology, Royal Infirmary of Edinburgh, NHS Lothian, Edinburgh, UK.

References
1. Everhart JE, Kruszon-Moran D, Perez-Perez GI, Tralka TS, McQuillan G. Seroprevalence and ethnic differences in Helicobacter pylori infection among adults in the United States. J Infect Dis. 2000;181:1359–63.
2. Ford AC, Axon AT. Epidemiology of Helicobacter pylori infection and public health implications. Helicobacter. 2010;15 Suppl 1:1–6.
3. Mandeville KL, Krabshuis J, Ladep NG, Mulder CJ, Quigley EM, Khan SA. Gastroenterology in developing countries: issues and advances. World J Gastroenterol. 2009;15:2839–54.
4. Parsonnet J, Hansen S, Rodriguez L, Gelb AB, Warnke RA, Jellum E, et al. Helicobacter pylori infection and gastric lymphoma. N Engl J Med. 1994;330: 1267–71.
5. Qadri Q, Rasool R, Gulzar GM, Naqash S, Shah ZA. H. pylori Infection, Inflammation and Gastric Cancer. J Gastrointest Cancer. 2014;45:126–32.
6. Panic N, Mastrostefano E, Leoncini E, Persiani R, Arzani D, Amore R, et al. Susceptibility to Helicobacter pylori infection: results of an epidemiological investigation among gastric cancer patients. Mol Biol Rep. 2014;41:3637–50.
7. Hsu WY, Lin CH, Lin CC, Sung FC, Hsu CP, Kao CH. The relationship between Helicobacter pylori and cancer risk. Eur J Intern Med. 2014;25:235–40.
8. Chen YS, Xu SX, Ding YB, Huang XE, Deng B. Helicobacter pylori Infection and the Risk of Colorectal Adenoma and Adenocarcinoma: an Updated Meta-analysis of Different Testing Methods. Asian Pac J Cancer Prev. 2013; 14:7613–9.
9. Peek Jr RM, Fiske C, Wilson KT. Role of innate immunity in Helicobacter pylori-induced gastric malignancy. Physiol Rev. 2010;90:831–58.
10. Gisbert JP, Calvet X, Cosme A, Almela P, Feu F, Bory F, et al. Long-term follow-up of 1,000 patients cured of Helicobacter pylori infection following an episode of peptic ulcer bleeding. Am J Gastroenterol. 2012;107:1197–204.
11. Ford AC, Forman D, Hunt RH, Yuan Y, Moayyedi P. Helicobacter pylori eradication therapy to prevent gastric cancer in healthy asymptomatic infected individuals: systematic review and meta-analysis of randomised controlled trials. BMJ. 2014;348:g3174.
12. Malfertheiner P, Megraud F, O'Morain CA, Atherton J, Axon AT, Bazzoli F, et al. Management of Helicobacter pylori infection–the Maastricht IV/Florence Consensus Report. Gut. 2012;61:646–64.
13. Hunt R, Fallone C, Veldhuyzan van Zanten S, Sherman P, Smaill F, Flook N, et al. Canadian Helicobacter Study Group Consensus Conference: Update on the management of Helicobacter pylori–an evidence-based evaluation of six topics relevant to clinical outcomes in patients evaluated for H pylori infection. Can J Gastroenterol. 2004;18:547–54.
14. Chey WD, Wong BC. American College of Gastroenterology guideline on the management of Helicobacter pylori infection. Am J Gastroenterol. 2007; 102:1808–25.
15. National Institute for Health and Care Excellence. Dyspepsia: Managing Dyspepsia in Adults in Primary Care. CG17. London: National Institute for Health and Care Excellence; 2004. Newcastle upon Tyne UK: Crown 2004.
16. Giorgio F, Principi M, De Francesco V, Zullo A, Losurdo G, Di Leo A, et al. Primary clarithromycin resistance to Helicobacter pylori: Is this the main reason for triple therapy failure? World J Gastrointest Pathophysiol. 2013;4: 43–6.
17. Sasaki M, Ogasawara N, Utsumi K, Kawamura N, Kamiya T, Kataoka H, et al. Changes in 12-Year First-Line Eradication Rate of Helicobacter pylori Based on Triple Therapy with Proton Pump Inhibitor, Amoxicillin and Clarithromycin. J Clin Biochem Nutr. 2010;47:53–8.
18. Scottish Intercollegiate Guidelines Network (SIGN). Dyspepsia. Edinburgh: SIGN; 2003. SIGN publication no.68.
19. Smith V, Devane D, Begley CM, Clarke M. Methodology in conducting a systematic review of systematic reviews of healthcare interventions. BMC Med Res Methodol. 2011;11:15.
20. Scottish Intercollegiate Guidelines Network (SIGN). Critical appraisal: notes and checklists. http://www.sign.ac.uk/methodology/checklists.html. Accessed 02 Feb 2014.
21. Lumley T. Network meta-analysis for indirect treatment comparisons. Stat Med. 2002;21:2313–24.
22. Mills EJ, Thorlund K, Ioannidis JP. Demystifying trial networks and network meta-analysis. BMJ. 2013;346:f2914.
23. Lunn DJ, Thomas A, Best N, Spiegelhalter D. WinBUGS - A Bayesian modelling framework: Concepts, structure, and extensibility. Stat Comput. 2000;10:325–37.
24. Wang Z, Xiong G, Wu S. Comparing the efficacy of esomeprazole and omeprazole combined with antibiotics in Helicobacter pylori eradication: A meta-analysis. Chin J Gastroenterol. 2006;11:598–601.
25. Zhang ZF, Zhao G, Liu LN. Effectiveness and safety of proton pump inhibitor and levofloxacin based first-line triple therapy in the eradication of Helicobacter pylori: a meta-analysis. Zhonghua Yi Xue Za Zhi. 2008;88: 2722–5.
26. Gou QY, Shi RH, Yu RB. Levofloxacin containing triple therapy vs standard triple therapy for eradication of Helicobacter pylori: A Meta-analysis. [Chinese]. Shi Jie Hua Ren Xiao Hua Za Zhi. 2014;22:5207–11.
27. Gisbert JP, Gonzalez L, Calvett X. Systematic review and meta-analysis: Proton pump inhibitor vs. ranitidine bismuth citrate plus two antibiotics in Helicobacter pylori eradication. Helicobacter. 2005;10:157–71.
28. Gisbert JP, De La Morena F. Systematic review and meta-analysis: Levofloxacin-based rescue regimens after Helicobacter pylori treatment failure. Aliment Pharmacol Ther. 2006;23:35–44.
29. Saad RJ, Schoenfeld P, Kim HM, Chey WD. Levofloxacin-based triple therapy versus bismuth-based quadruple therapy for persistent Helicobacter pylori infection: a meta-analysis. Am J Gastroenterol. 2006;101:488–96.
30. Li Y, Huang X, Yao L, Shi R, Zhang G. Advantages of moxifloxacin and levofloxacin-based triple therapy for second-line treatments of persistent Helicobacter pylori infection: a meta analysis. Wien Klin Wochenschr. 2010; 122:413–22.
31. Wu C, Chen X, Liu J, Li M-Y, Zhang Z-Q, Wang Z-Q. Moxifloxacin-containing triple therapy versus bismuth-containing quadruple therapy for second-line treatment of Helicobacter pylori infection: a meta-analysis. Helicobacter. 2011;16:131–8.
32. Di Caro S, Fini L, Daoud Y, Grizzi F, Gasbarrini A, De Lorenzo A, et al. Levofloxacin/amoxicillin-based schemes vs quadruple therapy for helicobacter pylori eradication in second-line. World J Gastroenterol. 2012; 18:5669–78.
33. Dong J, Yu X-F, Zou J. Azithromycin-containing versus standard triple therapy for Helicobacter pylori eradication: a meta-analysis. World J Gastroenterol. 2009;15:6102–10.
34. Yuan W, Yang K, Ma B, Li Y, Guan Q, Wang D, et al. Moxifloxacin-based triple therapy versus clarithromycin-based triple therapy for first-line treatment of Helicobacter pylori infection: a meta-analysis of randomized controlled trials. Intern Med. 2009;48:2069–76.
35. Ye CL, Liao GP, He S, Pan YN, Kang YB, Zhang ZY. Levofloxacin and proton pump inhibitor-based triple therapy versus standard triple first-line therapy for Helicobacter pylori eradication. Pharmacoepidemiol Drug Saf. 2014;23: 443–55.

36. Peedikayil MC, Alsohaibani FI, Alkhenizan AH. Levofloxacin-based first-line therapy versus standard first-line therapy for Helicobacter pylori eradication: meta-analysis of randomized controlled trials. PLoS One. 2014;9:e85620.

37. Xiao SP, Gu M, Zhang GX. Is levofloxacin-based triple therapy an alternative for first-line eradication of Helicobacter pylori? A systematic review and meta-analysis. Scand J Gastroentero. 2014;49:528–38.

38. Gene E, Calvet X, Azagra R, Gisbert JP. Triple vs. quadruple therapy for treating Helicobacter pylori infection: a meta-analysis. Aliment Pharmacol Ther. 2003;17:1137–43.

39. Venerito M, Krieger T, Ecker T, Leandro G, Malfertheiner P. Meta-analysis of bismuth quadruple therapy versus clarithromycin triple therapy for empiric primary treatment of Helicobacter pylori infection. Digestion. 2013;88:33–45.

40. Gisbert JP, Khorrami S, Calvet X, Gabriel R, Carballo F, Pajares JM. Meta-analysis: proton pump inhibitors vs. H2-receptor antagonists–their efficacy with antibiotics in Helicobacter pylori eradication. Aliment Pharmacol Ther. 2003;18:757–66.

41. Ren Q, Ma B, Yang K, Yan X. Lafutidine-based triple therapy for Helicobacter pylori eradication. Hepatogastroenterology. 2010;57:1074–81.

42. McNicholl AG, Linares PM, Nyssen OP, Calvet X, Gisbert JP. Meta-analysis: esomeprazole or rabeprazole vs. first-generation pump inhibitors in the treatment of Helicobacter pylori infection. Aliment Pharmacol Ther. 2012;36:414–25.

43. Gisbert JP, Khorrami S, Calvet X, Pajares JM. Systematic review: Rabeprazole-based therapies in Helicobacter pylori eradication. Aliment Pharmacol Ther. 2003;17:751–64.

44. Gisbert JP, Pajares JM. Esomeprazole-based therapy in Helicobacter pylori eradication: a meta-analysis. Dig Liver Dis. 2004;36:253–9.

45. Gisbert JP, Khorrami S, Calvet X, Pajares JM. Pantoprazole based therapies in Helicobacter pylori eradication: a systematic review and meta-analysis. Eur J Gastroenterol Hepatol. 2004;16:89–99.

46. Wang X, Fang JY, Lu R, Sun DF. A meta-analysis: comparison of esomeprazole and other proton pump inhibitors in eradicating Helicobacter pylori. Digestion. 2006;73:178–86.

47. Zhang G, Zou J, Liu F, Bao Z, Dong F, Huang Y, et al. The efficacy of moxifloxacin-based triple therapy in treatment of Helicobacter pylori infection: a systematic review and meta-analysis of randomized clinical trials. Braz J Med Biol Res. 2013;46:607–13.

48. Gisbert JP, Calvet X. Update on non-bismuth quadruple (concomitant) therapy for eradication of Helicobacter pylori. Clin Exp Gastroenterol. 2012;5:23–34.

49. Lv ZF, Wang FC, Zheng HL, Wang B, Xie Y, Zhou XJ, et al. Meta-analysis: is combination of tetracycline and amoxicillin suitable for Helicobacter pylori infection? World J Gastroenterol. 2015;21:2522–33.

50. Luther J, Higgins PDR, Schoenfeld PS, Moayyedi P, Vakil N, Chey WD. Empiric quadruple vs. triple therapy for primary treatment of Helicobacter pylori infection: Systematic review and meta-analysis of efficacy and tolerability. Am J Gastroenterol. 2010;105:65–73.

51. Vergara M, Vallve M, Gisbert JP, Calvet X. Meta-analysis: comparative efficacy of different proton-pump inhibitors in triple therapy for Helicobacter pylori eradication. Aliment Pharmacol Ther. 2003;18:647–54.

52. Ford AC, Malfertheiner P, Giguere M, Santana J, Khan M, Moayyedi P. Adverse events with bismuth salts for Helicobacter pylori eradication: systematic review and meta-analysis. World J Gastroenterol. 2008;14:7361–70.

53. Graham DY, Hammoud F, El-Zimaity HMT, Kim JG, Osato MS, El-Serag HB. Meta-analysis: proton pump inhibitor or H2-receptor antagonist for Helicobacter pylori eradication. Aliment Pharmacol Ther. 2003;17:1229–36.

54. Nishizawa T, Nishizawa Y, Yahagi N, Kanai T, Takahashi M, Suzuki H. Effect of supplementation with rebamipide for Helicobacter pylori eradication therapy: a systematic review and meta-analysis. J Gastroenterol Hepatol. 2014;29 Suppl 4:20–4.

55. Fock KM, Katelaris P, Sugano K, Ang TL, Hunt R, Talley NJ, et al. Second Asia-Pacific Consensus Guidelines for Helicobacter pylori infection. J Gastroenterol Hepatol. 2009;24:1587–600.

56. Hunt RH, Xiao SD, Megraud F, Leon-Barua R, Bazzoli F, van der Merwe S, et al. Helicobacter pylori in developing countries. World Gastroenterology Organisation Global Guideline. J Gastrointestin Liver Dis. 2011;20:299–304.

10

Malignant transformation of a gastric hyperplastic polyp in a context of *Helicobacter pylori*-negative autoimmune gastritis

Kenichi Yamanaka[1*], Hiroyuki Miyatani[1], Yukio Yoshida[1], Takehiro Ishii[1], Shinichi Asabe[1], Osamu Takada[2], Mitsuhiro Nokubi[3] and Hirosato Mashima[1]

Abstract

Background: Gastric foveolar hyperplastic polyps (GFHPs) are common findings in clinical practice. GFHPs commonly arise in a background of chronic atrophic gastritis, including autoimmune gastritis (type A gastritis), and have a potential risk of malignant transformation.

Case presentation: In 2005, a 55-year-old Japanese woman underwent upper endoscopy at another hospital and was found to have a pedunculated polyp (10 mm in diameter) on the greater curvature of the lower gastric body. On biopsy, the polyp was diagnosed as a GFHP. Nine years later, the polyp had grown to 20 mm in diameter, and the biopsy specimen taken at this time showed tubular adenocarcinoma. On admission to our hospital, the serum *Helicobacter Pylori* (*H. pylori*) immunoglobulin G antibody and stool *H. pylori* antigen were both negative. Anti-gastric parietal cell antibody was positive, as was the anti-intrinsic factor antibody, and the fasting serum gastrin level was markedly increased. In 2014, en bloc resection of the pedunculated polyp was performed by endoscopic submucosal dissection. The final histological diagnosis was adenocarcinoma of the stomach with submucosal and lymphatic invasion. Subsequently, additional radical distal gastrectomy was performed. At the latest follow-up (12 months postoperatively), no recurrence was noted.

Conclusions: We here reported a rare case of malignant transformation of GFHP arising in a context of type A gastritis. To our knowledge, there are no previous reports on malignant transformation of GFHP with submucosal and lymphatic invasion arising in a background of type A gastritis in the English literature. Further, there is currently no effective treatment other than endoscopic or surgical treatment for such cases. Given the potential risk of malignant transformation due to hypergastrinemia, we consider that endoscopic treatment should be considered as a first-line therapy when a malignant growth is suspected.

Keywords: Gastric hyperplastic foveolar polyp, Autoimmune gastritis, *Helicobacter pylori*, Gastric carcinoma, Case report

* Correspondence: yken211@omiya.jichi.ac.jp
[1]Department of Gastroenterology, Jichi Medical University, Saitama Medical Center, Saitama 330-8503, Japan
Full list of author information is available at the end of the article

Background

Gastric foveolar hyperplastic polyps (GFHPs) are common findings in clinical practice. They do not regress or disappear spontaneously and are associated with a risk of malignant transformation in 0.6–4.5 % of cases [1–5]. GFHPs commonly arise in a background of chronic atrophic gastritis, including both type B gastritis, associated with *Helicobacter Pylori* (*H. pylori*) infection, as well as type A gastritis (autoimmune gastritis) [6]. In Japan, type B gastritis accounts for > 76 % of all gastritis cases [7, 8]. A previous study reported that eradication of *H. pylori* led to regression and disappearance of gastric hyperplastic polyps in approximately 70 % of patients [9]. In this context, *H. pylori* eradication therapy is recommended in Japan. However, *H. pylori* eradication therapy is not effective for all cases, particular for GFHPs arising in a background of autoimmune gastritis (type A gastritis). With the increased prevalence and effectiveness of *H. pylori* eradication therapy, the clinical impact of autoimmune gastritis, and thereby also of GFHPs, is rising. There is currently no effective treatment other than endoscopic or surgical treatment for GFHPs arising in a background of *H. pylori*-negative type A gastritis. Therefore, endoscopic treatment is recommended as the first-line therapy when a malignant growth is suspected.

Case presentation

In November 2005, a 55-year-old Japanese woman underwent upper endoscopy at another hospital and was found to have a pedunculated polyp, measuring 10 mm in diameter, on the greater curvature of the lower gastric body (Fig. 1a). On biopsy, it was diagnosed as a GFHP. At the moment of the first diagnosis, there was only an endoscopic report and the endoscopic appearance could be compatible with an atrophic mucosa. In January 2013, upper endoscopy was repeated, which revealed that the polyp had grown to 12 mm in diameter with a slightly rounded head (Fig. 1b). Biopsy was not performed at the time.

In June 2014, the patient underwent positron emission tomography-computed tomography to evaluate the treatment effect on her right breast cancer, for which she had undergone surgery and received chemotherapy and radiation therapy at the age of 53 years. There was an abnormal accumulation in the lower gastric body (Fig. 2). Subsequent upper endoscopy showed that the polyp had grown to 20 mm in diameter, and the surface of the head was slightly reddish and tense (Fig. 1c). The biopsy specimen obtained from the head of the polyp was histologically diagnosed as tubular adenocarcinoma and was determined to be unrelated to the breast cancer. It was suggested that the polyp became malignant during the nine years of follow-up, and the patient was referred to our institution for further evaluation and treatment.

Physical examination

On physical examination, scars from the right breast mastectomy with bilateral axillary lymph node dissection were noted. No other remarkable findings were observed.

Laboratory data (Table 1)

No abnormalities were found in the blood counts or liver and renal function tests. The serum *H. pylori* immunoglobulin G antibody and stool *H. pylori* antigen were both negative. The anti-gastric parietal cell antibody was positive (80-fold increase), as was the anti-intrinsic factor antibody. The fasting serum gastrin level was markedly increased at > 3000 pg/ml (normal range, < 200 pg/ml). The serum pepsinogenI level and pepsinogen I/II ratio were both low (Table 1).

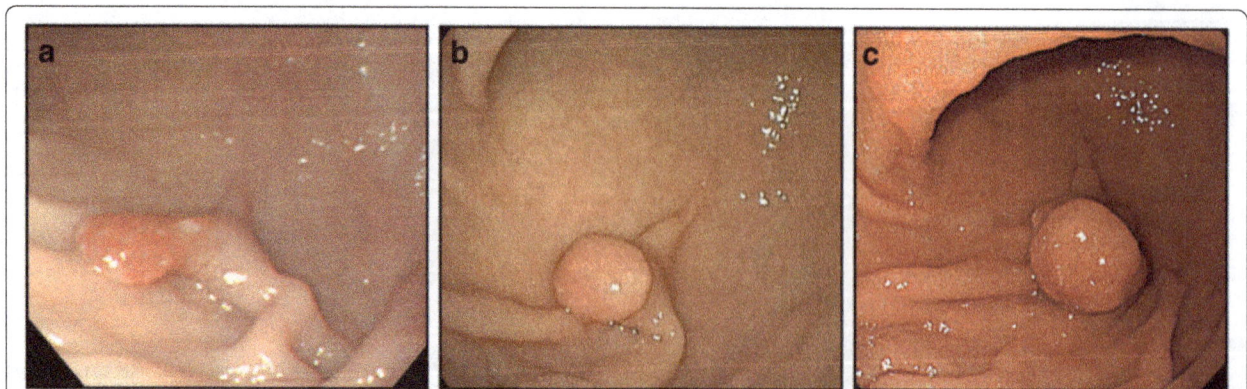

Fig. 1 Endoscopy findings. **a**. In 2005, a pedunculated polyp measuring approximately 10 mm in diameter was observed on the greater curvature of the lower gastric body. The surface of the polyp was slightly reddish. On biopsy, the lesion was diagnosed as a hyperplastic foveolar polyp. **b**. In 2013, the pedunculated polyp on the greater curvature of the lower gastric body had grown to 12 mm in diameter. The head of the polyp was more rounded compared to the image taken in 2005. **c**. In 2014, the pedunculated polyp on the greater curvature of the lower gastric body had grown to 20 mm in diameter. The head of the polyp was slightly reddish, more rounded, and tense

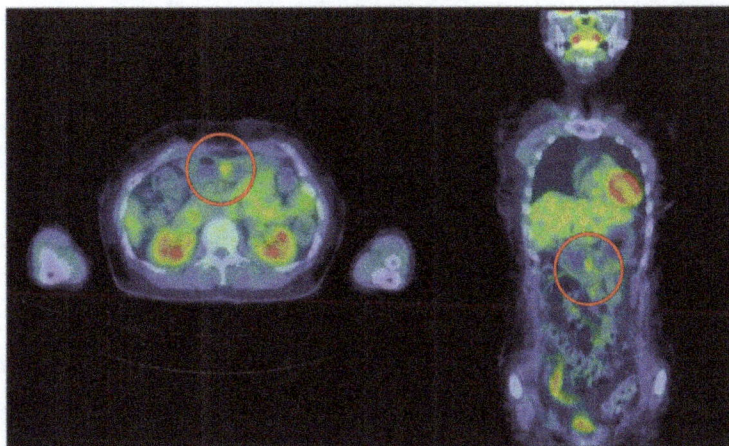

Fig. 2 Positron emission tomography-computed tomography findings. A well-circumscribed mass was observed in the lower gastric body, with a maximum standardized uptake value of 2.7

Medication
The patient was not taking any medication at the time.

Positron emission tomography-computed tomography (July 2014) (Fig. 2)
A well-circumscribed mass with a maximum standardized uptake value of 2.7 was observed in the lower gastric body. There were no findings suggesting the presence of gastrinoma.

Clinical course
In August 2014, en bloc resection of the pedunculated polyp, measuring 20 mm in diameter, on the greater curvature of the lower gastric body was performed by endoscopic submucosal dissection (Fig. 3).

Histopathological examination showed tumor lesions, which had well-defined borders with hyperplastic glands (Fig. 4a, b). The tumor lesions were strongly positive for p53 and Ki-67, while the hyperplastic lesions were not (Fig. 4c). Submucosal invasion was observed in the stalk, with an invasion depth of 300 μm (Fig. 4d). In D2-40-positive and cluster of differentiation 34-negative lymph ducts, cells with acidophilic cytoplasm and large nuclei were observed. The cells were positive for keratin, indicating lymphovascular invasion (Fig. 4e). As a result the final histological diagnosis was adenocarcinoma of the stomach, tubular adenocarcinoma > papillary adenocarcinoma, size of resected lesion 20 mm in size, submucosal invasion of 0.3 mm, venous invasion (-), lymphatic invasion (+).

Table 1 Laboratory data

Hematological analysis	Value	Unit	Blood chemistry	Value	Unit
White blood cell count	4800	/μl	TP	7.3	g/dl
Hemoglobin	11.9	g/dl	Alb	4.4	g/dl
Hematocrit	37.8	%	T-bil	0.81	mg/dl
Platelets	19.5×10^4	/μl	D-bil	0.24	mg/dl
			AST	34	U/L
Tumor markers			ALT	25	U/L
Carcinoembryonic antigen	1.3	ng/ml	LDH	197	U/L
Cancer antigen-15-3	17.1	U/ml	γ-GTP	16	IU/l
			BUN	11	mg/dl
Anti-parietal cell antibody	80	fold	Cre	0.55	mg/dl
Anti-intrinsic factor antibody	+		Gastrin	>3000	pg/dl
Pepsinogen I	7.6	ng/ml	Vit B12	208	pg/ml
Pepsinogen II	16.3	ng/ml			
Pepsinogen I/II/ ratio	<0.5	ng/ml			

Abbreviations: *TP* total protein, *Alb* albumin, *T-bil* total bilirubin, *d-bil* direct bilirubin, *AST* aspartate aminotransferase, *ALT* alanine aminotransferase, *LDH* lactate dehydrogenase, *γ-GTP* gamma-glutamyl transpeptidase, *BUN* blood urea nitrogen, *Cre* creatinine, *Vit* vitamin

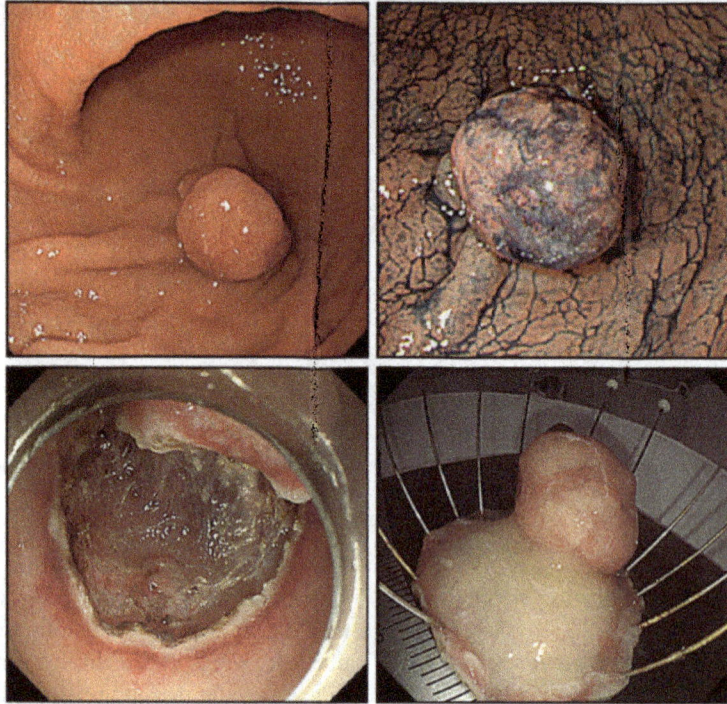

Fig. 3 Endoscopic submucosal dissection. En bloc endoscopic submucosal dissection was performed for the pedunculated polyp, measuring 20 mm in diameter, on the greater curvature of the lower gastric body

Consequently, additional radical distal gastrectomy was performed. Examination of the surgical specimens showed a scar resulting from the endoscopic submucosal dissection on the anterior wall of the gastric body. There were no residual tumor cells or lymph node metastasis. Examination of the background mucosa showed that the proper gastric glands in the pyloric region were preserved, while those in the mucosa of the gastric body were atrophic and showed intestinal metaplasia and pseudo-pyloric metaplasia (Fig. 5). In the OLGA staging system, the corpus and the antrum were scored as 2 and 0, respectively, indicating stageII gastritis at the time of surgery [10, 11]. Chromogranin A staining revealed enterochromaffin-like cell hyperplasia (linear hyperplasia and micronodular hyperplasia) (Fig. 5b, arrows indicate micronodular hyperplasia). *H. pylori* infection was negative (Fig. 5).

Conclusions

The classification of chronic gastritis into types A and B was proposed by Strickland et al. [12]. However, currently, there are no established diagnostic criteria for the diagnosis of type A gastritis. Traditionally, type A gastritis has been diagnosed based on the anti-gastric parietal and anti-intrinsic factor antibody findings, presence of corpus-predominant atrophic gastritis, and serum gastrin levels, with Ban et al. stating that asymptomatic type A gastritis could be diagnosed by anti-gastric parietal

antibody [13]. The prevalence of autoimmune gastritis is unclear [13, 14]. In the early stage, the diagnosis of type A gastritis is difficult even with a biopsy, since the symptoms of anemia due to malabsorption of vitamin B12 and iron usually develop at a later stage. In the present case, we considered that the patient was not infected with *H. pylori*, because her serum *H. pylori* immunoglobulin G antibody, stool *H. pylori* antigen, and histological examination were all negative. On the other hand, the patient was positive for anti-gastric parietal cell and anti-intrinsic factor antibodies, and had a markedly elevated level of serum gastrin and reduced pepsinogenI level and pepsinogenI/II ratio. Moreover, the patient had corpus-predominant atrophic gastritis, OLGA stageII, and enterochromaffin-like cell hyperplasia. Taken together, these findings led to the diagnosis of type A chronic atrophic gastritis. Although we did not have the sufficient histological data from the first endoscopy performed in 2005, mild corpus atrophy was detected at that time. Rugge et al. reported that in 116 patients with autoimmune gastritis, 87 cases (75.0 %) remained and 25 cases (21.6 %) progressed to a higher OLGA gastritis stage during a mean follow-up period of 54 months (range, 24–108 months) [11]. Considering the gastritis stage in 2014, the present case can thus be speculated to have been at stageI orII in 2005. Type A gastritis is characterized by the presence of hypergastrinemia associated with reduced gastric acid secretion. Gastrin is a peptide hormone synthesized and released mainly from G

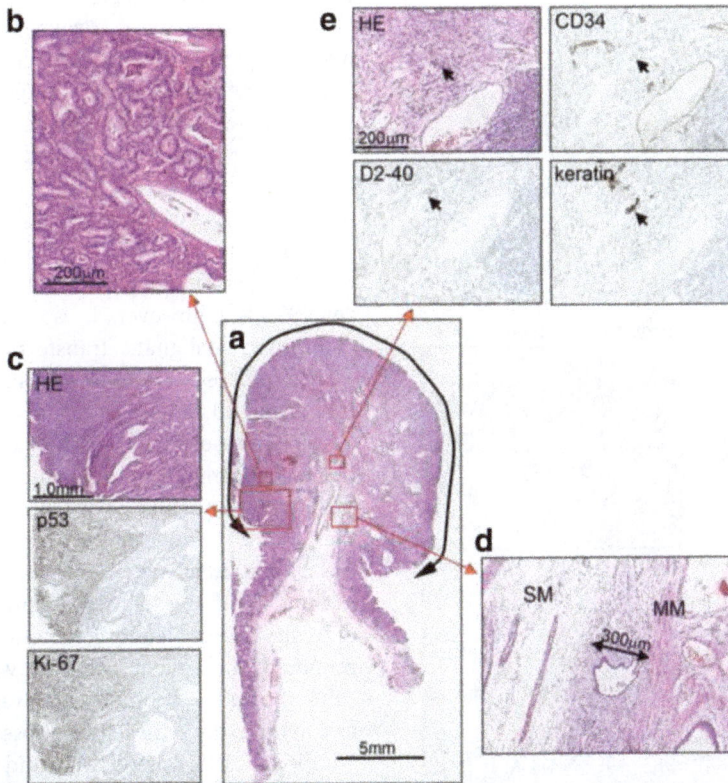

Fig. 4 Histological findings. **a.** Hematoxylin and eosin (HE) staining. **b.** High magnification image of the boxed area. **c.** HE, p53, and Ki-67 stainings of the border between the hyperplastic glands and the tumor glands. The tumor lesions were strongly positive for p53 and Ki-67. **d.** Submucosal invasion in the stalk, with an invasion depth of 300 μm (MM, muscularis mucosae; SM, submucosal layer). **e.** HE, cluster of differentiation 34 (CD34), D2-40, and keratin staining. In CD34-negative and D2-40-positive lymph ducts, keratin-positive cells with acidophilic cytoplasm and large nuclei were observed, indicating lymphatic invasion (*arrows*)

cells in the gastric antrum, which plays a role in the regulation of gastric acid secretion and gastrointestinal motility [15]. Furthermore, it is known to exert trophic actions on digestive cells [16, 17]. In the present patient, it was suggested that the GFHP had grown during the nine-year follow-up period, owing to her hypergastrinemia; her serum gastrin level was > 3000 pg/ml before undergoing distal gastrectomy, but decreased to 74 pg/ml 48 h after the surgery.

The process of cancer development is considered to be a multistage process (hyperplasia → dysplasia → carcinoma); that is, as the polyp grows and becomes more dysplastic, the risk of cancer increases [2, 5, 18, 19]. The most important risk factors of malignant transformation in chronic atrophic gastritis include age over 50 years, severe atrophy, and the presence of intestinal metaplasia extension [20]. The present patient fit the first and third risk factors. Rugge et al. reported that the risk of cancer was restricted to case of high-risk gastritis stage (OLGA stages III-IV) and that it was associated mainly with concomitant *H. pylori* infection [11]. However, malignant transformation in type A gastritis associated with hypergastrinemia might be induced at an earlier gastritis

stage. Several genetic alterations have been revealed in hyperplastic polyps, including abnormal expression of tumor suppressor p53, K-ras mutations, and microsatellite instability [18, 21]. Shibahara et al. conducted a study of gastric hyperplastic polyps and reported that increased expression of p53 was observed in dysplastic and carcinoma cells but not in the normal or hyperplastic cells, and that the expression of Ki67 was higher in the carcinoma and dysplastic cells than in the hyperplastic cells. They suggested that examinations of p53 and Ki67 were useful markers of malignant transformation of gastric hyperplastic polyps [22]. Yao et al. and Zea-Iriarte et al. also suggested that p53 plays an important role in the malignant transformation of gastric hyperplastic polyps [19, 23]. In the present case, the expression of p53 was strongly positive in the carcinoma cells and Ki67 was positive in approximately 50 % of the carcinoma cells, while these stainings were much decreased in the non-transformed cells (Fig. 4b).

The reported incidence of malignant transformation of GFHP ranges from 0.6 to 4.5 % [1–5], and Fujino et al. reported that the mean diameter of GFHPs with malignant transformation was as large as 23.4 ± 10.2 mm [24].

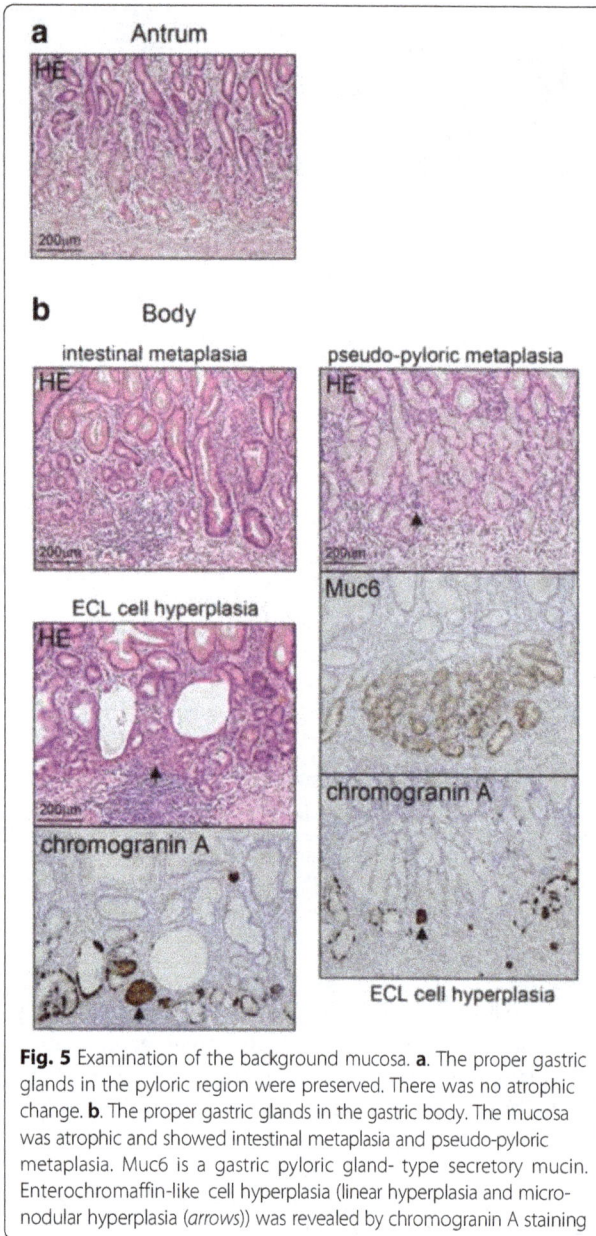

Fig. 5 Examination of the background mucosa. **a**. The proper gastric glands in the pyloric region were preserved. There was no atrophic change. **b**. The proper gastric glands in the gastric body. The mucosa was atrophic and showed intestinal metaplasia and pseudo-pyloric metaplasia. Muc6 is a gastric pyloric gland- type secretory mucin. Enterochromaffin-like cell hyperplasia (linear hyperplasia and micro-nodular hyperplasia (arrows)) was revealed by chromogranin A staining

Regarding the histological type, most previously reported cases were differentiated adenocarcinomas, while a few were poorly-differentiated adenocarcinomas or signet ring cell carcinomas [25–28]. The GFHP in the present patient was 20 mm in diameter and histologically diagnosed as differentiated adenocarcinoma (Fig. 4).

The diagnostic criteria of malignant GFHP proposed by Nakamura et al. in 1985 are as follows [29]: 1) coexistence of benign and malignant parts in the same polyp; 2) existence of sufficient evidence that the benign area has previously been a benign polyp; and 3) existence of sufficient cellular and structural atypia in the malignant area to be diagnosed as cancer. The patient in the present study met these criteria and was therefore diagnosed with malignant

transformation of GFHP over nine years. GFHPs with carcinoma have been reported to have the following macroscopic characteristics: pedunculated form, larger size (>20 mm), reddish color, irregular or nodular surface, white-coated, and bleeding tendency [2, 23, 25, 30, 31]. Our patient displayed four of these macroscopic features, including pedunculated form, a diameter > 20 mm, growth tendency, and a white-coated lesion.

It has been reported that magnifying endoscopy with narrow band imaging is useful for the diagnosis of cancer [32–34]; however, it is not sufficiently useful for diagnosing malignant transformation of gastric hyperplastic polyps [23]. Ahn et al. reported that GFHPs measuring 10 mm or larger in diameter should be endoscopically resected [35], whereas Tanabe et al. reported the disappearance of a 20 mm hyperplastic polyp with malignant transformation after *H. pylori* eradication therapy [36]. The lesion in the present patient was diagnosed as tubular adenocarcinoma on biopsy. Endoscopic estimation of the invasion depth of the carcinoma was difficult; hence, endoscopic submucosal dissection, a minimally invasive procedure, was performed. The results showed a submucosal invasion depth of 0.3 mm and lymph duct invasion. Subsequently, we performed additional distal gastrectomy and lymph node dissection. There was no distant metastasis, and we considered that complete removal of the tumor was achieved. At the time of this report, the patient has been followed-up for 12 months after surgery with no recurrence.

To our knowledge, there are only a few previous cases, limited to Japan, of malignant GFHP with submucosal invasion requiring surgical treatment [37, 38], and there are no previous reports on malignant transformation of GFHP with submucosal invasion and lymphatic invasion arising in a background of type A gastritis in the English literature. Thus, the present case is considered very rare and to provide valuable information. Importantly, there is currently no effective treatment other than endoscopic or surgical treatment for GFHPs, secondary to type A gastritis. Moreover, as this type of polyp has a potential risk of malignant transformation due to hypergastrinemia, endoscopic or surgical treatment should be considered when malignant transformation is suspected.

Abbreviation
GFHP: Gastric foveolar hyperplastic polyp

Acknowledgements
None.

Funding
None.

Authors' contributions

YK, MH, YY, IT, TO, NM, and MH performed the research; YK designed the research, analyzed the data, and wrote the paper; AS revised the manuscript critically. All authors read and approved the final manuscript.

Competing interests

The authors declare that they have no competing interests.

Consent for publication

Written consent was obtained from the patient.

Author details

[1]Department of Gastroenterology, Jichi Medical University, Saitama Medical Center, Saitama 330-8503, Japan. [2]Department of Surgery, Jichi Medical University, Saitama Medical Center, Saitama 330-8503, Japan. [3]Department of Pathology, Jichi Medical University, Saitama Medical Center, Saitama 330-8503, Japan.

References

1. Abraham SC, Singh VK, Yardley JH, Wu TT. Hyperplastic polyps of the stomach: associations with histologic patterns of gastritis and gastric atrophy. Am J Surg Pathol. 2001;25:500–7.
2. Daibo M, Itabashi M, Hirota T. Malignant transformation of gastric hyperplastic polyps. Am J Gastroenterol. 1987;82:1016–25.
3. Orlowska J, Jarosz D, Pachlewski J, Butruk E. Malignant transformation of benign epithelial gastric polyps. Am J Gastroenterol. 1995;90:2152–9.
4. Hattori T. Morphological range of hyperplastic polyps and carcinomas arising in hyperplastic polyps of the stomach. J Clin Pathol. 1985;38:622–30.
5. Terada T. Malignant transformation of foveolar hyperplastic polyp of the stomach: a histopathological study. Med Oncol. 2011;28:941–4.
6. Coati I, Fassan M, Farinati F, Graham DY, Genta RM, Rugge M. Autoimmune gastritis: pathologist's viewpoint. World J Gastroenterol. 2015;21:12179–89.
7. Ljubicić N, Banić M, Kujundzić M, Antić Z, Vrkljan M, Kovacević I, et al. The effect of eradicating Helicobacter pylori infection on the course of adenomatous and hyperplastic gastric polyps. Eur J Gastroenterol Hepatol. 1999;11:727–30.
8. Bonilla Palacios JJ, Miyazaki Y, Kanayuma S, Yasunaga Y, Matsuzawa Y. Serum gastrin, pepsinogens, parietal cell and Helicobacter pylori antibodies in patients with gastric polyps. Acta Gastroenterol Latinoam. 1994;24:77–82.
9. Okusa T, Takashimizu I, Fujiki K, Suzuki S, Shimoi K, Horiuchi T, et al. Disappearance of hyperplastic polyps in the stomach after eradication of Helicobacter pylori. A randomised, clinical trial. Ann Intern Med. 1998;129:712–5.
10. Rugge M, Correa P, Di Mario F, El-Omar E, Fiocca R, Geoboes K, et al. OLGA staging for gastritis: a tutorial. Dig Liver Dis. 2008;40:650–8.
11. Rugge M, Fassan M, Pizzi M, Zorzetto V, Maddalo G, Realdon S, et al. Autoimmune gastritis: histology phenotype and OLGA staging. Aliment Pharmacol Ther. 2012;35:1460–6.
12. Strickland RG, Mackay IR. A reappraisal of nature and significance of chronic atrophic gastritis. Am J Dig Dis. 1973;18:426–40.
13. Toh BH. Diagnosis and classification of autoimmune gastritis. Autoimmun Rev. 2014;13:459–62.
14. Toh BH, Chan J, Kyaw T, Alderuccio F. Cutting edge issues in autoimmune gastritis. Clin Rev Allergy Immunol. 2012;42:269–78.
15. Dockray GJ, Varro A, Dimaline R, Wang T. The gastrins: their production and biological activities. Annu Rev Physiol. 2001;63:119–39.
16. Smith AM, Watson SA. Review article: gastrin and colorectal cancer. Aliment Pharmacol Ther. 2000;14:1231–47.
17. Rozengurt E, Walsh JH. Gastrin, CCK, signaling, and cancer. Annu Rev Physiol. 2001;63:49–76.
18. Dijkhuizen SM, Entius MM, Clement MJ, Polak MM, Van den Berg FM, Craanen ME, et al. Multiple hyperplastic polyps in the stomach: evidence for clonality and neoplastic potential. Gastroenterology. 1997;112:561–6.
19. Yao T, Kajiwara M, Kuroiwa S, Iwashita A, Oya M, Kabashima A, et al. Malignant transformation of gastric hyperplastic polyps: alteration of phenotypes, proliferative activity, and p53 expression. Hum Pathol. 2002;33:1016–22.

20. Vannella L, Lahner E, Annibale B. Risk of gastric neoplasias in patients with chronic atrophic gastritis: a critical reappraisal. World J Gastroenterol. 2012;18:1279–85.
21. Nogueria AM, Carneiro F, Seruca R, Cirnes L, Veiga I, Machado JC, et al. Microsatellite instability in hyperplastic and adenomatous polyps of the stomach. Cancer. 1999;86:1649–56.
22. Shibahara K, Haraguchi Y, Sasaki I, Kiyonari H, Oishi T, Iwashita A, et al. A case of gastric hyperplastic polyp with malignant transformation. Hepatogastroenterology. 2005;52:319–21.
23. Zea-Iriarte WL, Sekine I, Itsuno M, Makiyama K, Naito S, Nakayama T, et al. Carcinoma in gastric hyperplastic polyps. A phenotypic study. Dig Dis Sci. 1996;41:377–86.
24. Fujino M, Yamamoto Y, Morozumi A, Kawai T. Malignant transformation of gastric polyps. Nihon Rinsho. 1991;49:155–9 [article in Japanese].
25. Zea-Iriarte WL, Itsuno M, Makiyama K, Hara K, Haraguchi M, Ajioka Y. Signet ring cell carcinoma in hyperplastic polyp. Scand J Gastroenterol. 1995;30:604–8.
26. Fry LC, Lazenby AL, Lee DH, Mönkemüller K. Signet-ring-cell adenocarcinoma arising from a hyperplastic polyp. Gastrointest Endosc. 2005;61:493–5.
27. Gotoh Y, Fujimoto K, Sakata Y, Fujisaki J, Nakano S. Poorly differentiated adenocarcinoma in a gastric hyperplastic polyp. South Med J. 1996;89:453–4.
28. Hirasaki S, Suzuki S, Kanzaki H, Fujita K, Matsumura S, Matsumoto E. Minute signet ring cell carcinoma occurring in gastric hyperplastic polyp. World J Gastroenterol. 2007;13:5779–80.
29. Nakamura T, Nakano G. Histological classification and malignant change in gastric polyps. J Clin Pathol. 1985;38:754–64.
30. Mitsufuji S, Tsuchihashi Y, Isetani K, Tokita K, Maruyama K, Hosokawa Y, et al. A ten-year observation of malignant changes in a hyperplastic polyp of the stomach–a cellular kinetic study using bromodeoxyuridine (BrdU). Gan No Rinsho. 1990;36:1035–41 [article in Japanese].
31. Yamaguchi K, Shiraishi G, Maeda S, Kitamura K. Adenocarcinoma in hyperplastic polyp of the stomach. Am J Gastroenterol. 1990;85:327–8.
32. Hirano H, Yoshida T, Yoshimura H, Fukuoka M, Ohkubo E, Tachibana S, et al. Poorly differentiated adenocarcinoma with signet-ring cell carcinoma in a hyperplastic polyp of the stomach: report of a case. Surg Today. 2007;37:901–4.
33. Yao K, Oishi T, Matsui T, Yao T, Iwashita A. Novel magnified endoscopic findings of microvascular architecture in intramucosal gastric cancer. Gastrointest Endosc. 2002;56:279–84.
34. Yao K, Takaki Y, Matsui T, Iwashita A, Anagnostopoulos GK, Kaye P, et al. Clinical application of magnification endoscopy and narrow-band imaging in the upper gastrointestinal tract: new imaging techniques for detecting and characterizing gastrointestinal neoplasia. Gastrointest Endosc Clin N Am. 2008;18:415–33.
35. Ahn JY, da Son H, Choi KD, Roh J, Lim H, Choi KS, et al. Neoplasms arising in large gastric hyperplastic polyps: endoscopic and pathologic features. Gastrointest Endosc. 2014;80:1005–13.
36. Tanabe H, Hara H, Ohkubo C, Miyokawa N, Sano H. Disappearance of gastric adenocarcinoma in hyperplastic polyp after eradication of Helicobacter pylori. Nihon Shokakibyo Gakkai Zasshi. 2005;102:559–63 [article in Japanese].
37. Nimura H, Kashiwagi H, Mitsumori N, Arai Y, Yonezawa J, Kaise M, et al. The easy endoscopic polypectomy of gastric hyperplastic polyp should not be carried out. Shokaki Geka. 2007;30:569–79 [article in Japanese].
38. Yamashita S, Kaise M. Malignant transformation in a case of gastric hyperplastic polyp. Shokaki Naishikyo. 2015;27:101–5 [article in Japanese].

11

Triple therapy versus sequential therapy for the first-line *Helicobacter pylori* eradication

Ji Young Chang, Ki-Nam Shim*, Chung Hyun Tae, Ko Eun Lee, Jihyun Lee, Kang Hoon Lee, Chang Mo Moon, Seong-Eun Kim, Hye-Kyung Jung and Sung-Ae Jung

Abstract

Background: The eradication rate of *Helicobacter pylori* (*H. pylori*) with triple therapy which was considered as standard first-line treatment has decreased to 70–85%. The aim of this study is to compare 7-day triple therapy versus 10-day sequential therapy as the first line treatment.

Methods: Data of 1240 *H. pylori* positive patients treated with triple therapy or sequential therapy from January 2013 to December 2015 were analyzed retrospectively. The patients who had undertaken previous *H. pylori* eradication therapy or gastric surgery were excluded.

Results: There were 872 (74.3%) patients in the triple therapy group, and 302 (25.7%) patients in the sequential therapy group. There was no significant difference between the two groups regarding age, residence, comorbidities or drug compliance, but several differences were noted in endoscopic characteristics and indication for the treatment. The eradication rate of *H. pylori* by intention to treat analysis was 64.3% in the triple therapy group, and 81.9% in the sequential therapy group ($P = 0.001$). In per protocol analysis, *H. pylori* eradication rate in the triple therapy and sequential therapy group was 81.9 and 90.3, respectively ($P = 0.002$). There was no significant difference in overall adverse events between the two groups ($P = 0.706$). For the rescue therapy, bismuth-containing quadruple therapy showed comparable treatment efficacy after sequential therapy, as following triple therapy.

Conclusions: The eradication rate of triple therapy was below the recommended threshold. Sequential therapy could be effective and tolerable candidate for the first-line *H. pylori* eradication therapy.

Keywords: *Helicobacter pylori*, Anti-bacterial agents, First-line triple therapy, Sequential therapy

Background

The prevalence of *Helicobacter pylori* (*H. pylori*) infection has decreased over the past decade, changed from 66.9 to 54.4% between 1998 and 2011, but its prevalence is still high in Korea [1]. *H. pylori* infection is a known risk factor of upper gastrointestinal diseases, such as chronic gastritis, peptic ulcer disease, mucosa-associated lymphoid tissue (MALT) lymphoma, and gastric cancer [2, 3]. Eradication of *H. pylori* reduces the recurrence rate of peptic ulcer disease or recurrent gastric cancer after endoscopic resection of early gastric cancer, and it also induces the remission of MALT lymphoma [4–6]. Therefore, *H. pylori* eradication has critical role in

promoting national health in Korea, where 95% of confirmed *H. pylori* strains have highly virulent East Asian-type cytotoxin-associated gene A which is potent in causing gastric cancer [7, 8].

Triple therapy (TT) consists of proton-pump inhibitor (PPI), clarithromycin, and amoxicillin has been considered as standard first-line treatment for *H. pylori* in Korea since 1998 [9]. Recently updated Korean guideline also recommended TT as the first-line regimen [10]. However, the efficacy of TT has decreased progressively. The recent nationwide survey reported the decreasing trend of eradication rate of TT which was 84.9–87.5% from 2001 to 2007, but 80.0–81.4% from 2008 to 2010 ($P < 0.0001$) [11]. The most important factor of reduced efficacy of TT is increasing antibiotic resistance of *H. pylori*, especially to clarithromycin [12]. The primary resistance rate to clarithromycin increased from

* Correspondence: shimkn@ewha.ac.kr
Department of Internal Medicine, Ewha Womans University School of Medicine, Ewha Medical Research Institute, 1071 Anyangcheon-ro, Yangcheon-gu, Seoul 158-710, South Korea

23.7 to 71.2%, whereas amoxicillin increased from 6.3 to 14.9% during the period of 2003–2012 [13].

Therefore, several protocols have been suggested in order to overcome treatment failure of TT, including the extending of treatment duration, the use of four-drug regimen such as sequential therapy (SET), concomitant therapy, hybrid therapy, and the prescription of novel antibiotics such as levofloxacin [14]. Reasonable treatment regimens need to attain *H. pylori* eradication rate of higher than 80.0% by intention to treat (ITT) analysis, and higher than 90.0% by per protocol (PP) analysis [15, 16]. Several previous meta-analyses reported the superiority of SET than TT [17, 18], whereas other studies revealed conflicting results [19, 20].

In Ewha Womans University Medical Center, SET has been tried as an alternative first-line treatment *for H. pylori* since 2013. So, we aimed to compare 7-day TT with 10-day SET as the first line treatment in our medical center. We also evaluated the adverse events of the two regimens, clinical factors associated with successful eradication, and effectiveness of the second line treatment after these two treatments.

Methods

Study subjects

From January 2013 to December 2015, 1240 patients who were older than 18-year old, diagnosed with *H. pylori* infection and treated with TT or SET at Ewha Womans University Hospital were enrolled retrospectively. *H. pylori* infection was confirmed by histology, rapid urease test (HP Kit™, Jongkeundang, Korea), C-urea breath test or serum *H. pylori* anti-body test. At least 4 weeks after treatment, *H. pylori* eradication was demonstrated by any of these tests. The patients who had undertaken previous *H. pylori* eradication therapy or gastric surgery were excluded.

We evaluated demographic information, residence area, current status of smoking and alcohol consumption, comorbidities, endoscopic diagnosis, indication for *H. pylori* eradication, drug compliance, and treatment-related adverse events through medical records review. Endoscopic findings and the results of endoscopic biopsies were also reviewed retrospectively. For detailed analysis, drug compliance was divided into two categories; good or poor compliance. Good compliance was defined if the patient took more than 80% of the prescribed medicine, and who took less than 80% of prescribed medicine was belonged to poor compliance group. For the PP analysis, patients who were poorly compliant or lost to follow-up were excluded.

Standard TT for seven days consists of twice a day amoxicillin (1000 mg), clarithromycin (500 mg), and standard dose of PPI. SET for 10 days consists of twice a day amoxicillin (1000 mg), standard dose of PPI for 5 days, followed by twice a day clarithromycin (500 mg), metronidazole (500 mg), and standard dose of PPI for another 5 days.

This study was approved by the Institutional Review Board of our medical center (IRB number; 2016-04-051-002).

Statistical analyses

All statistical analyses were performed with using SPSS program, version 22.0. Continuous variables were reported as the mean with the standard deviation. To analyze the baseline clinical characteristics, adverse events and eradication rates between the two groups, Student t-test or the Mann-Whitney U test was used for continuous variables, and the chi-square or the Fisher's exact test was used for categorical variables. *H. pylori* eradication rates were demonstrated by ITT and PP analyses. Univariate and multivariate logistic regression were performed for evaluating independent associated factors with successful *H. pylori* eradication. The P value of < 0.05 was considered as statistical significance.

Results

Baseline characteristics

A total of 1240 patients received *H. pylori* eradication therapy from January 2013 to December 2015. After excluding 66 patients who had previous *H. pylori* eradication or gastric surgery, 1174 patients were included finally. There were 872 patients in the TT group and 302 patients in the SET group. A detailed flowchart of the enrolled patients is shown in Fig. 1. The baseline characteristics of the study population are summarized in Table 1. There was no significant difference between the two groups regarding age, residence, comorbidities or drug compliance. But, more males and more patients who were diagnosed with *H. pylori* infection by histology were included in the SET group than the TT group. Several differences were found in the endoscopic

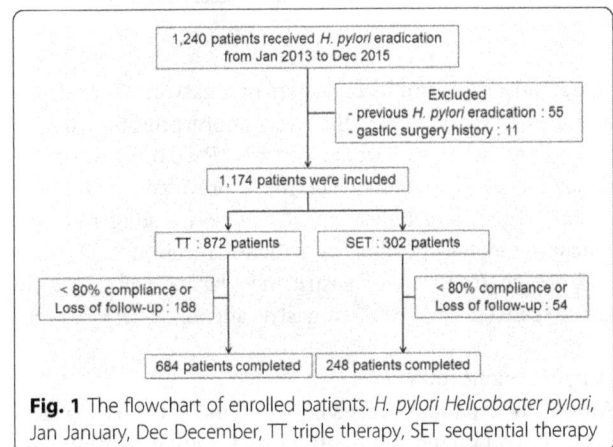

Fig. 1 The flowchart of enrolled patients. *H. pylori* Helicobacter pylori, Jan January, Dec December, TT triple therapy, SET sequential therapy

Table 1 Baseline clinical characteristics

	TT	SET	P value
	N = 872 (74.3%)	N = 302 (25.7%)	
Age (mean ± SD)	52.26 ± 13.52	51.83 ± 12.17	0.607
Male	477 (54.7)	192 (63.6)	0.007
Residence			0.510
Seoul	695 (79.7)	246 (81.5)	
Another area	177 (20.3)	56 (18.5)	
Smoking	217 (24.9)	113 (37.4)	<0.001
Alcohol	389 (41.3)	91 (39.2)	<0.001
Diabetes mellitus	98 (11.2)	33 (10.9)	0.882
Hypertension	185 (21.2)	71 (23.5)	0.405
Chronic kidney disease	12 (1.4)	4 (1.3)	0.999
Chronic liver disease	24 (2.8)	7 (2.3)	0.685
Ischemic heart disease	23 (2.6)	12 (4.0)	0.239
Compliance > 80%	707 (81.1)	256 (84.8)	0.150
H. pylori test			<0.001
Histology	293 (33.6)	182 (60.3)	
Rapid urease test	586 (64.9)	116 (38.4)	
Urea breath test	8 (0.9)	2 (0.7)	
Serology	5 (0.6)	2 (0.7)	
Endoscopic diagnosis			
Chronic gastritis	201 (23.1)	31 (10.3)	<0.001
Atrophy or metaplasia	332 (38.1)	141 (46.7)	0.009
Gastric ulcer	274 (31.4)	119 (39.4)	0.011
Duodenal ulcer	331 (38.0)	89 (29.5)	0.008
Duodenitis	52 (6.0)	18 (6.0)	0.998
Indication of H. pylori eradication			
Peptic ulcer disease	522 (59.9)	148 (49.0)	0.001
Endoscopic resection of EGC	21 (2.4)	24 (7.9)	<0.001
Endoscopic resection of adenoma	36 (4.1)	24 (7.9)	0.009
MALT lymphoma	4 (0.5)	2 (0.7)	0.651
H. pylori gastritis	83 (9.5)	23 (7.6)	0.320
Atrophy or metaplasia	130 (14.9)	61 (20.2)	0.032

TT triple therapy, SET sequential therapy, SD standard deviation, H. pylori Helicobacter pylori, EGC early gastric cancer, MALT mucosa associated lymphoid tissue

characteristics - atrophy or metaplastic gastritis ($P = 0.009$), and gastric ulcers ($P = 0.011$) were more prevalent in the SET group, whereas chronic gastritis ($P < 0.001$) and duodenal ulcers ($P = 0.008$) were more prevalent in the TT group. In terms of indication of *H. pylori* eradication, significantly higher portion of patients received SET after endoscopic resection of gastric neoplasms such as early gastric cancers ($P < 0.001$) or gastric adenomas ($P = 0.009$).

H. pylori eradication rates
Among 872 patients receiving first-line TT, 684 (78.4%) patients completed the treatment with good compliance.

In the SET group, 248 (82.1%) patients completed the treatment with good compliance in total of 302 patients. The eradication rate of SET was significantly higher than TT by both ITT ($P = 0.001$) and PP ($P = 0.002$) analyses. The TT showed the eradication rate of 64.3 and 81.9% by ITT and PP analyses, respectively. The overall eradication rate of SET was 81.9 in ITT, and 90.3% in PP analysis (Fig. 2).

Clinical factors related to the *H. pylori* eradication
Possible clinical factors related to successful *H. pylori* eradication were also analyzed. But, there were no statistically significant factors to predict successful eradication in both univariate and multivariate analyses (Table 2).

Comparison of treatment-related adverse events
During the treatment, 33 (3.8%) patients in the TT group, and 10 (3.3%) patients in the SET group had treatment-related adverse events. The most common adverse event was diarrhea (1.3% versus (vs.) 1.7%; TT vs. SET), followed by nausea or vomiting in both groups. But, there was no significant difference in the rate of specific adverse event as well as overall adverse events between the two groups (Table 3).

Second-line eradication therapy after first-line eradication failure
A detailed flow-chart of second-line eradication therapy after failure of first-line eradication therapy is shown in Fig. 3. Among 124 (18.1%) patients who failed in first-line TT, 109 patients received second-line eradication therapy; 28.4% for bismuth-containing quadruple therapy (BCQT) for 7 days (BCQT-7), 68.8% for BCQT for 14 days (BCQT-14), and 2.8% of patients for TT for 7 days. Data from the patients who received second-line TT could not be included for further analyses because of poor compliance or loss of follow-up. The eradication rate in patients who received BCQT-7 after failing

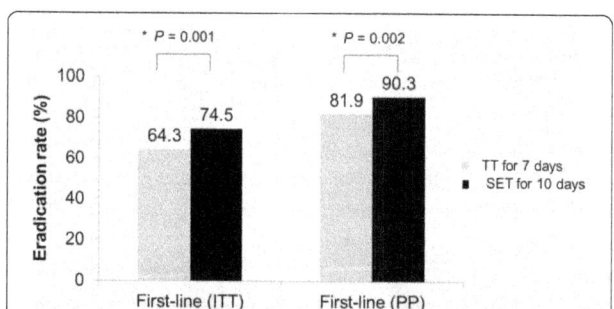

Fig. 2 Comparison of eradication rate of *Helicobacter pylori* with first-line triple therapy with sequential therapy. The eradication rate of SET was significantly higher than TT by both ITT ($P = 0.001$) and PP ($P = 0.002$) analyses. TT triple therapy, SET sequential therapy, ITT intention to treat, PP per protocol

Table 2 Clinical factors related to successful *Helicobacter pylori* eradication

	TT			SET		
	OR	95% CI	*P* value	OR	95% CI	*P* value
Univariate analyses						
Male gender	0.941	0.637 – 1.391	0.761	1.039	0.436 – 2.477	0.932
Age < 50 years	0.724	0.481 – 1.089	0.121	1.634	0.702 – 3.807	0.255
Residence – Seoul	0.819	0.509 – 1.320	0.413	1.154	0.375 – 3.553	0.803
Alcohol	0.942	0.628 – 1.415	0..775	0.909	0.391 – 2.115	0.824
Smoking	0.883	0.553 – 1.411	0.602	0.802	0.329 – 1.955	0.628
Diabetes mellitus	1.375	0.770 – 2.455	0.281	1.190	0.330 – 4.289	0.790
Hypertension	0.933	0.579 – 1.502	0.775	1.131	0.426 – 2.999	0.805
Indication						
Peptic ulcer disease	0.690	0.456 – 1.043	0.079	1.559	0.567 – 4.284	0.389
Malignant disease	0.647	0.297 – 1.410	0.273	1.604	0.461 – 5.581	0.458
Multivariate analysis						
Male gender	0.941	0.635 – 1.394	0.761	1.013	0.419 – 2.449	0.976
Age < 50 years	0.718	0.476 – 1.083	0.114	1.708	0.717 – 4.068	0.227
Residence – Seoul	0.792	0.490 – 1.282	0.343	1.203	0.280 – 3.831	0.750
Indication						
Peptic ulcer disease	0.679	0.447 – 1.030	0.069	1.538	0.554 – 4.272	0.409
Malignant disease	0.607	0.277 – 1.330	0.212	1.877	0.517 – 6.817	0.338

TT triple therapy, *SET* sequential therapy, *OR* odds ratio, *CI* confidence interval

first-line TT was 71.0 and 84.0% by ITT and PP analysis; eradication rate for BCQT-14 after TT was 85.3 and 95.5% by ITT and PP analysis, respectively. Twenty-four (9.7%) patients failed at their first-line SET, and 22 patients received BCQT-14 which showed the eradication rate of 72.7% in ITT and 84.2% in PP analysis. We found no significant differences in the overall eradication rates, compliance, adverse events between any of these three groups (Table 4).

The most common complication after second-line treatment was nausea or vomiting in all of three groups.

After failure of second-line eradication therapy in the SET group, two patients refused further treatment, and one patient received third-line eradication therapy consisted with twice a day standard dose of PPI, amoxicillin (1000 mg), and levofloxacin (500 mg) for 7 days. But, eradication of *H. pylori* also failed after third-line treatment.

Discussion

Our study revealed that the eradication rate of TT was below the recommended threshold by both of ITT and

Table 3 Adverse events during first-line *Helicobacter pylori* eradication therapy

	TT	SET	*P* value
	N = 872 (74.3%)	N = 302 (25.7%)	
Total	33 (3.8)	10 (3.3)	0.706
Diarrhea	11 (1.3)	5 (1.7)	0.574
Nausea or vomiting	9 (1.0)	3 (1.0)	0.999
Abdominal pain	8 (0.9)	0 (0)	0.122
Skin rash	1 (0.1)	1 (0.3)	0.448
Metallic taste	1 (0.1)	0 (0)	0.999
Others[a]	5 (0.6)	2 (0.7)	0.999

TT triple therapy, *SET* sequential therapy, *H. pylori* Helicobacter pylori
[a] Others included dyspepsia, bloating, and dizziness

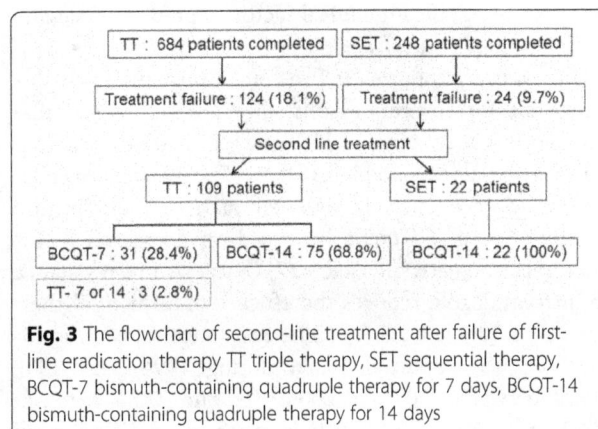

Fig. 3 The flowchart of second-line treatment after failure of first-line eradication therapy TT triple therapy, SET sequential therapy, BCQT-7 bismuth-containing quadruple therapy for 7 days, BCQT-14 bismuth-containing quadruple therapy for 14 days

Table 4 Comparisons of second-line treatment after failure of first-line eradication therapy

	TT → BCQT-7	TT → BCQT-14	SET → BCQT-14	P value
Eradication rate, % (n)				
ITT	71 (22/31)	85.3 (64/75)	72.7 (16/22)	0.162
PP	84 (21/25)	95.5 (64/67)	84.2 (16/19)	0.076
Compliance > 80%, % (n)	80.6 (25)	89.3 (67)	86.4 (19)	0.511
Adverse events, % (n)	25.8 (8)	22.7 (17)	18.2 (4)	0.839

TT triple therapy, *SET* sequential therapy, *BCQT-7* bismuth-containing quadruple therapy for 7 days, *BCQT-14* bismuth-containing quadruple therapy for 14 days, *ITT* intention to treat, *PP* per protocol

PP analyses. This result is in accordance with the most recent meta-analysis for treatment of *H. pylori*, which concluded that SET was superior than TT showing the overall eradication rate of TT for 69.8 and 77.0%, and SET for 79.7 and 85.0% by ITT and PP analyses, respectively [14]. The most important cause of decreased efficacy of TT is considered as increasing antibiotic resistant rate, especially to clarithromycin [21]. The eradication rate of *H. pylori* was significantly different depending on the resistance or sensitivity to clarithromycin of the strain; 67.9% for clarithromycin-resistant strains and 95.5% for the clarithromycin-sensitive strains [12].

Previous studies proposed several clinical factors associated with *H. pylori* eradication failure including, age, gender, smoking, previous antibiotics usage [22, 23]. The most recent study in Korea reported that female gender could be associated with treatment failure, based on the fact that *H. pylori* strain with point mutation in the 23S rRNA were preferentially infected in women which could result in treatment failure with clarithromycin [24]. Also, smoking may increase treatment failure by reducing antibiotics delivery to gastric mucosa, because smoking decreases gastric blood flow and mucus secretion and smoking itself is an indicator for poor compliance [24–26]. However, we could not find any statistically significant clinical factor to predict successful eradication of *H. pylori*.

Our study supports SET as an alternative first-line treatment for several reasons. First, SET achieved reasonable target by both of ITT and PP analyses, whereas TT showed unacceptable efficacy. The reason for relatively higher efficacy of SET for *H. pylori* eradication compared with TT could be based on decreased resistance rate to metronidazole [27], because the resistance to nitroimidazole reduces the efficacy of sequential therapy up to 50% [21, 28, 29]. The resistance rate to metronidazole was reported 40.5% during 1994–1999 [30], 49.6% between 2003 and 2005 [31], and 27.5% between 2003 and 2009 [12] in Korea. And clarithromycin

resistance is thought to have less effect on the efficacy of SET than on TT [32]. Second, treatment-related adverse events of SET were tolerable in most of the patients. There was no patient who discontinued the treatment due to treatment-related adverse event in our study. Also, no significant differences were found regarding overall complication rates or incidence of individual complication between two groups. Third, drug compliance in the SET group was comparable with that of the TT group. There has been concern about complex administration schedule and higher complication rates of SET than TT [14] which could directly influence on drug compliance and possibly lower drug efficacy. But, our study revealed good compliance of the SET group, almost 85.0%, which was not statistically different from the TT group and showed no significant difference regarding adverse events between the two groups. In our medical center, all physicians explained possible treatment-related complications before prescribing medication with sufficient time, and this was also thought to be the cause of good compliance of SET. Fourth, we suggested reasonable treatment option in cases of treatment failure of first-line SET. One of the major concerns of four-drug regimen is choice of second-line treatment when first-line eradication therapy failed, because there could be more chances of acquiring antibiotic resistance [33]. According to the Maastricht IV Consensus Report, BCQT is recommended as optimal second-line treatment [34], and 2013 revised Korean guidelines also recommends BCQT for second-line option after failure of first-line TT [10]. However, there is no definite guideline for the second-line treatment after failure of SET. According to our results, BCQT could be good second-line treatment option after failure of first-line SET.

This study has several limitations. First, test for *H. pylori* identification or antibiotic sensitivity test was not performed which could clarify direct influence of antibiotic susceptibility on eradication rate. Antibiotic resistance rate, especially clarithromycin resistance is significant factor for determining the efficacy of *H. pylori* eradication with TT or SET [24]. Thus, these kinds of tests are the best way to reduce eradication failure arising from antibiotic resistance [21]. But, it is very difficult to test all patients in the general clinics, and cost-effectiveness is another problem [21]. In a recent prospective study evaluating the efficacy of SET and amoxicillin/tetracycline containing bismuth quadruple therapy (PBAT) for the first-line eradication in the patients from nine different provinces, SET did not reach the 90% eradication rate in the PP analysis despite SET was more effective than PBAT [35]. This discordance with our result could be explained by the difference of local antibiotic resistance. In Korea, it has been reported that antibiotics resistance of *H. pylori* is differ according to the geographic region. In Seoul where our institution is located, resistance rate to clarithromycin is known to be 14.8%, however above study included the provinces in which showed higher resistance rate compared to Seoul such as Busan (42.1%) or Gyeonggi (32.5%) [27], and that might be the cause for the decreased efficacy of SET. The dicision for the appropriate empirical antibiotic therapy should be made based on the data of recentlly updated local antibiotic resistance [11], and therfore nationwide updated data for antibiotic resistance of H. pylori should be surveyed.

Second, as this study was conducted retrospectively, there were limitations to obtain detailed medical information such as previous medication history including antibiotics or PPI which could have an influence on eradication failure or diagnosis of H. pylori infection. Also, treatment-related adverse events in our study might be down-estimated for the same reason. Compared with previous studies which reported SET-related adverse event rates from 23.3 [14] to 48.0% [32], there was relatively small number of complications in our study (3.3%).

Third, this study enrolled the patients only in the single-center, and the majority of them resided in Seoul. So applying the results of this study to another area could have limitation. However, this study has strength in terms of its large number of study subjects and assessment of the efficacy of rescue therapy after failure of first-line eradication therapy.

Conclusions

The eradication rate of TT was below the recommended threshold. However, SET showed acceptable eradication rate by both ITT ($P = 0.001$) and PP ($P = 0.002$) analyses with comparable adverse events. SET also has reasonable second-line treatment option, BCQT after failure of first-line SET. Therefore, SET could be effective and tolerable candidate for the first-line H. pylori eradication therapy.

Abbreviations
BCQT: Bismuth-containing quadruple therapy; H. pylori: Helicobacter pylori; ITT: Intention to treat; MALT: Mucosa-associated lymphoid tissue; PP: Per protocol; PPI: Proton-pump inhibitor; SET: Sequential therapy; TT: Triple therapy; vs.: Versus

Acknowledgements
Not applicable.

Funding
No external funding.

Authors' contributions
JC- data collection, organization, analysis and interpretation of data, writing and revision of the manuscript.; KS- design the study, analysis and

interpretation of data, progress guidance and responsible for the whole study; CT- analysis and interpretation of data; KL- help JC collecting data; JL- help JC collecting data; KL- help JC collecting data; CM- analysis and interpretation of data; SK- analysis and interpretation of data; HJ- analysis and interpretation of data; SJ- analysis and interpretation of data. All authors have read and approved the final manuscript.

Competing interests
The authors declare that they have no competing interests.

Consent for publication
Not applicable.

References
1. Lim SH, Kwon JW, Kim N, Kim GH, Kang JM, Park MJ, Yim JY, Kim HU, Baik GH, Seo GS, et al. Prevalence and risk factors of helicobacter pylori infection in Korea: nationwide multicenter study over 13 years. BMC Gastroenterol. 2013;13:104.
2. Moss SF, Malfertheiner P. Helicobacter and gastric malignancies. Helicobacter. 2007;12 Suppl 1:23–30.
3. Yamada T, Searle JG, Ahnen D, Aipers DH, Greenberg HB, Gray M, et al. Helicobacter pylori in Peptic Ulcer Disease. JAMA. 1994;272:65–69.
4. Leodolter A, Kulig M, Brasch H, Meyer-Sabellek W, Willich SN, Malfertheiner P. A meta-analysis comparing eradication, healing and relapse rates in patients with helicobacter pylori-associated gastric or duodenal ulcer. Aliment Pharmacol Ther. 2001;15:1949–58.
5. Wotherspoon AC, Doglioni C, Diss TC, Pan L, Moschini A, de Boni M, Isaacson PG. Regression of primary low-grade B-cell gastric lymphoma of mucosa-associated lymphoid tissue type after eradication of Helicobacter pylori. Lancet. 1993;342:575–7.
6. Bae SE, Jung HY, Kang J, Park YS, Baek S, Jung JH, Choi JY, Kim MY, Ahn JY, Choi KS, et al. Effect of Helicobacter pylori eradication on metachronous recurrence after endoscopic resection of gastric neoplasm. Am J Gastroenterol. 2014;109:60–7.
7. Lee SY. New guidelines for Helicobacter pylori treatment: comparisons between Korea and Japan. Korean J Gastroenterol. 2014;63:151–7.
8. Abe T, Kodama M, Murakami K, Matsunari O, Mizukami K, Inoue K, Uchida M, Okimoto T, Fujioka T, Uchida T, et al. Impact of helicobacter pylori CagA diversity on gastric mucosal damage: an immunohistochemical study of east-Asian-type CagA. J Gastroenterol Hepatol. 2011;26:688–93.
9. Korean H. Diagnosis and treatment of Helicobacter pylori infection in Korea. Korean J Gastroenterol. 1998;32:275–89.
10. Kim SG, Jung HK, Lee HL, Jang JY, Lee H, Kim CG, Shin WG, Shin ES, Lee YC. Korean college of helcobacter and upper gastrointestinal research. Guidelines for the diagnosis and treatment of helicobacter pylori infection in Korea, 2013 revised edition. Korean J Gastroenterol. 2013;62:3–26.
11. Shin WG, Lee SW, Baik GH, Huh KC, Lee SI, Chung JW, Jung WT, Park MI, Jung HK, Kim HU, et al. Eradication rates of helicobacter pylori in Korea over the past 10 years and correlation of the amount of antibiotics use: nationwide survey. Helicobacter. 2016;21:266–78.
12. Hwang TJ, Kim N, Kim HB, Lee BH, Nam RH, Park JH, Lee MK, Park YS, Lee DH, Jung HC, et al. Change in antibiotic resistance of helicobacter pylori strains and the effect of A2143G point mutation of 23S rRNA on the eradication of H. Pylori in a single center of Korea. J Clin Gastroenterol. 2010;44:536–43.
13. Lee JW, Kim N, Kim JM, Nam RH, Chang H, Kim JY, Shin CM, Park YS, Lee DH, Jung HC. Prevalence of primary and secondary antimicrobial resistance of Helicobacter pylori in Korea from 2003 through 2012. Helicobacter. 2013;18:206–14.
14. Lee SW, Kim HJ, Kim JG. Treatment of helicobacter pylori infection in Korea: a systematic review and meta-analysis. J Korean Med Sci. 2015;30:1001–9.
15. Lam SK, Talley NJ. Report of the 1997 Asia pacific consensus conference on the management of helicobacter pylori infection. J Gastroenterol Hepatol. 1998;13:1–12.
16. Kim N, Kim JJ, Choe YH, Kim HS, Kim JI, Chung IS. Korean college of helicobacter and upper gastrointestinal research; korean association of gastroenterology. Diagnosis and treatment guidelines for helicobacter pylori infection in Korea. Korean J Gastroenterol. 2009;54:269–78.

17. Kim JS, Kim BW, Ham JH, Park HW, Kim YK, Lee MY, Ji JS, Lee BI, Choi H. Sequential therapy for *helicobacter pylori* infection in Korea: systematic review and meta-analysis. Gut Liver. 2013;7:546–51.

18. Chung JW, Ha M, Yun SC, Kim JH, Lee JJ, Kim YJ, Kim KO, Kwon KA, Park DK, Lee DH. Meta-analysis: sequential therapy is superior to conventional therapy for *helicobacter pylori* infection in Korea. Korean J Gastroenterol. 2013;62:267–71.

19. Choi WH, Park DI, Oh SJ, Baek YH, Hong CH, Hong EJ, Song MJ, Park SK, Park JH, Kim HJ, et al. Effectiveness of 10 day-sequential therapy for *Helicobacter pylori* eradication in Korea. Korean J Gastroenterol. 2008;51:280–4.

20. Park S, Chun HJ, Kim ES, Park SC, Jung ES, Lee SD, Jang JS, Kwon YD, Keum B, Seo YS. M1053 The 10-day sequential therapy for *Helicobacter pylori* eradication in Korea: less effective than expected. Gastroenterology. 2009;136(5):A-339–40.

21. Kim SY, Jung SW. *Helicobacter pylori* eradication therapy in Korea. Korean J Gastroenterol. 2011;58:67–73.

22. Byun YH, Jo YJ, Kim SC, Lee JS, Shin WY, Park YS, Kim SH, Lee HH, Song MH. Clinical factors that predicts successful eradication of *Helicobacter pylori*. Korean J Gastroenterol. 2006;48:172–9.

23. Cho DK, Park SY, Kee WJ, Lee JH, Ki HS, Yoon KW, Cho SB, Lee WS, Joo YE, Kim HS, et al. The trend of eradication rate of *Helicobacter pylori* infection and clinical factors that affect the eradication of first-line therapy. Korean J Gastroenterol. 2010;55:368–75.

24. Kim SE, Park MI, Park SJ, Moon W, Choi YJ, Cheon JH, Kwon HJ, Ku KH, Yoo CH, Kim JH, et al. Trends in *Helicobacter pylori* eradication rates by first-line triple therapy and related factors in eradication therapy. Korean J Intern Med. 2015;30:801–7.

25. Moayyedi P, Chalmers DM, Axon AT. Patient factors that predict failure of omeprazole, clarithromycin, and tinidazole to eradicate *Helicobacter pylori*. J Gastroenterol. 1997;32:24–7.

26. Suzuki T, Matsuo K, Ito H, Sawaki A, Hirose K, Wakai K, Sato S, Nakamura T, Yamao K, Ueda R, et al. Smoking increases the treatment failure for *Helicobacter pylori* eradication. Am J Med. 2006;119:217–24.

27. Kim JY, Kim NY, Kim SJ, Baik GH, Kim GH, Kim JM, Nam RH, Kim HB, Lee DH, Jung HC, et al. Regional difference of antibiotic resistance of *Helicobacter pylori* strains in Korea. Korean J Gastroenterol. 2011;57:221–9.

28. Beek D, De Craen A. A systematic review of *Helicobacter pylori* eradication therapy—the impact of antimicrobial resistance on eradication rates. Aliment Pharmacol Ther. 1999;13:1047–55.

29. Megraud F. *H pylori* antibiotic resistance: prevalence, importance, and advances in testing. Gut. 2004;53:1374–84.

30. Kim JJ, Reddy R, Lee M, Kim JG, El-Zaatari FA, Osato MS, Graham DY, Kwon DH. Analysis of metronidazole, clarithromycin and tetracycline resistance of *Helicobacter pylori* isolates from Korea. J Antimicrob Chemother. 2001;47:459–61.

31. Kim N, Kim JM, Kim CH, Park YS, Lee DH, Kim JS, Jung HC, Song IS. Institutional difference of antibiotic resistance of *Helicobacter pylori* strains in Korea. J Clin Gastroenterol. 2006;40:683–7.

32. Liou JM, Chen CC, Chen MJ, Chen CC, Chang CY, Fang YJ, Lee JY, Hsu SJ, Luo JC, Chang WH, et al. Sequential versus triple therapy for the first-line treatment of *Helicobacter pylori*: a multicentre, open-label, randomised trial. Lancet. 2013;381:205–13.

33. Olofsson SK, Cars O. Optimizing drug exposure to minimize selection of antibiotic resistance. Clin Infect Dis. 2007;45:S129–36.

34. Malfertheiner P, Megraud F, O'Morain CA, Atherton J, Axon AT, Bazzoli F, Gensini GF, Gisbert JP, Graham DY, Rokkas T, et al. Management of *helicobacter pylori* infection-the Maastricht IV/Florence consensus report. Gut. 2012;61:646–64.

35. Lee JY, Kim N, Park KS, Kim HJ, Park SM, Baik GH, Shim KN, Oh JH, Choi SC, Kim SE, et al. Comparison of sequential therapy and amoxicillin/tetracycline containing bismuth quadruple therapy for the first-line eradication of *Helicobacter pylori*: a prospective, multi-center, randomized clinical trial. BMC Gastroenterol. 2016;16:79.

12

Higher frequency of cagA EPIYA-C Phosphorylation Sites in *H. pylori* strains from first-degree relatives of gastric cancer patients

Dulciene MM Queiroz[2], Cícero ISM Silva[1], Maria HRB Goncalves[1], Manuel B Braga-Neto[1], Andréa BC Fialho[1], André MN Fialho[2], Gifone A Rocha[2], Andreia MC Rocha[2], Sérgio A Batista[2], Richard L Guerrant[3], Aldo AM Lima[4] and Lucia LBC Braga[1*]

Abstract

Background: To evaluate the prevalence of more virulent *H. pylori* genotypes in relatives of gastric cancer patients and in patients without family histories of gastric cancer.

Methods: We evaluated prospectively the prevalence of the infection by more virulent *H. pylori* strains in 60 relatives of gastric cancer patients comparing the results with those obtained from 49 patients without family histories of gastric cancer. *H. pylori* status was determined by the urease test, histology and presence of *H. pylori* ureA. The cytotoxin associated gene (*cag*A), the *cag*A-EPIYA and vacuolating cytotoxin gene (*vac*A) were typed by PCR and the *cag*A EPIYA typing was confirmed by sequencing.

Results: The gastric cancer relatives were significant and independently more frequently colonized by *H. pylori* strains with higher numbers of CagA-EPIYA-C segments (OR = 4.23, 95%CI = 1.53–11.69) and with the most virulent s1m1 *vac*A genotype (OR = 2.80, 95%CI = 1.04–7.51). Higher numbers of EPIYA-C segments were associated with increased gastric corpus inflammation, foveolar hyperplasia and atrophy. Infection by s1m1 *vac*A genotype was associated with increased antral and corpus gastritis.

Conclusions: We demonstrated that relatives of gastric cancer patients are more frequently colonized by the most virulent *H. pylori cag*A and *vac*A genotypes, which may contribute to increase the risk of gastric cancer.

Keywords: Helicobacter pylori, Gastric cancer, H. pylori CagA-EPIYA, H. pylori/vacA

Background

Helicobacter pylori, a Gram-negative bacterium that infects the stomach of approximately half the world's population, is associated with the development of gastro-duodenal diseases including gastric and duodenal peptic ulcer, distal gastric adenocarcinoma and mucosa-associated lymphoid tissue lymphoma [1]. It is estimated that individuals infected with *H. pylori* have more than two-fold increased risk of developing gastric cancer compared with non-infected ones [2] although Japanese studies might suggest that nearly all gastric cancer is related to *Helicobacter* [3]. Why only 1 to 5% of *H. pylori*-infected persons develop gastric cancer remains unknown and it seems to depend on the relationship between environmental, host genetics and bacterial virulence factors.

Several studies have shown an increased risk of developing gastric cancer in relatives of patients with the disease [2,4]. Similarly, an increased prevalence of precancerous gastric lesions has been observed in relatives of gastric cancer patients [5]. However, molecular mechanisms by which *H. pylori* triggers the process leading to gastric carcinoma remain largely unknown.

The most investigated *H. pylori* virulence determinant, the *cag*-PAI (cytotoxin associated gene pathogenicity island), encodes a type IV secretion system (T4SS) that is responsible for the entrance of an effector protein,

* Correspondence: lucialib@terra.com.br
[1]Clinical Research Unity – Department of Internal Medicine, University Hospital Walter Cantídio – Federal University of Ceará, P.O. Box: 60430270, Fortaleza, Ceará, Brazil
Full list of author information is available at the end of the article

CagA, into host gastric epithelial cells [6,7]. Once translocated, CagA localizes to the inner surface of the plasma membrane where it is phosphorylated on the tryrosine residues within phosphorylation motifs in carboxy-terminal variable region of the protein by multiple members of the src-family tyrosine kinases. Once phosphorylated, CagA forms a physical complex with SHP-2 phosphatase and triggers abnormal cellular signals, which enhance the risk of damaged cells acquiring precancerous genetic changes [8,9].

The phosphorylation motifs, defined as a sequence of five amino acids (Glu-Pro-Ile-Tyr-Ala), are classified as EPIYA-A, EPIYA-B, EPIYA-C and EPIYA-D, according to amino acid sequences flanking the motifs. CagA proteins nearly always possess EPIYA-A and -B segments, that are followed by none, one, two or three C segments in strains circulating in the Western countries, or a D segment, in East Asia strains [10,11]. It has also been shown that infection with CagA strains having high number of EPIYA-C segments imparts a greater risk of precancerous gastric lesions and cancer [12-15].

Another virulence factor of H. pylori is a protein known as vacuolating cytotoxin A (VacA), which causes cytoplasmatic vacuolization in gastric epithelial cells, increasing the plasma cell and mitochondrial membrane permeability leading to apoptosis. The production of the cytotoxin is associated with the cag-PAI but depends on the vacA genotype [16-18]. The vacA is a polymorphic gene with two main signal region genotypes s1 and s2, and two different alleles in the mid region of the gene named m1 and m2. Infection with strains possessing the s1m1 genotype has been associated with precancerous gastric hypochlorhydria [17] and gastric carcinoma [19].

In a recent study conducted in Fortaleza, Northeastern, Brazil, in an area of high prevalence of gastric cancer and H. pylori infection, our group has shown a high prevalence of either pangastritis or precancerous lesions in relatives of gastric cancer patients infected with H. pylori [20].

Furthermore, Argent et al., (2008) observed an association between vacA s1m1 genotype of H. pylori strains and low gastric acid secretion in first-degree relatives of gastric cancer patients from Scotland [21]. Otherwise, the authors did not find associations between CagA positive status and or number of tyrosine phosphorylated motifs and gastric lesions in that population.

Since geographical differences have been observed among studies that evaluated association between H. pylori virulence factors and diseases, the aim of this cross-sectional prospective study was to evaluate the CagA EPIYA motifs of H. pylori strains in first-degree relatives of gastric cancer patients comparing the results with those obtained from a control group composed of subjects with no family history of gastric cancer. Because the s1m1

genotype of the vacA H. pylori was seen to be more frequently observed in the strains of gastric cancer patients, we also evaluated the vacA mosaicism in the strains.

Methods

The study was approved by the Ethical Committee of Research of the University of Ceará, and informed consent was obtained from each subject.

Patients

Sixty H. pylori-positive first-degree relatives [42 female; mean age 40.42 ± 11.80; (4 brothers and 13 sisters; mean age 56.24 ± 11.80 years, 14 sons and 29 daughters; mean age 34.51 ± 7.66)] of gastric cancer patients from outpatient follow-up at Walter Cantídio Hospital were invited to participate. The control group was composed of 49 (32 female; mean age 43.20 ± 12.59) H. pylori-positive patients who concurrently underwent upper gastrointestinal endoscopy for investigation of dyspepsia at the same Hospital. They did not have family history of gastric cancer, and were social class matched with the study group. Patients with history of gastric surgery, active gastrointestinal bleeding, use of steroids, immunosuppressive drugs, NSAIDs, proton pump inhibitors or who were treated for H. pylori eradication were excluded from the study. Relatives and controls were not included if they were under 18 or above 81 years old.

Biopsy fragment collection

Gastric fragments were obtained during endoscopy from five different sites as recommended by the Updated Sydney System for classification of gastritis [22]. Additionally, two fragments were collected from the antral mucosa for the rapid urease test and for DNA to investigate the presence of H. pylori genes. H. pylori infection was confirmed by positive results in at least two tests including a rapid urease test, histological analysis and presence of ureA gene of H. pylori.

Histology

Endoscopic biopsy samples of the gastric mucosa were fixed in 10% formalin and embedded in paraffin wax, and 4-μm-sections were stained with hematoxylin-eosin for routine histology. Gastritis was classified according to the Updated Sydney system. The samples of the gastric mucosa were also stained with Giemsa for detection of H. pylori.

DNA extraction

The antral gastric DNA was extracted using the QIAmp (QIAGEN, Hilden, Germany) kit according to the manufacturer's recommendations with minor modifications [23]. The DNA concentration was determined by spectrophotometry using NanoDrop 2000 (Thermo Scientific, Wilmington, NC) and stored at −20°C until use.

The presence of *H. pylori* specific *ure*A gene was evaluated according to methodology reported by Clayton *et al.*, [24]. The standard Tx30a *H. pylori* strain was used as a positive control, and an *Escherichia coli* strain and distilled water were both used as negative controls.

The thermocycler GeneAmp PCR System 9700 (Applied Biosystems, Foster City, CA) was used for all reactions. The amplified products were electrophoresed in 2% agarose gel, stained with ethidium bromide, and analyzed in an ultraviolet light transilluminator.

vacA and cagA detection

PCR amplification of the *vac*A signal sequence and mid region was performed by using the oligonucleotide primers described by Atherton *et al.*, [15]. The strains were initially classified as type s1 or s2 and type m1 or m2. All *H. pylori* strains with s1 were further characterized into s1a, s1b or s1c [25,26].

The *cag*A gene was amplified by means of two previously described set of primer pairs [27,28]. A *H. pylori* strain from our collection (1010–95), known to be *vac*A s1m1 and *cag*A-positive, was used as a positive control, and the s2m2 *vac*A genotype, *cag*A-negative standard Tx30a *H. pylori* strain and distilled water were both used as negative controls. The *H. pylori* strains were considered to be *cag*A-positive when at least one of the two reactions was positive.

Amplification of the 3' variable region of cagA

For the PCR amplification of the 3' variable region of the *cag*A gene (that contains the EPIYA sequences), 20 to 100 ng of DNA were added to 1% Taq DNA polymerase buffer solution (KCl 50 mM and Tris−HCl 10 mM, pH, 8.0), 1.5 mM $MgCl_2$, 100 µM of each deoxynucleotide, 1.0 U Platinum Taq DNA polymerase (Invitrogen, São Paulo, Brazil), and 10 pmol of each primer, for a total solution volume of 20 µL. The primers used were previously described by Yamaoka *et al.* [29]. The reaction conditions were: 95°C for 5 minutes, followed by 35 cycles of 95°C for 1 minute, 50°C for 1 minute, and 72°C for 1 minute, ending with 72°C for 7 minutes. The reaction yielded products of 500 to 850 bp as follows: EPIYA-AB: 500 bp; EPIYA-ABC: 640 bp; EPIYA-ABCC: 740 bp and EPIYA-ABCCC: 850 bp (Figure 1).

We also used the method described by Argent *et al.* [30] for the PCR amplification of the 3' variable region of the *cag*A gene that contains the EPIYA sequences in order to improve the accuracy of our results.

Sequencing of the 3' variable region of cagA

A subset of samples was randomly selected for sequencing in order to confirm the PCR results. PCR products were purified with the Wizard SV Gel and PCR Clean-up System (Promega, Madison, MI) according to the manufacturer's recommendations. Purified products were sequenced using a BigDye Terminator v3.1 Cycle Sequencing kit in an ABI 3130 Genetic Analyzer (Applied Biosystems, Foster City, CA). The sequences obtained were aligned using the CAP3 Sequence Assembly Program (available from: http://pbil.univ-lyon1.fr/cap3.php). After alignment, nucleotide sequences were transformed into amino acid sequences using the Blastx program (available from: http://blast.ncbi.nlm.nih.gov/Blast.cgi) and compared to sequences deposited into the GenBank (http://www.ncbi.nlm.nih.gov/Genbank/).

Statistical analysis

Data were analyzed with SPSS (Inc. Chicago, IL), version 17.0. The risk of relatives of gastric carcinoma to be infected by more virulent strains, with increased number of EPIYA-C motifs and s1m1 *vac*A genotype, was initially evaluated in univariate analysis. For that, *cag*A strains were stratified in those possessing at least one EPIYA−C segment and those with more than one EPIYA-C segment and the most virulent *vac*A s1m1 genotype was compared with s1m2 plus s2m2. Variables with a *p*-value less-than or equal to 0.25 were included in the final model of logistic regression, controlling for the influences of age and sex. Odds Ratio (OR) and 95% confidence intervals (CI) were calculated. The logistic model fitness was evaluated with the Hosmer-Lemeshow test [31]. Association of the number of EPIYA-C segments and the presence of *vac*A virulent genotypes with the degree of gastric inflammation, atrophy and intestinal metaplasia was done by the two-tailed Mann−Whitney Test. The level of significance was set at a *p* value ≤0.05.

Results

The presence of *H. pylori* specific *ure*A gene was detected in the gastric mucosa of all 109 studied subjects.

cagA status of the patients

*cag*A positivity was observed in the gastric fragments from 51 (85.00%) of 60 gastric cancer relatives and in those from 43 (87.76%) of 49 controls, without difference between the groups (*p* = 0.68; OR = 1.26, 95%CI = 0.37 − 4.40).

The number of EPIYA-C segments

The EPIYA pattern of all *cag*A-positive strains from both relatives of gastric cancer patients and controls were successfully typed. The Yamaoka methodology allowed the detection of mixed strain infection. The concordance between the methods used was almost 100%. The results were confirmed by sequencing of the 3' variable region of *cag*A in 30 randomly selected PCR products.

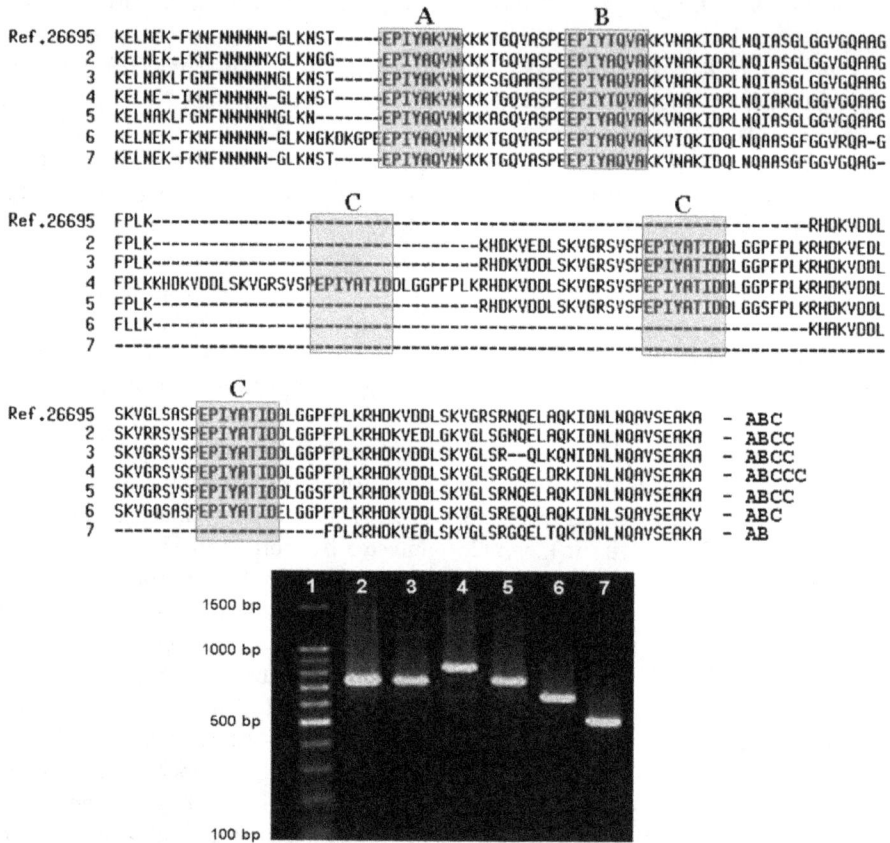

Figure 1 Electrophoresis of representative samples with different CagA EPIYA patterns seen in relatives of gastric cancer patients and controls. Columns 2, 3 e 5: EPIYA-ABCC (740 bp); column 4: EPIYA-ABCCC (850 bp); column 6: EPIYA-ABC (640 bp) and Column 7: EPIYA-AB (500 bp). Upper: partial alignment of amino acid sequencing of the carboxy-terminal CagA strains and a reference strain (*H. pylori* 26695).

Four patterns of EPIYA motifs were found: AB, ABC, ABCC, and ABCCC. No Asian EPIYA-D motif was observed. The distribution of the EPIYA genotypes is shown in the Table 1.

*vac*A mosaicism distribution

The distribution of *vac*A genotypes is shown in the Table 2. In 59 cases (54.13%) the *vac*A genotype was

s1m1, in 35 (32.11%) it was s1m2 and 6 (5.50%) s2m2. In three (2.75%) cases two *vac*A genotypes were observed and in six (5.50%) only the signal sequence (s1) was detected. DNA was not enough to genotype m allele in four among these cases and in two, m was not typable. In all cases with s1 strains they were genotyped as s1b, except in one case who was colonized by s1a and s1b strains.

Table 1 Distribution of EPIYA genotypes in the gastric cancer relatives (n = 51) and controls (n = 43) colonized by a *cag*A-positive strains

EPIYA Genotype	Control group n (%)	Gastric cancer relatives	
		Siblings n (%)	offspring n (%)
EPIYA-AB	03 (7.0)	0	0
EPIYA-ABC	32 (74.4)	09 (60.0)	20 (55.5)
EPIYA-ABCC	07 (16.3)	04 (26.7)	12 (33.2)
EPIYA-ABCCC	01 (2.3)	01 (6.7)	02 (5.6)
EPIYA-ABC + ABCC	0	01 (6.7)	02 (5.6)
Total	43 (100.0)	15 (100.0)	36 (100.0)

Table 2 Distribution of *vac*A alleles of *H. pylori* strains of relatives of gastric cancer patients (n = 55) and control group (n = 48)

*vac*A Genotypes[1]	Control group n (%)	Gastric cancer relatives	
		Siblings n (%)	Offspring n (%)
s1m1	23 (47.92)	10 (66.67)	26 (65.00)
s1m2	21 (43.75)	04 (26.67)	10 (25.00)
s2m2	03 (6.25)	01 (6.67)	02 (5.00)
Mixed[2]	01 (2.08)	0	02 (5.00)
Total	48 (100)	15 (100)	40 (100)

[1]Only *vac*A s1 genotype was identified in 6 cases (1 control, 2 siblings and 3 offsprings of gastric cancer relatives); [2]Mixed infection by s1m1 and s2m2 or s1m1 and s1m2 (two cases).

Infection by the most toxigenic *vac*A genotype (s1m1) was more frequently observed in the gastric cancer relatives (65.45%) than in the controls (47.92%). When s and m alleles were individually evaluated, no difference in the frequency of s1 allele was observed between the groups, but m1 allele was more frequently observed in the gastric cancer relatives.

Association among the number of EPIYA-C motifs and the *vac*A s1m1 genotype and family history of gastric cancer

The relatives of gastric cancer patients were significantly and independently more frequently colonized by *H. pylori* strains with increased number CagA-EPIYA-C segments and with the most virulent s1m1 *vac*A genotype even after adjustment for age and gender (Table 3).

No difference was observed between siblings and off-spring in respect to infection by strains containing an increased number of EPIYA-C motifs ($p = 0.98$; OR = 1.20, 95%CI = 0.30 – 4.86) and the *vac*A genotypes s1m1 vs. s1m2 and s2m2 ($p = 0.84$; OR = 0.92, 95%CI = 0.22 – 3.97) as shown in the Tables 1 and 2.

Associations among the number of EPIYA-C segments and *vac*A genotypes and gastric histological alterations

The degrees of corpus gastritis ($p = 0.04$), antrum activity ($p = 0.01$) and corpus activity were significantly higher in the relative of gastric cancer patients than in the control group.

A higher number of EPIYA-C segments was associated with gastric corpus inflammation ($p = 0.04$), gastric corpus foveolar hyperplasia ($p = 0.05$) and gastric corpus atrophy ($p = 0.05$) in the relatives of gastric cancer patients.

Infection by the most virulent *vac*A s1m1 genotype was associated with more marked antral ($p = 0.03$) and corpus ($p = 0.05$) gastritis, when both groups were evaluated together.

Discussion

H. pylori infection is recognized as the most important risk factor for distal gastric cancer. Furthermore, the increased rates of the disease in relatives of gastric

Table 3 Covariables associated with gastric cancer in the first-degree relatives of gastric cancer patients in comparison with subjects without family history of gastric cancer

Variables	Univariate analysis	Multivariate analysis		
	p	OR	95% CI	*p*
Gender	0.27	–	–	–
Age	0.30	–	–	–
> 1 EPIYA-C motif	0.01	4.23	1.53 – 11.69	0.006
s1m1 *vac*A allele	0.17	2.80	1.04 – 7.51	0.04

The Hosmer-Lemeshow test was fit (8 degrees of freedom, p > 0.20, with 10 steps).

cancer points to host genetics and/or share of the most *H. pylori* virulence strains as risk factors.

In this study, we demonstrated that relatives of gastric cancer patients are more frequently colonized by *H. pylori* strains with the most virulent *vac*A genotype, s1m1, and by CagA-positive strains possessing a higher number of EPIYA-C segments than the *H. pylori* strains of the patients without a family history of the disease.

Although no previous study has demonstrated that gastric cancer relatives are more frequently colonized by more virulent *H. pylori* strains, infection by *vac*A s1m1 was associated with low gastric acid secretion, a precancerous condition, in first-degree relatives of Scottish gastric cancer patients [21]. Otherwise, no association between the gastric acid secretion and the number of CagA EPIYA-C segments was observed by the authors [21].

CagA is the first bacterial oncoprotein to be identified [32]. The protein is delivered into the gastric epithelial cell through a bacterial T4SS and localizes to the inside of the cell membrane, where it is phosphorylated by host cell kinases. Upon phosphorylation, the EPIYA-C segment interacts with SHP-2 phosphatase, a bona fide oncoprotein that is associated with a series of human cancers. The higher the number of EPIYA-C segments, the higher the affinity for SHP-2 which is required for a full activation of ERK/MAPK pathway.

Infection with CagA strains possessing higher number of EPIYA-C segments has been associated with precancerous gastric lesions and gastric cancer in Caucasian [11-13,30] and Brazilian populations [15].

It is well established that *H. pylori* infection is predominantly acquired in childhood and that the infection often persists for life unless treated. Epidemiological data and genetic analysis of *H. pylori* strains have demonstrated that the strains are usually acquired within the family. In fact, infected mother and infected siblings are the main risk factors for the acquisition of the infection [33,34] and genetic fingerprint methods have demonstrated genetic homogeneity in the *H. pylori* strains within the families. Based on these findings and the results of the present study, we may hypothesize that first degree relatives of gastric cancer patients may share more virulent *H. pylori* strains that may increase the risk of gastric cancer.

As noted above, first-degree relatives of gastric cancer patients also share the same or similar genetic background that may increase the risk of gastric cancer. Polymorphisms in genes coding pro-inflammatory cytokines, such as interleukin 1 beta (IL-1β), interleukin-1 receptor antagonist (IL1Ra) and tumor necrosis factor-alpha (TNF-α) are accepted as risk factors of gastric cancer, depending on the geographic region [35-39]. It has also been demonstrated that having increasing number of pro-inflammatory genotypes [36,37], as well as a concomitant infection by more virulent *H. pylori* strains progressively increases the risk of gastric precancerous lesions and cancer [39].

Conclusions

In conclusion, we demonstrated that relatives of gastric cancer patients are more frequently colonized by the most virulent *H. pylori cag*A and *vac*A genotypes, which may, in addition to human genetic predispositions, further increase their risk of gastric cancer, thus providing additional reasons to better understand these infections and perhaps their targeted eradicative treatment.

Competing interests
The authors declare no-confllict-of-interest.

Authors' contributions
DMMQ supervised laboratory work and analyzed the data critical writing and reviewing manuscript., SAB performed DNA extraction, PCR and sequencing and statistical analysis, GAR and AMCR, participated in implementation of the study and wrote the manuscript, CISMS and MHB performed DNA extraction, PCR and database management, MBN, ABF and AMN participated in implementation of the study, data collection, database management and statistical analysis. RLG and AAML performed critical analysing of the data and reviewing of the manuscript. LLBCB participated in conception, design, implementation, coordination of the study and contributed to manuscript writing critical writing and reviewing. All authors have read and approved the final version of the manuscript.

Acknowledgements
This work was supported by Instituto Nacional de Ciências e Tecnologia em Biomedicina do Semiárido Brasileiro (INCT) and CNPq, Brazil. We are grateful to Professor Barry J Marshall for critical reading of the manuscript.
Results of the study was presented as abstract at Digestive Disease Week, DDW 2011, Chicago USA.

Author details
[1]Clinical Research Unity – Department of Internal Medicine, University Hospital Walter Cantídio – Federal University of Ceará, P.O. Box: 60430270, Fortaleza, Ceará, Brazil. [2]Laboratory of Research in Bacteriology, Federal University of Minas Gerais, Belo Horizonte, Minas Gerais, Brazil. [3]Center for Global Health, University of Virginia, Charlottesville, VA, USA. [4]Department of Physiology and Pharmacology, Federal University of Ceará, Fortaleza, Ceará, Brazil.

References
1. Parsonnet J, Friedman GD, Vandersteen DO: *Helicobacter pylori* and the risk of gastric carcinoma. *N Engl J Med* 1991, **25**:1127–1131.
2. Brenner H, Arndt V, Stürmer T, Stegmaier C, Ziegler H, Dhom G: Individual and joint contribution of family history and *Helicobacter pylori* infection to the risk of gastric carcinoma. *Cancer* 2000, **88**:274–279.
3. Uemura N, Okamoto S: Effect of *Helicobacter pylori* eradication on subsequent development of cancer after endoscopic resection of early gastric cancer in Japan. *Gastroenterol Clin North Am* 2000, **29**:819–827.
4. Chang YW, Han YS, Lee DK, Kim HJ, Lim HS, Moon JS, *et al*: Role of *Helicobacter pylori* infection among offspring or siblings of gastric cancer patients. *Int J Cancer* 2002, **101**:469–474.
5. Jablonska M, Chlumska A: Genetic factors in the development of gastric precancerous lesions – a role of *Helicobacter pylori? Int J Cancer* 2001, **95**:477–481.
6. Segal ED, Cha J, Lo J, Falkow S, Tompkins LS: Altered states: Involvement of phosphorylated CagA in the induction of host cellular growth changes by *Helicobacter pylori. Proc Natl Acad Sci USA* 1999, **96**:14559–14564.
7. Odenbreit S, Püls J, Sedlmaier B, Gerland E, Fischer W, Haas R: Translocation of *Helicobacter pylori* CagA into gastric epithelial cells by type IV secretion. *Science* 2000, **287**:1497–1500.
8. Higashi H, Tsutsumi R, Muto S, Sugiyama T, Azuma T, Asaka M, *et al*: SHP-2 tyrosine phosphatase as an intracellular target of *Helicobacter pylori* CagA protein. *Science* 2002, **295**:683–686.
9. Naito M, Yamazaki T, Tsutsumi R, Higashi H, Onoe K, Yamazaki S, *et al*: Influence of EPIYA-repeat polymorphism on the phosphorylation-dependent biological activity of *Helicobacter pylori* CagA. *Gastroenterology* 2006, **130**:1181–1190.
10. Hatakeyama M: Oncogenic mechanisms of the *Helicobacter pylori* CagA protein. *Nat Rev Cancer* 2004, **4**:688–694.
11. Argent RH, Hale JL, El-Omar EM, Atherton JC: Differences in *Helicobacter pylori* CagA tyrosine phosphorylation motif patterns between western and East Asian strains, and influences on interleukin-8 secretion. *J of Med Microb* 2008, **57**:1062–1067.
12. Yamaoka Y, El-Zimaity HMT, Gutierrez O, Figura N, Kim JK, Kodama T, *et al*: Relationship between the cagA 3 ' repeat region of *Helicobacter pylori*, gastric histology, and susceptibility to low pH. *Gastroenterology* 1999, **117**:342–349.
13. Basso D, Zambon CF, Letley DP, Stranges A, Marchet A, Rhead JL, *et al*: Clinical relevance of *Helicobacter pylori cag*A and *vac*A gene polymorphisms. *Gastroenterology* 2008, **135**:91–99.
14. Sicinschi LA, Correa P, Peek RM, Camargo MC, Piazuelo MB, Romero-Gallo J, *et al*: CagA C-terminal variations in *Helicobacter pylori* strains from Colombian patients with gastric precancerous lesions. *Clin Microbiol Infect* 2010, **16**:369–378.
15. Batista SA, Rocha GA, Rocha AM, Saraiva IE, Cabral MM, Oliveira RC, *et al*: Higher number of *Helicobacter pylori* CagA EPIYA C phosphorylation sites increases the risk of gastric cancer, but not duodenal ulcer. *BMC Microbiol* 2011, **11**:61.
16. Atherton JC, Cao P, Peek RM Jr, Tummuru MK, Blaser MJ, Cover TL: Mosaicism in vacuolating cytotoxin alleles of Helicobacter pylori. Association of specific vacA types with cytotoxin production and peptic ulceration. *J Biol Chem* 1995, **270**:17771–177777.
17. Willihite DC, Blanke SR: *Helicobacter pylori* vauolating cytotoxin induces activation of the proapoptotic enters cells, localizes to the mithochondria, and induces mithochondrial membrane permeability changes correlated to toxin channel activity. *Cell Microbiol* 2004, **6**:143–154.
18. Yamasaki E, Wada A, Kumatori A, Nakagawa I, Funao J, Nakayama M, *et al*: *Helicobacter pylori* vacuolating cytotoxin induces activation of the proapoptotic proteins Bax and Bak, leading to cytochrome c release and cell death, independent of vacuolation. *J Biol Chem* 2006, **281**:11250–11259.
19. Ashour AA, Magalhães PP, Mendes EN, Collares GB, de Gusmão VR, Queiroz DM, *et al*: Distribution of vacA genotypes in *Helicobacter pylori* strains isolated from Brazilian adult patients with gastritis, duodenal ulcer or gastric carcinoma. *FEMS Immunol Med Microbiol* 2002, **33**:173–178.
20. Motta CR, Cunha MP, Queiroz DM, Cruz FW, Guerra EJ, Mota RM, *et al*: Gastric precancerous lesions and *Helicobacter pylori* infection in relatives of gastric cancer patients from northeastern Brazil. *Digestion* 2008, **78**:3–8.
21. Argent RH, Thomas RJ, Aviles-Jimenez F, Letley DP, Limb MC, El-Omar EM, Atheton JC: Toxigenic *Helicobacter pylori* infection precedes hypochlorydria in cancer relatives, and *H. pylori* evolves in these families. *Clin Canc Res* 2008, **14**:2227–2235.
22. Dixon MF, Genta RM, Yardley JH, Correa P: Classification and grading of gastritis. The updated Sydney System. International Workshop on the Histopathology of Gastritis, Houston 1994. *Am J Surg Pathol* 1996, **20**:1161–1181.
23. Monteiro MA, Chan KH, Rasko DA, Taylor DE, Zheng PY, Appelmelk BJ, *et al*: Simultaneous expression of type 1 and type 2 Lewis blood group antigens by *Helicobacter pylori* lipopolysaccharides. Molecular mimicry between *h. pylori* lipopolysaccharides and human gastric epithelial cell surface glycoforms. *J Biol Chem* 1998, **273**:11533–11543.
24. Clayton CL, Kleanthous H, Coates PJ, Morgan DD, Tabaqchali S: Sensitive Detection of *Helicobacter-pylori* by Using Polymerase Chain-Reaction. *J Clin Microbiol* 1992, **30**:192–200.
25. van Doorn LJ, Figueiredo C, Sanna R, Plaisier A, Schneeberger P, de Boer W, *et al*: Clinical relevance of the cagA, vacA, and iceA status of *Helicobacter pylori. Gastroenterology* 1998, **115**:58–66.
26. Atherton JC, Cover TL, Wells RJ, Morales MR, Hawley CJ, Blaser MJ: Simple accurate PCR-based system for typing vauolating cytotoxin alleles of *Helicobacter pylori. J Clin Microbiol* 1999, **37**:2979–2982.

27. Kelly SM, Pitcher MC, Farmery SM, Gibson GR: Isolation of *Helicobacter pylori* from feces of patients with dyspepsia in the United Kingdom. *Gastroenterology* 1994, **107**:1671–1674.

28. Peek RM Jr, Miller GG, Tham KT, Perez-Perez GI, Cover TL, Atherton JC, *et al*: Detection of *Helicobacter pylori* gene expression in human gastric mucosa. *J Clin Microbiol* 1995, **33**:28–32.

29. Yamaoka Y, Kodama T, Kashima K, Graham DY, Sepulveda AR: Variants of the 3' region of the *cag*A gene in *Helicobacter pylori* isolates from patients with different *H. pylori*-associated diseases. *J Clin Microbiol* 1998, **36**:2258–2263.

30. Argent RH, Kidd M, Owen RJ, Thomas RJ, Limb MC, Atherton JC: Determinants and consequences of different levels of CagA phosphorylation for clinical isolates of *Helicobacter pylori*. *Gastroenterology* 2004, **127**:514–523.

31. Hosmer DW, Lemeshow S (Eds): *Applied Logistic Regression, JH*. New York: Wiley Interscience Publication; 2000.

32. Hatakeyama M: Anthorpological and clinical implications for structural diversity of the *Helicobacter pylori* CagA oncoprotein. *Cancer Sci* 2011, **102**:36–43.

33. Rocha GA, Rocha AM, Silva LD, Santos A, Bocewicz AC, Queiroz R, Rde M, *et al*: Transmission of *Helicobacter pylori* infection in families of preschool-aged children from Minas Gerais, Brazil. *Trop Med Int Health* 2003, **8**:987–991.

34. Kivi M, Johansson AL, Reilly M, Tindberg Y: *Helicobacter pylori* status in family members as risk factors for infection in children. *Epidemiol Infect* 2005, **133**:645–652.

35. El-Omar EM, Carrington M, Chow WH, McColl KE, Bream JH, Young HA, *et al*: Interleukin-1 polymorphisms assocaited with increased risk of gastric cancer. *Nature* 2000, **404**:398–402.

36. El-Omar EM, Rabkin CS, Gammon MD, Vaughan TL, Risch HA, Schoenberg JB, *et al*: Increased risk of noncardia gastric cancer associated with porinfalmmatory cytokine genes polymorhisms. *Gastroenterology* 2003, **124**:1193–1201.

37. Machado JC, Figueiredo C, Canedo P, Pharoah P, Carvalho R, Nabais S, *et al*: A proinflammatory genetic profile increases the risk for chronic atrophic gastritis and gastric carcinoma. *Gastroenterology* 2003, **125**:364–371.

38. Rocha GA, Guerra JB, Rocha AMC, Saraiva IEB, da Silva DA, de Oliveira CA, *et al*: IL1RN polymorphic gene and cagA-positive status independently increase the risk of noncardia gastric carcinoma. *Int J Cancer* 2005, **115**:678–683.

39. Figueiredo C, Machado JC, Pharoah P, Seruca R, Sousa S, Carvalho R, *et al*: *Helicobacter pylori* and interleukin 1 genotyping: an opportunity to identify high-risk individuals for gastric carcinoma. *J Natl Cancer Instit* 2002, **94**:1680–1687.

13

Additional corpus biopsy enhances the detection of *Helicobacter pylori* infection in a background of gastritis with atrophy

Hung-Chieh Lan[1,3], Tseng-Shing Chen[1*], Anna Fen-Yau Li[2], Full-Young Chang[1] and Han-Chieh Lin[1]

Abstract

Background: The best sites for biopsy-based tests to evaluate *H. pylori* infection in gastritis with atrophy are not well known. This study aimed to evaluate the site and sensitivity of biopsy-based tests in terms of degree of gastritis with atrophy.

Methods: One hundred and sixty-four (164) uninvestigated dyspepsia patients were enrolled. Biopsy-based tests (i.e., culture, histology Giemsa stain and rapid urease test) and non-invasive tests (anti-*H. pylori* IgG) were performed. The gold standard of *H. pylori* infection was defined according to previous criteria. The sensitivity, specificity, positive predictive rate and negative predictive rate of biopsy-based tests at the gastric antrum and body were calculated in terms of degree of gastritis with atrophy.

Results: The prevalence rate of *H. pylori* infection in the 164 patients was 63.4%. Gastritis with atrophy was significantly higher at the antrum than at the body (76% vs. 31%; $p<0.001$). The sensitivity of biopsy-based test decreased when the degree of gastritis with atrophy increased regardless of biopsy site (for normal, mild, moderate, and severe gastritis with atrophy, the sensitivity of histology Giemsa stain was 100%, 100%, 88%, and 66%, respectively, and 100%, 97%, 91%, and 66%, respectively, for rapid urease test). In moderate to severe antrum or body gastritis with atrophy, additional corpus biopsy resulted in increased sensitivity to 16.67% compare to single antrum biopsy.

Conclusions: In moderate to severe gastritis with atrophy, biopsy-based test should include the corpus for avoiding false negative results.

Keywords: Gastritis with atrophy, Biopsy-based test, Biopsy site, *Helicobacter pylori*

Background

Helicobacter pylori (H. pylori) and gastritis with atrophy are both risk factors for gastric cancer [1]. Around one-third of infected patients are estimated to have gastritis with atrophy [2] and the regression of these pre-neoplasm lesions may occur after successful eradication [3-5]. As such, *H. pylori* eradication in patients with gastritis with atrophy is recommended by current guidelines [1,6,7].

Although eradication is essential for this group of patients, the accurate identification of *H. pylori* against a background of gastritis with atrophy remains difficult [8]. False negative results occur even under more reliable *H. pylori* diagnostic tests like histology Giemsa stain [9]. False negative status, or the so-called sampling error, may result from patchy bacterial colonization through the stomach and altered distribution because of gastritis with atrophy and intestinal metaplasia. Thus, it is important to set a recommended biopsy site.

The updated Sydney Classification had set the gold standard for gastric biopsy more than 10 years ago [10]. According to this Classification, five biopsy sites should be collected: one specimen each should be obtained from the lesser and the greater curvature of the antrum, both within 2–3 cm form the pylorus; from the lesser curvature of the corpus about 4 cm proximal to the

* Correspondence: tschen@vghtpe.gov.tw
[1]Division of Gastroenterology, Department of Medicine, Taipei Veterans General Hospital and National Yang-Ming University, #201 Shih-Pai Road, Section 2, Taipei, Taiwan, ROC
Full list of author information is available at the end of the article

angulus; from the middle portion of the greater curvature of the corpus, approximately 8 cm from the cardia; and one from incisura angularis. However, for the consideration of patient's comfort and operator's convenience, this kind of extensive approach is uncommon in our daily practice. Studies on the most practical biopsy site for diagnosing *H. pylori* infection have conflicting results. Antrum biopsy is recommended by Genta et al. [11] while others recommend at least one corpus biopsy [12,13]. Hazell et al. and Woo et al. found it necessary to take both antral and corpus biopsies [14,15]. According to current guidelines, there is no optimal site when performing a biopsy-based test in a general condition, much less in those with gastritis with atrophy [16].

It is suggested that as gastritis with atrophy progresses, the mid corpus is the last area involved and is the last "lodgeable" mucosa for *H. pylori* in the stomach [17,18]. Additional corpus biopsy is suggested in these situations [12] but the exact additional benefit is not well known.

This prospectively designed study used the combination method as gold standard to investigate the correlation among sensitivity of biopsy-based test, biopsy location, degree of gastritis with atrophy, and *H. pylori* prevalence rate.

Methods
Patient population
Dyspeptic patients scheduled for upper gastrointestinal endoscopy were recruited. Patients with any of the following conditions were excluded: (1) ulcer complications (e.g., bleeding, stenosis, or perforation); (2) previous stomach surgery; (3) gastric neoplasms; (4) use of any substituted benzimidazoles and bismuth-containing preparations within the last 7 days prior to the start of the study; (5) past or current treatment with anti-*H. pylori* therapy; or (6) severe systemic diseases. All patients provided prior informed consent and received invasive and non-invasive tests for *H. pylori*. The local Ethics Committee on Human Test approved the study.

Endoscopy and biopsy sampling
According to the updated Sydney system, the biopsy sampling protocol required that more than five biopsy samples were obtained: two from the antral mucosa; one from the mucosa of the angularis incisura; two from the oxyntic area. For the consideration of patients' comfort and operator's convenience, we modified this recommendation. Two biopsy sites with multiple biopsies were applied to our endoscopy biopsy protocol. Three sets of biopsy specimens each from the greater curvature of the mid-body and lesser curvature of the antrum near the incisura were obtained during endoscopy for urease, histologic, and culture tests.

Rapid urease test
One biopsy from the greater curvature of the mid-body and one from the lesser curvature near the incisura were obtained for the urease test (CLO test; Delta West, Bentley, Australia). Antral and body biopsy specimens were evaluated separately, and the test was considered positive when the color changed from orange to pink within 24 hours.

Histologic evaluation of the biopsy samples
Biopsy specimens from the antrum and the body were fixed in formalin and assessed for the presence of *H. pylori* by a modified Giemsa stain, and for the degree of inflammatory cell infiltration, atrophy, and intestinal metaplasia by hematoxylin and eosin staining. The antrum and body histologic features of gastric mucosa were graded according to the updated Sydney System (0, none; 1, mild; 2, moderate; and 3, severe) [10]. In addition, the degree of gastritis activity was evaluated in Giemsa-negative patients with positive for either rapid urease test or serology. Also, the activity of gastritis was recorded according to the updated Sydney System. (1–4 points with 1 representing "normal", 2 to 4 representing "mildly, moderately and markedly active gastritis", respectively). Those who got two or more points on the pathological review were regarded as active gastritis which is an indirect sign of *H. pylori* infection. An experienced pathologist (Anna Fen-Yau Li) who was blinded to the results of other tests for *H. pylori* evaluated all histologic sections.

Culture
In culture, the biopsy sample was homogenized with 0.3 mL broth, plated on chocolate agar, and incubated at 37°C in a micro-aerobic (15% CO_2 and 5% O_2) incubator until the colony appeared, which was usually 3 days. The negative plates were kept for 7 days. The growth of *H. pylori* was confirmed by the characteristic morphology (Gram-negative and curved) and positive catalase, oxidase, and urease reactions observed.

Serologic evaluation
Serum specimens were tested for the presence of IgG antibodies against *H. pylori* using a quantitative ELISA test (HEL-pTEST II; AMRAD, Kew, Australia) according to the manufacturer's instructions. A specimen was considered positive if it contained >50 units/mL and negative if it contained ≤50 units/mL.

Serum pepsinogen levels

For serology studies, blood was drawn immediately after endoscopy and collected and stored at –70°C until assay. Fasting serum Pepsinogen I was measured in all patients by radioimmunoassay (Pepsik; Sorin Biomedica, Saluggia, Italy) according to the manufacturer's instructions, while basal Pepsinogen II levels were determined using a specific enzyme immunoassay (BIOHIT Plc, Helsinki, Finland).

Gold standard definition

To define the gold standard of active *H. pylori* infection, we modified the approach used by Shin et al. before [8]. A patient was classified as current *H. pylori* infection based on either a positive culture or, in the case of a negative culture, both positive histology and positive urease test (Group A). A patient was classified as *H. pylori*-negative when the culture, histologic examination, urease test, and serology were all negative (Group E). When either the histologic examination (Giemsa stain or presence of active gastritis) or urease test was positive, the results were classified based on the results of serology test. When IgG antibodies to *H. pylori* were detected, the results were considered "probably positive" (Group B). When IgG antibodies were not detected, the results were regarded as being "probably negative" (Group C). When a patient was serologically positive but negative on all biopsy-based tests, this was interpreted as either a past *H. pylori* infection or a false-positive result and the patient was classified as negative for current *H. pylori* infection (Group D). Groups A and B were defined as gold standard positive while Groups C, D, and E were gold standard negative.

Statistical analysis

Standard methods were used to calculate the sensitivity, specificity, and positive and negative predictive values, their 95% confidence intervals, and their test validity. Chi-square tests were used to compare variables (i.e., number of cases who had moderate-to-marked gastritis with atrophy at the antrum and corpus). To examine the decreasing trend in the prevalence of histology, as influenced by the severity of glandular atrophy, chi-square test for trend was applied. All statistical analyses and database collection were performed using the Statistical Package for Social Sciences (SPSS 17.0 for Windows, SPSS. Inc., Chicago, IL, USA).

Results

Subjects characteristics

A total of 164 patients were enrolled in this study. Regardless of the biopsy site, a total of 328 biopsy specimens were received for histologic evaluation (Figure 1).

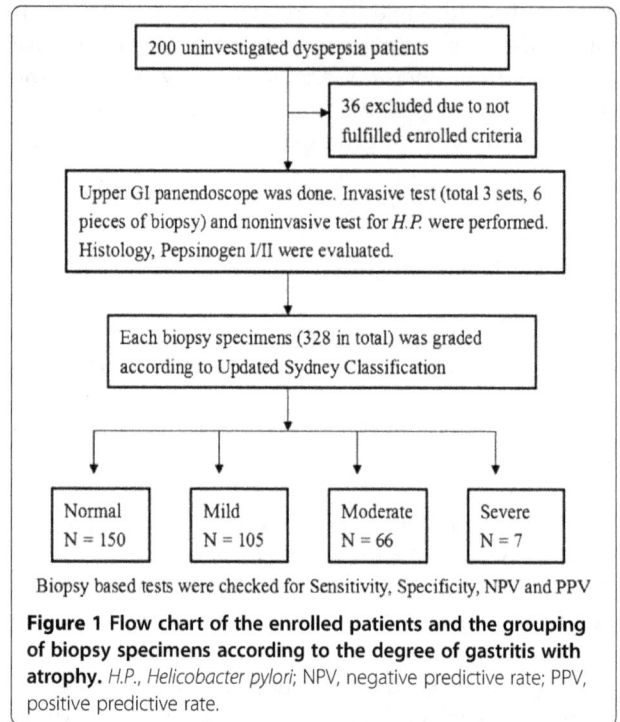

Figure 1 Flow chart of the enrolled patients and the grouping of biopsy specimens according to the degree of gastritis with atrophy. *H.P.*, *Helicobacter pylori*; NPV, negative predictive rate; PPV, positive predictive rate.

Using the pre-defined gold standard, the results of the four diagnostic tests for detecting current *H. pylori* infection in all subjects (n=164) were shown in Figure 2. Culture was positive in 87 patients. Among the patients who were culture negative, 16 were positive for both

H. pylori culture	CLO	Histology	Active gastritis	Serology	No. patients	Group
+	+	+		+	72	
+	+	+		-	15	
+		+		+	0	
+	+			+	0	
+	-	-		+	0	A
+	-	-		-	0	
-	+	+		+	14	
-	+	+		-	2	
-	+	-		+	1	
-		+		+	0	B
-	+		+		0	
-	-	-	+	+	0	
-	+	-		-	0	
-	-	+		-	0	C
-	-	-		+	2	D
-	-	-		-	58	E
Total					164	

Figure 2 Diagnostic tests for Helicobacter pylori detection: Group A, definitely positive (n=103); Group B, probably positive (n=1); Group C, probably negative (n=0); Group D, past *H. pylori* infection or false positive (n=2); Group E, definitely negative (n=58); CLO, indicates rapid urease test on biopsy specimens; Histology, refers to *H. pylori* positive based on modified Giemsa staining; Active gastritis, refers to presence or absence of active gastritis (an indirect sign of active *H. pylori* infection).

the CLOtest and histology. These 103 patients were regarded as true positives (Group A). Moreover, one patient was positive on serology and positive on either the CLOtest or histology testing (Giemsa stain or presence of active gastritis), so this patient was classified as probably *H. pylori* positive (Group B). No patient was positive for a single biopsy-based test, so there was no probably negative patient (Group C). Two patients were positive on serology only (with titers of 67 unit/ml and 171 unit/ml, respectively). Their gastritis activity of the biopsy specimens were reviewed again. None of them showed active gastritis in the pathological review (both of them got 1 point at their antrum and body biopsy specimens). They were considered either a past *H. pylori* infection or a false positive (Group D). Fifty-eight patients were negative on all tests and were considered true negative (Group E).

When Groups A and B were considered as *H. pylori* positive and groups C, D, and E as *H. pylori* negative, the patients' characteristics, including numbers of *H. pylori* infection, mean ratio of Pepsinogen I/II, and numbers of peptic ulcer and gastritis with atrophy were shown in Table 1. The overall *H. pylori* infection rate was 63.4% and the mean Pepsinogen I/II ratio was 2.37. According to Updated Sydney Classification, 50 patients (31.5%) had moderate-to-severe antrum gastritis with atrophy, and 23 (14.0%) had moderate-to-severe body gastritis with atrophy. Compared to the body, the antrum had significantly higher percentage of gastritis with atrophy (Figure 3). The antrum also had significantly higher percentage of intestinal metaplasia (antrum 11.6% vs. body 0%, $p<0.001$).

Sensitivity of biopsy based tests and degree of gastritis of atrophy

Regardless of biopsy site, the biopsy specimens (n=328) were grouped according to the degree of gastritis with atrophy. Of these, 208 specimens were collected from the "defined infection" patients (Groups A and B). In these biopsy specimens, 101 had normal histology while 70 had mild, 34 had moderate, and 3 had severe gastritis with atrophy. The sensitivity of histology Giemsa stain and rapid urease test in these specimens were evaluated (Figure 4) As the degree of gastritis with atrophy progressed, the sensitivities of these two biopsy-based test decreased (sensitivity of histology Giemsa stain in normal, mild, moderate, and severe gastritis with atrophy was 100%, 100%, 88%, and 66%, respectively, while the sensitivity of rapid urease test was 100%, 97%, 91%, and 66%, respectively).

Sensitivity of biopsy based tests and biopsy sites

Using the pre-defined gold standard, the sensitivities and specificities of the diagnostic tests, depending on

Table 1 Demographic characteristics of patients (n=164)

Age-year, mean (range)	43.51	(20–70)
Gender-no. (%)		
Male	85	(51.8)
Female	79	(48.2)
PgI/PgII ratio (range)		
-Mean	2.37	(0.46–11.51)
H. pylori status		
Infection	104	(63.4)
Non-infection	60	(36.6)
Total histology		
specimens and *H. pylori* status		
Infection	208	(63.4)
Non infection	120	(36.6)
Peptic ulcer, no. (%)		
GU	7	(4.2)
DU	53	(32.3)
Antrum gastritis with atrophy		
Normal to mild	114	(69.5)
Moderate to severe	50	(31.5)
Body gastritis with atrophy		
Normal to mild	141	(86.0)
Moderate to severe	23	(14.0)
Antrum intestinal metaplasia		
Normal	145	(88.4)
Intestinal metaplasia	19	(11.6)
Body intestinal metaplasia		
Normal	164	(100.0)
Intestinal metaplasia	0	(0)

grade of antrum and body atrophy, were presented in Tables 2 and 3. In moderate to severe antrum gastritis with atrophy (n=50), single antrum biopsy for CLOtest yielded fair sensitivity (84%; 95% CI: 63.08-94.75%), which was lower than single body biopsy or combination of body and antrum (100%; 95% CI: 83.42-100%). There was a similar finding in histology (sensitivity of single antrum biopsy, 84% vs. 96% in single body biopsy or combination of body and antrum). However, when the degree of antrum gastritis with atrophy was normal-to-mild, the sensitivity of both biopsy-based tests, regardless of biopsy site, was between 97.47% and 100% (Table 2).

In moderate-to-severe body gastritis with atrophy (n=23), single antrum biopsy for CLOtest yielded fair sensitivity (83.33%; 95% CI: 50.88-97.06%), which was lower than single body biopsy or combination of body and antrum (100%; 95% CI: 69.87-100%). A similar finding was found in histology Giemsa stain (sensitivity of

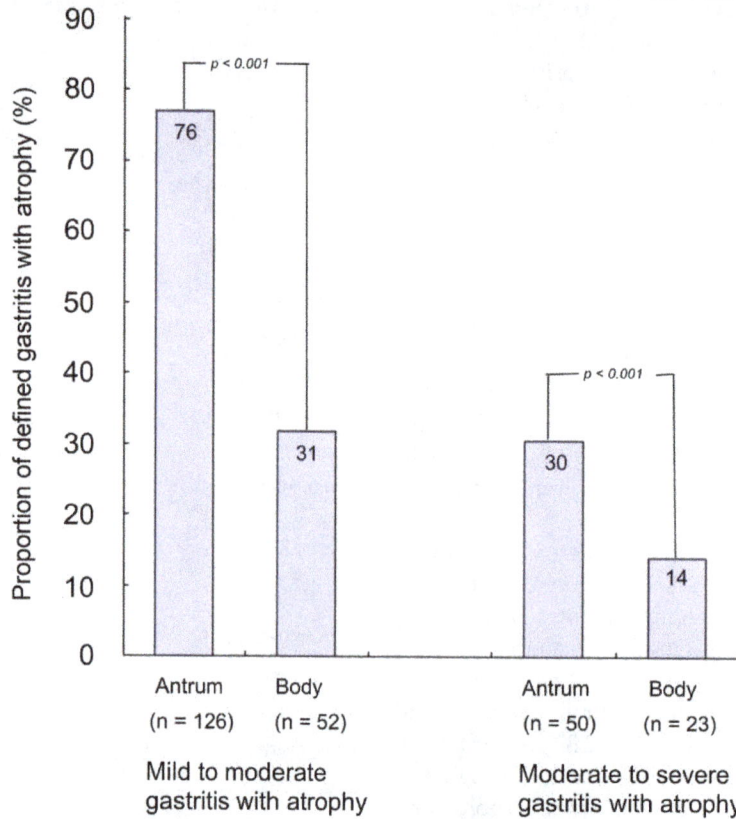

Figure 3 The proportion of mild-severe and moderate-severe gastritis with atrophy based on biopsy site. The *p* value was calculated using the chi-square test.

single antrum biopsy, 83.33% vs. 91.67% in single body biopsy or combination of body and antrum). However, when the degree of body gastritis with atrophy was normal to mild (n=141), the sensitivity of both biopsy based tests, regardless of biopsy site, was between 95.66% and 100% (Table 3).

The prevalence rate of *H. pylori* infection between normal, mild, moderate, and severe gastritis with atrophy were evaluated. As the degree of gastritis with atrophy increased, the prevalence rate of *H. pylori* infection decreased (Figure 5). As the degree of antrum gastritis with atrophy increased, the prevalence rate of *H. pylori* infection decreased significantly (*p*=0.027; chi-square test for trends). A similar trend was found in body gastritis with atrophy, with a trend of decreasing *H. pylori* infection rate (*p*=0.216).

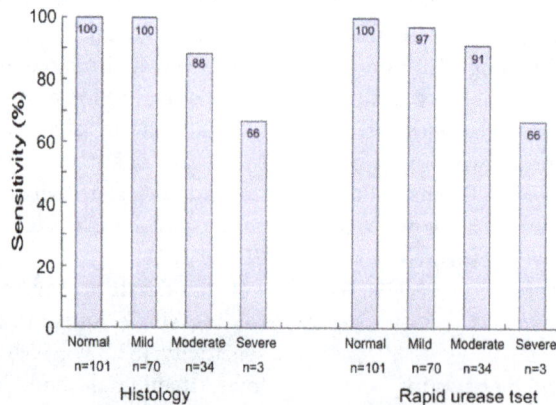

Figure 4 The sensitivity of biopsy-based tests (histology Giemsa stain and rapid urease test) according to grade of mucosal atrophy.

Table 2 *H. pylori* **sensitivity and specificity depending on the grade of antrum gastritis with atrophy**

Ca degree of gastritis with atrophy at antrum	Normal to mild	Moderate to severe
n=164	n=114	n=50
CLOtest Antrum		
Sensitivity	97.47 (90.31-99.56)	84.00 (63.08-94.75)
Specificity	100.00 (87.68-100.00)	100.00 (83.42-100.00)
PPV	100.00 (94.08-100.00)	100.00 (80.76-100.00)
NPV	94.59 (80.47-99.06)	86.20 (67.43-95.49)
Accuracy	98.25	
CLOtest Body		
Sensitivity	100.00 (94.22-100.00)	100.00 (83.42-100.00)
Specificity	100.00 (87.68-100.00)	100.00 (83.42-100.00)
PPV	100.00 (94.22-100.00)	100.00 (83.42-100.00)
NPV	100.00 (87.68-100.00)	100.00 (83.42-100.00)
Accuracy	100.00	100.00
CLOtest Antrum + Body		
Sensitivity	100.00 (94.22-100.00)	100.00 (83.42-100.00)
Specificity	100.00 (87.68-100.00)	100.00 (83.42-100.00)
PPV	100.00 (94.22-100.00)	100.00 (83.42-100.00)
NPV	100.00 (87.68-100.00)	100.00 (83.42-100.00)
Accuracy	100.00	100.00
Histology Antrum		
Sensitivity	98.73 (92.18-99.93)	84.00 (63.08-94.75)
Specificity	100.00 (87.68-100.00)	100.00 (83.42-100.00)
PPV	100.00 (94.15-100.00)	100.00 (80.76-100.00)
NPV	97.22 (83.80-99.85)	86.20 (67.43-95.49)
Accuracy	99.12	92.00
Histology Body		
Sensitivity	100.00 (94.22-100.00)	96.00 (77.68-99.79)
Specificity	100.00 (87.68-100.00)	100.00 (83.42-100.00)
PPV	100.00 (94.22-100.00)	100.00 (82.83-100.00)
NPV	100.00 (87.68-100.00)	96.15 (78.42-99.80)
Accuracy	100.00	98.00
Histology Antrum + Body		
Sensitivity	100.00 (94.22-100.00)	96.00 (77.68-99.79)
Specificity	100.00 (87.68-100.00)	100.00 (83.42-100.00)
PPV	100.00 (94.22-100.00)	100.00 (82.83-100.00)
NPV	100.00 (87.68-100.00)	96.15 (78.42-99.80)
Accuracy	100.00	98.00

Discussion

Biopsy-based tests are important diagnostic tools for *H. pylori*. However, the optimal biopsy site is still unknown, especially in cases of gastritis with atrophy. Current guidelines only recommend combining antrum and body biopsies for rapid urease test in the circumstance of antibiotics or proton pump inhibitors exposure. Sampling from the angularis, corpus, and antrum for histology was ever suggested in the same situation [16]. Reviewing recent studies, there is little practical information about the adequate biopsy numbers and suitable biopsy sites. Single and multiple specimens at the antrum alone, at the

Table 3 *H. pylori* **sensitivity and specificity depending on grade of body gastritis with atrophy**

Ca degree of gastritis with atrophy at body n=164	Normal to mild n=141	Moderate to severe n=23
CLOtest Antrum		
Sensitivity	95.66 (88.62-98.60)	83.33 (50.88-97.06)
Specificity	100.00 (90.94-100.00)	100.00 (67.86-100.00)
PPV	100.00 (94.79-100.00)	100.00 (65.55-100.00)
NPV	92.45 (80.93-97.55)	84.61 (53.66-97.29)
Accuracy	97.16	91.30
CLOtest Body		
Sensitivity	100.00 (95.00-100.00)	100.00 (69.87-100.00)
Specificity	100.00 (90.94-100.00)	100.00 (67.85-100.00)
PPV	100.00 (95.00-100.00)	100.00 (69.87-100.00)
NPV	100.00 (90.94-100.00)	100.00 (67.85-100.00)
Accuracy	100.00	100.00
CLOtest Antrum + Body		
Sensitivity	100.00 (95.00-100.00)	100.00 (69.87-100.00)
Specificity	100.00 (90.94-100.00)	100.00 (67.85-100.00)
PPV	100.00 (95.00-100.00)	100.00 (69.87-100.00)
NPV	100.00 (90.94-100.00)	100.00 (67.85-100.00)
Accuracy	100.00	100.00
Histology Antrum		
Sensitivity	96.74 (90.09-99.15)	83.33 (50.88-97.06)
Specificity	100.00 (90.94-100.00)	100.00 (67.86-100.00)
PPV	100.00 (94.84-100.00)	100.00 (65.55-100.00)
NPV	94.23 (83.08-98.50)	84.61 (53.66-97.29)
Accuracy	97.87	91.30
Histology Body		
Sensitivity	100.00 (95.00-100.00)	91.67 (59.75-99.56)
Specificity	100.00 (90.94-100.00)	100.00 (67.86-100.00)
PPV	100.00 (95.00-100.00)	100.00 (67.86-100.00)
NPV	100.00 (90.94-100.00)	91.67 (59.75-99.56)
Accuracy	100.00	95.65
Histology Antrum + Body		
Sensitivity	100.00 (95.00-100.00)	91.67 (59.75-99.56)
Specificity	100.00 (90.94-100.00)	100.00 (67.86-100.00)
PPV	100.00 (95.00-100.00)	100.00 (67.86-100.00)
NPV	100.00 (90.94-100.00)	91.67 (59.75-99.56)
Accuracy	100.00	95.65

body alone, or in combination of antrum and body had been described and applied (Table 4). These diagnostic approaches seem largely arbitrarily [8,16,19-28]. In order to clarify the exact benefit of these biopsy sites, a gold standard is necessary.

In 2009, Shin et al. modified *H. pylori* diagnostic methods and set a validated gold standard according to combination tests results [8]. Since the combination method is the preferred approach in patients with gastritis with atrophy, the defined gold standard may best correlate with active *H. pylori* infection. Our study follows this approach to determine the best biopsy site with highest sensitivity against a background of gastritis with atrophy.

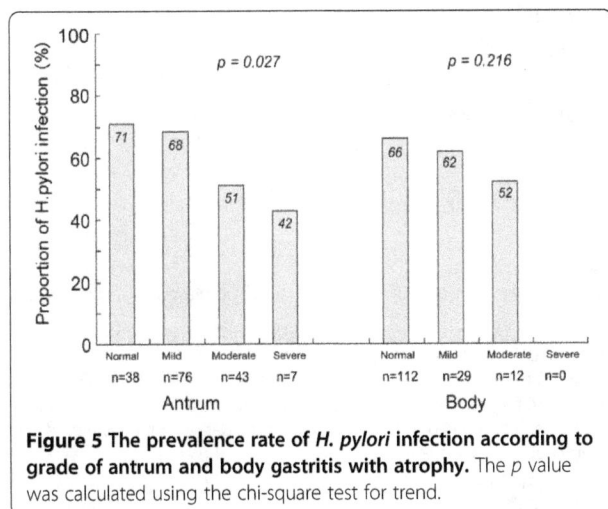

Figure 5 The prevalence rate of *H. pylori* infection according to grade of antrum and body gastritis with atrophy. The *p* value was calculated using the chi-square test for trend.

The present study has several findings. First, making a biopsy at the antrum increases the risk of obtaining atrophic gastric mucosa, which is associated higher frequency of false negative results. Second, when body gastritis with atrophy develops, antrum atrophy exists already. Third, antrum biopsy alone has decreased sensitivity when there is moderate-to-severe antrum gastritis with atrophy (CLOtest up to 16% and histology up to 12%) and moderate-to-severe body gastritis with atrophy (CLOtest up to 16.67% and histology up to 8.34%).

First, the frequency of antrum gastritis with atrophy is higher than that of the body. This is consistent with previous studies [22,29]. It is believed that gastritis with atrophy progresses from the antrum initially and extends to the body in the advanced stage [12,17,18]. Thus, the prevalence rate of antrum gastritis with atrophy is significantly higher than that of the body. As such, taking a biopsy at the antrum may yield higher chances of atrophic gastric mucosa than taking one from the body.

Regardless of biopsy site, if the degree of gastritis with atrophy in each specimen is considered, sensitivity decreases as the severity of gastritis with atrophy progresses (Figure 3). This is similar to the findings of Kim et al. [22]. These false negative subjects could be proven to be *H. pylori* infected after combining with other diagnostic methods. Such phenomenon is explained by the increasing rate of sampling error as gastritis with atrophy progresses [29]. Thus, biopsy at antrum increases the risk of getting atrophic gastric mucosa that is associated with higher frequency of false negatives.

Second, applying the aforementioned conclusion on biopsy site and on the degree of gastritis with atrophy, it is interesting to find an opposite results between antrum atrophy and body atrophy. Theoretically, biopsy site at the atrophic area yields poorer sensitivity so single antrum biopsy done in antrum atrophy subjects results in less sensitivity. However, this principle does not apply in single body biopsy performed in body atrophy cases. Instead, the present study reveals a general rule that antrum biopsy results in lower sensitivity in either antrum or body atrophy. This is because when body gastritis with atrophy occurs, antrum atrophy exists already [17,18,29]. In fact, most of the patients here with

Table 4 Studies on the diagnostic tests of *H. pylori* and the respective biopsy sites chosen, published between November 2005 and February 2011

Authors	Country and population studied	Sampling site of Histology stain	Sampling site of Rapid urease test	Age range of subjects (years)	Numbers of subjects	Numbers of *H. pylori*-positive %
Choi et al. [22]	Korea, health check-up examinees	*1LA1LB	1LA	Mean 47.8	515	53.2
Hsu et al. [23]	Taiwan, dyspepsia	-	1LA vs. 1LA1GB	Mean 55.0-57.8	355	33.5
Vaira et al. [24]	Italy, dyspepsia	2A	2A	Median 52	1000	45.3
Goh et al. [25]	Malaysia, dyspepsia	1A1B	1A1B	Mean 50.7	206	53.9
Shin et al. [8]	Korea, gastritis with atrophy	2A2B	1A1B	Mean 57.7	651	41.2
Siddique et al. [26]	Kuwait, endoscopy evaluation	-	1A vs. 2A vs. 3A vs. 4A	Mean 36.1	100	-
Yoo et al. [21]	Korea, dyspepsia	2A2B	1LA1LB	Mean 56.8	430	-
Yakoob et al. [27]	Pakistan, dyspepsia	2A	2A	Mean 43	109	57.0
Kim et al. [28]	Korea, gastric cancer	2LA2LB2GB	1GB	Median 61	194	84.0
Tang et al. [29]	Taiwan, bleeding	2B2U	2A	Mean 63.5	324	53.7
Roma-Giannikou et al. [30]	Greece	1A	1A	Mean 10.4	254	-
Chey et al. [15]	Guideline	1GA1GB1Ag	1AgB1GA	-	-	-

*1A, one piece from the antrum; 1B, one piece from the body; 2A2B, two pieces from the antrum and 2 from the body; 1LA, one piece from the lesser curvature of the antrum; 1LB, one piece from the lesser curvature of the body; 1GA, one piece from the great curvature of the antrum;1GB, one piece from the great curvature of the body; 1AgB, one piece from the body angularis; 2U, two pieces from the ulcer margin.

moderate-to-severe body atrophy (n=23) also have moderate-to-severe antrum atrophy (20/23).

Third, single body biopsy discloses an increased sensitivity as compared with single antrum biopsy in a background of moderate-to-severe antrum gastritis with atrophy (CLOtest up to 16% and histology up to 12%). Similar finding is founded when corpus biopsy is taken in moderate-to-severe body gastritis with atrophy (with a increased sensitivity in CLOtest up to 16.67% and histology up to 8.34%). In contrast, single antrum and single corpus has comparable sensitivity when gastritis with atrophy is normal-to-mild (CLOtest 97.47–95.66 and histology 96.74–98.73). Poor colonization of *H. pylori* in the atrophic mucosa and intestinal metaplasia have been well discussed [9,12]. When performing biopsy-based test in a background of gastritis with atrophy, sampling errors, insufficient bacterial load [9], bacterial migration, bacterial clearance [12], bacterial patchy distribution, and poor mucosal colonization in areas of intestinal metaplasia are common causes of false negative results. Furthermore, as the gastritis with atrophy progresses, the prevalence of *H. pylori* infection decreases. Single specimen sampling at the antrum may miss this relative small but risky patients. And this approach may miss those who could get benefit from eradication. Therefore, the present study recommends additional corpus biopsy to avoid false negative results in moderate-to-severe gastritis with atrophy.

This study has several potential limitations. First, it was conducted in a *H. pylori* endemic area, such that the interpretation and application of the study results should consider the local *H. pylori* prevalence rate. Second, in evaluating gastritis with atrophy by histology, the sampling method used was based on the modified Updated Sydney Classification. The latest approach method to evaluate gastritis with atrophy is OLGA staging, which is composed of multiple antrum and body biopsy specimens [30]. The average grade of antrum and body gastritis with atrophy in these specimens was evaluated while staging was based on the degree and extent of gastritis with atrophy. In this study, only one piece at the antrum and one at the body was used to represent the whole antrum and body mucosal condition. This may be inadequate. However, compared to histology, non-invasive methods like Pepsinogen I/II ratio also disclosed lower values in moderate-to-severe gastritis with atrophy (mean Pepsinogen I/II ratio, 1.96 in moderate-to-severe antrum gastritis with atrophy and 1.79 in moderate-to-severe body gastritis with atrophy). This may eliminate the concern of inadequate sampling in the present study. Third, though we used visual analogue scale to score the gastritis with atrophy, grading of antrum atrophy is most difficult for pathologists since kappa values are very low and this wound be our limitation [10].

Conclusion
Biopsy-based test should include corpus specimen in cases of moderate-to-severe gastritis with atrophy to avoid false negative results.

Abbreviations
H. pylori: Helicobacter pylori.

Competing interests
The authors have no potential conflicts (financial, professional, or personal).

Authors' contributions
HC Lin, TS Chen and HC Lan designed the project. TS Chen, FY Chang and AFY Lee performed the experiments. HC Lan wrote the manuscript. TS Chen and HC Lan contributed to the discussion of the data and the revision of the manuscript. All readers read and approved the final manuscript.

Authors' information
Writing Assistance: Gene Alzona Nisperos, MD.

Acknowledgments
This study was supported by the Taiwan Otsuka Pharmaceutical Company Ltd.

Author details
[1]Division of Gastroenterology, Department of Medicine, Taipei Veterans General Hospital and National Yang-Ming University, #201 Shih-Pai Road, Section 2, Taipei, Taiwan, ROC. [2]Department of Pathology and Laboratory Medicine, Taipei Veterans General Hospital and National Yang-Ming University, Taipei, Taiwan, ROC. [3]Division of General Medicine, Department of Medicine, Taipei City Hospital, Taipei, Taiwan, ROC.

References
1. Malfertheiner P, Megraud F, O'Morain CA, Atherton J, Axon AT, Bazzoli F, Gensini GF, Gisbert JP, Graham DY, Rokkas T, El-Omar EM, Kuipers EJ: **Management of *Helicobacter pylori* infection–the Maastricht IV/ Florence Consensus Report.** *Gut* 2012, **61**:646–664.
2. Kuipers EJ, Uyterlinde AM, Pena AS, Roosendaal R, Pals G, Nelis GF, Festen HP, Meuwissen SG: **Long-term sequelae of *Helicobacter pylori* gastritis.** *Lancet* 1995, **345**:1525–1528.
3. Ito M, Haruma K, Kamada T, Mihara M, Kim S, Kitadai Y, Sumii M, Tanaka S, Yoshihara M, Chayama K: ***Helicobacter pylori* eradication therapy improves atrophic gastritis and intestinal metaplasia: a 5-year prospective study of patients with atrophic gastritis.** *Aliment Pharmacol Ther* 2002, **16**:1449–1456.
4. Ohkusa T, Fujiki K, Takashimizu I, Kumagai J, Tanizawa T, Eishi Y, Yokoyama T, Watanabe M: **Improvement in atrophic gastritis and intestinal metaplasia in patients in whom *Helicobacter pylori* was eradicated.** *Ann Intern Med* 2001, **134**:380–386.
5. Rokkas T, Pistiolas D, Sechopoulos P, Robotis I, Margantinis G: **The long-term impact of *Helicobacter pylori* eradication on gastric histology: a systematic review and meta-analysis.** *Helicobacter* 2007, **12**(Suppl2):32–38.
6. Malfertheiner P, Megraud F, O'Morain C, Bazzoli F, El-Omar E, Graham D, Hunt R, Rokkas T, Vakil N, Kuipers EJ: **Current concepts in the management of *Helicobacter pylori* infection: the Maastricht III Consensus Report.** *Gut* 2007, **56**:772–781.
7. Malfertheiner P, Megraud F, O'Morain C, Hungin AP, Jones R, Axon A, Graham DY, Tytgat G: **Current concepts in the management of *Helicobacter pylori* infection–the Maastricht 2-2000 Consensus Report.** *Aliment Pharmacol Ther* 2002, **16**:167–180.
8. Shin CM, Kim N, Lee HS, Lee HE, Lee SH, Park YS, Hwang JH, Kim JW, Jeong SH, Lee DH, Jung HC, Song IS: **Validation of diagnostic tests for *Helicobacter pylori* with regard to grade of atrophic gastritis and/or intestinal metaplasia.** *Helicobacter* 2009, **14**:512–519.
9. Korstanje A, van Eeden S, Offerhaus GJ, Sabbe LJ, den Hartog G, Biemond I, Lamers CB: **The 13-carbon urea breath test for the diagnosis of

Helicobacter pylori infection in subjects with atrophic gastritis: evaluation in a primary care setting. *Aliment Pharmacol Ther* 2006, 24:643–650.

10. Dixon MF, Genta RM, Yardley JH, Correa P: Classification and grading of gastritis. The updated Sydney system. International workshop on the histopathology of gastritis, Houston 1994. *Am J Surg Pathol* 1996, 20:1161–1181.

11. Genta RM, Graham DY: Comparison of biopsy sites for the histopathologic diagnosis of *Helicobacter pylori*: a topographic study of *H. pylori* density and distribution. *Gastrointest Endosc* 1994, 40:342–345.

12. Satoh K, Kimura K, Taniguchi Y, Kihira K, Takimoto T, Saifuku K, Kawata H, Tokumaru K, Kojima T, Seki M, Ido K, Fujioka T: Biopsy sites suitable for the diagnosis of *Helicobacter pylori* infection and the assessment of the extent of atrophic gastritis. *Am J Gastroenterol* 1998, 93:569–573.

13. Van IMC, Laheij RJ, de Boer WA, Jansen JB: The importance of corpus biopsies for the determination of *Helicobacter pylori* infection. *Neth J Med* 2005, 63:141–145.

14. Hazell SL, Hennessy WB, Borody TJ, Carrick J, Ralston M, Brady L, Lee A: *Campylobacter pyloridis* gastritis II: distribution of bacteria and associated inflammation in the gastro-duodenal environment. *Am J Gastroenterol* 1987, 82:297–301.

15. Woo JS, El-Zimaity HM, Genta RM, Yousfi MM, Graham DY: The best gastric site for obtaining a positive rapid urease test. *Helicobacter* 1996, 1:256–259.

16. Chey WD, Wong BC: American college of gastroenterology guideline on the management of *helicobacter pylori* infection. *Am J Gastroenterol* 2007, 102:1808–1825.

17. Correa P: Chronic gastritis: a clinico-pathological classification. *Am J Gastroenterol* 1988, 83:504–509.

18. Kimura K: Chronological transition of the fundic-pyloric border determined by step-wise biopsy of the lesser and greater curvatures of the stomach. *Gastroenterology* 1972, 63:584–592.

19. Choi J, Kim CH, Kim D, Chung SJ, Song JH, Kang JM, Yang JI, Park MJ, Kim YS, Yim JY, Lim SH, Kim JS, Jung HC, Song IS: Prospective evaluation of a new stool antigen test for the detection of *Helicobacter pylori*, in comparison with histology, rapid urease test, (13)C-urea breath test, and serology. *J Gastroenterol Hepatol* 2011, 26:1053–1059.

20. Goh KL, Cheah PL, Navaratnam P, Chin SC, Xiao SD: HUITAI rapid urease test: a new ultra-rapid biopsy urease test for the diagnosis of *Helicobacter pylori* infection. *J Dig Dis* 2007, 8:139–142.

21. Hsu WH, Wang SS, Kuo CH, Chen CY, Chang CW, Hu HM, Wang JY, Yang YC, Lin YC, Wang WM, Wu DC, Wu MT, Kuo FC: Dual specimens increase the diagnostic accuracy and reduce the reaction duration of rapid urease test. *World J Gastroenterol* 2010, 16(23):2926–2930.

22. Kim CG, Choi IJ, Lee JY, Cho SJ, Nam BH, Kook MC, Hong EK, Kim YW: Biopsy site for detecting *Helicobacter pylori* infection in patients with gastric cancer. *J Gastroenterol Hepatol* 2009, 24:469–474.

23. Roma-Giannikou E, Roubani A, Sgouras DN, Panayiotou J, Van-Vliet C, Polyzos A, Roka K, Daikos G: Endoscopic tests for the diagnosis of *helicobacter pylori* infection in children: validation of rapid urease test. *Helicobacter* 2010, 15:227–232.

24. Siddique I, Al-Mekhaizeem K, Alateeqi N, Memon A, Hasan F: Diagnosis of *Helicobacter pylori* improving the sensitivity of CLOtest by increasing the number of gastric antral biopsies: *J Clin Gastroenterol* 2008, 42:356–360.

25. Tang JH, Liu NJ, Cheng HT, Lee CS, Chu YY, Sung KF, Lin CH, Tsou YK, Lien JM, Cheng CL: Endoscopic diagnosis of *Helicobacter pylori* infection by rapid urease test in bleeding peptic ulcers: a prospective case–control study. *J Clin Gastroenterol* 2009, 43:133–139.

26. Vaira D, Vakil N, Gatta L, Ricci C, Perna F, Saracino I, Fiorini G, Holton J: Accuracy of a new ultrafast rapid urease test to diagnose *Helicobacter pylori* infection in 1000 consecutive dyspeptic patients. *Aliment Pharmacol Ther* 2010, 31:331–338.

27. Yakoob J, Jafri W, Abid S, Jafri N, Abbas Z, Hamid S, Islam M, Anis K, Shah HA, Shaikh H: Role of rapid urease test and histopathology in the diagnosis of *Helicobacter pylori* infection in a developing country. *BMC Gastroenterol* 2005, 5:38.

28. Yoo JY, Kim N, Park YS, Hwang JH, Kim JW, Jeong SH, Lee HS, Choe C, Lee DH, Jung HC, Song IS: Detection rate of *Helicobacter pylori* against a background of atrophic gastritis and/or intestinal metaplasia. *J Clin Gastroenterol* 2007, 41:751–755.

29. Kang HY, Kim N, Park YS, Hwang JH, Kim JW, Jeong SH, Lee DH, Jung HC, Song IS: Progression of atrophic gastritis and intestinal metaplasia drives *Helicobacter pylori* out of the gastric mucosa. *Dig Dis Sci* 2006, 51:2310–2315.

30. Rugge M, Meggio A, Pennelli G, Piscioli F, Giacomelli L, De Pretis G, Graham DY: Gastritis staging in clinical practice: the OLGA staging system. *Gut* 2007, 56:631–636.

14

Low rate of recurrence of *Helicobacter Pylori* infection in spite of high clarithromycin resistance in Pakistan

Javed Yakoob[1], Shahab Abid[1*], Wasim Jafri[1], Zaigham Abbas[1], Khalid Mumtaz[1], Saeed Hamid[1] and Rashida Ahmed[2]

Abstract

Background: The aim was to investigate the reinfection rate of *H. pylori* during a follow-up period of 12 months in adults who had undergone eradication therapy.

Methods: One hundred-twenty patients; 116 with gastritis, 3 with duodenal ulcer and 1 gastric ulcer, were studied. Their mean age was 41 ± 13 years (range 18–77) and male: female ratio of 2:1. *H. pylori* were cultured and antibiotic sensitivity was determined by Epsilometer test (E-test) for clarithromycin (CLR) and amoxicillin (AMX). Primers of *urease C* gene of *H. pylori* and Sau-3 and Hha I restriction enzymes were used for polymerase chain reaction-restriction fragment length polymorphism analysis (PCR-RFLP). ^{14}C urea breath test (^{14}C-UBT) was performed 4 weeks after the eradication therapy. The successfully treated patients were observed for 12 months with ^{14}C-UBT to assess *H. pylori* status. If ^{14}C-UBT was negative, it was repeated after every 12 weeks. If ^{14}C-UBT was positive, endoscopy was repeated with biopsies.

Result: The eradication therapy was successful in 102(85%) patients. Out of forty-seven *H. pylori* isolates cultured, clarithromycin sensitivity was present in 30(64%) and amoxicillin in 45(98%), respectively. Follow-up ^{14}C-urea breath tests of all 102 patients who eradicated *H. pylori* remained negative up to 9 months. However, in 6 patients, the ^{14}C-UBT confirmed recurrence at 12 months. The recurrence rate was 6%.

Conclusion: A low rate of recurrence of *H. pylori* infection was found in patients with dyspeptic symptoms. *H. pylori* isolates demonstrated a high invitro clarithromycin resistance.

Keywords: *Helicobacter pylori*, Clarithromycin resistance, Recurrence, Nonulcer dyspepsia

Background

Helicobacter pylori (*H. pylori*) is a Gram negative microorganism that has been categorized as a class I carcinogen [1]. It is associated with gastritis, gastric and duodenal ulcers, gastric adenocarcinoma, and mucosa-associated lymphoid tissue lymphoma [2]. Long term chronic gastritis associated with *H. pylori* is known to progress to glandular atrophy and intestinal metaplasia (IM) over a period of 12 years [3]. *Helicobacter pylori* gastritis may lead to multifocal atrophy and IM, gradually expanding from the antrum to the body [3]. A long term study with five year

follow up from China have reported no change in the degree of intestinal metaplasia (IM) and atrophy after successful eradication [3]. In other long term randomized controlled trials there was a significant regression of preneoplastic lesions such as atrophy and IM among those who had cleared the infection after five to six years of follow up [4,5]. A definite cure of peptic ulcer disease and prevention of ulcer complications, as well as cure of mucosa-associated lymphoid tissue (MALT) lymphoma is dependent on successful eradication of *H. pylori*.

Recurrence of *H. pylori* after a successful eradication is rare in developed countries and more frequent in developing countries [6]. Recrudescence is recolonization of the same strain while reinfection is colonization with a new strain. Reinfection is considered to be more likely

* Correspondence: shahab.abid@aku.edu
[1]Department of Medicine, Aga Khan University, Stadium Road, Karachi 74800, Pakistan
Full list of author information is available at the end of the article

to be responsible for most of the cases [6]. This differentiation is difficult and requires utilization of molecular fingerprinting techniques to confirm that the identified bacteria, before and after therapy, are genetically identical [7]. Recrudescence results from treatment failure while reinfection is considered a problem of heavy *H. pylori* contamination of the environment, drinking water, institutionalized patients, medical personnel or family members, especially in developing countries [6]. In developing countries, *H. pylori* infection is widespread.

Regional studies available from Bangladesh, India and Iran have shown varied recurrence rates [8-10]. In a recent study in Karachi in apparently healthy children, *H. pylori* seroprevalence in children aged 11–15 years was 54% [11]. *H. pylori* seropositivity increased with age and in low-middle socioeconomic status [11]. However, local studies addressing the issue of recurrence of *H. pylori* are not available. In this study we investigated the recurrence rate of *H. pylori* during a follow-up period of 12 months in adults who had undergone eradication therapy.

Methods

Patients

One hundred-twenty consecutive patients with dyspepsia attending the endoscopy suite of gastroenterology section of Aga Khan University Hospital were enrolled from April 2008–June 2010. There were eighty males and forty females (age range 17–80 years, mean age 41 ± 13 years; Table 1). An informed consent was taken from all patients and the Aga Khan University ethics review committee approved the study. Only those who were willing to comply with the follow-up schedule and gave informed consent were enrolled in the study. Pregnant and lactating women, patients with esophageal or gastric tumors and patients with liver cirrhosis and esophageal varices were excluded. In addition, those who had received antisecretory drugs, antibiotics, nonsteroidal anti-inflammatory drugs, corticosteroids or bismuth-containing drugs during the preceding 8 weeks were also excluded. All the patients were native residents of the city. Endoscopic examination was conducted using Olympus video endoscopes (Olympus Tokyo, Japan), and the presence of lesions in the esophageal and gastroduodenal mucosa was noted. Gastric biopsy specimens were obtained three each from the antrum and corpus for rapid urease test (RUT), histology, culture and PCR for *H. pylori* urease C gene. The biopsies from the antrum were obtained 2–3 cm from the pylorus, and from the body, midway between the antral-body junction and the cardia. Patients who were positive for *H. pylori* infection by means of ^{14}C-UBT with RUT or histology received treatment comprising of a proton pump inhibitor (esomeprazole) 20 mg BD (twice a day) for 10 days and clarithromycin 500 mg BD and amoxicillin 500 mg BD

Table 1 Patients characteristics

Age (years)	
Mean ± SD	41 ± 13
Range	18-77
Gender	
Male	80(67)*
Female	40(33)
Diagnosis	
Gastritis	116(97)
Gastric ulcer	1(1)
Duodenal ulcer	3(2)
Histology	
Grade 1	61(51)
Grade 2	54(45)
Grade 3	5(4)
Antibiotic susceptibility pattern	**n = 47**
Clarithromycin	
Sensitive	30(64)
Resistance	17(36)
Amoxicillin	
Sensitive	45(96)
Resistance	2(4)
***H. pylori* DNA fingerprint (PCR-RFLP)**	
Same on both sides	102(85)
Different on both sides	18(15)

*n (%) = number and percentage.

for 7 days. Two weeks after completion of treatment, ^{14}C-UBT was performed to document eradication of *H. pylori* infection. Patients with positive ^{14}C-UBT were excluded from the study while those with negative were followed up every 3 months by a ^{14}C-UBT for 12 months until it tested positive and was followed by endoscopy and biopsy.

Sample size

The required sample size is 103 individuals, calculated on the basis of an estimated prevalence of reinfection of 13% and bound on error of estimation specified to be at the most .065 (6.5%) and a confidence level of 95% [8].

Rapid urease test

The tissue specimens were used for the RUT (Pronto dry, Medical Instrument Corp, France) consisting of a dry filter paper enriched with urea, phenol red (a pH indicator), buffers and a bacteriostatic agent in a sealed plastic slide [12]. *H. pylori* urease enzyme present in the biopsy tissue sample decomposed urea to cause a pH rise that changed color of the dot from yellow to a bright magenta. Pronto Dry results were read in 30 minutes and one hour. The color change from yellow to pink was considered a positive result and no color change as negative for Pronto Dry.

Histological analysis

Formalin-fixed and paraffin-embedded gastric biopsy specimens were routinely processed. Gastritis activity was graded on a four-point scale of none (grade 0), mild (grade 1), moderate (grade 2), and severe (grade 3) according to the guidelines of the Sydney system [13]. The presence of H. pylori was assessed on modified Giemsa-stained sections.

^{14}C- Urea breath test

Patients swallowed 37 kBq (1 μCi) of an encapsulated form of 14C-urea/citric acid composition (Helicap, Noster System AB, Sweden) with water after endoscopy [14]. Breath samples were collected with a special dry cartridge system (Heliprobe Breath Card, Noster System AB, Sweden) after 10 min. Patients exhaled gently into the cartridge mouthpiece until the indicator membrane changed in color from orange to yellow. Breath card was inserted into a β-scintillation counter (Heliprobe-analyser, Noster System AB Stockholm, Sweden) and activity was counted for 250 s. Results were expressed both as counts per minute (HCPM) and as grade (0: not infected, CPM < 25; 1: equivocal, CPM 25–50; 2: infected, CPM > 50), which was suggested by the manufacturer according to the counts obtained from the cartridges. Grades 0 and 1 were considered negative for the detection of H. pylori. In a previous study the accuracy of ^{14}C-UBT was compared to histology and RUT. Accuracy of ^{14}C-UBT was 93% in comparison with histology while its positive and negative predictive values were 97% and 84%, respectively [14]. Comparison of ^{14}C-UBT with RUT gives an accuracy of 96%, with positive and negative predictive values of 95% and 97%, respectively [14].

Culture and identification of H. pylori

The specimens were transported immediately in sterile phosphate buffered saline to isolate H. pylori. Thus, within three hours of collection each specimen was homogenized and the resulting suspension was inoculated onto Columbia Blood Agar (Oxoid) medium and Dents supplement (containing vancomycin, trimethoprim and polymyxin) and incubated at 37°C under microaerophilic conditions for 4–7 days. Plates were then examined for bacterial growth and typical colonies were selected for identification. The identity of H. pylori was confirmed by Gram stain, urease and catalase test. One half of the homogenate was used for culture, and the other half was kept at −80°C for future DNA extraction. H. pylori isolates were defined as gram-negative spiral-shaped bacilli that were catalase positive and rapidly (less than 1 h)

urease positive. H. pylori NCTC 11637 (type strain) was used as a positive control for the culture conditions and identification tests.

Antibiotic susceptibility testing

Antibiotic susceptibility was determined on Mueller Hinton agar (Oxoid, UK) containing 10% defibrinated sheep blood and a cell suspension calibrated at 3 McFarland units by the Epsilometer (E-test) using clarithromycin and amoxicillin E-test strips (AB Biodisk, Solna, Sweden). Plates were read after 3 days of incubation at 37°C. The tests were carried out according to the manufacturer's instructions. H. pylori NCTC 11637 was used as a sensitive control.

Extraction of genomic DNA

DNA was extracted from gastric tissue as described before [15]. Samples were stored at −20°C before PCR amplification was performed. DNA content and purity was determined by measuring the absorbance at 260 nm and 280 nm using a spectrophotometer (Beckman DU-600, USA).

PCR amplification for H. pylori ure C gene

PCR was performed using extracted DNA as the template and urease gene C for primers. Forward primer (5'-TGGGACTGATGGCGTGAGGG-3') and reverse primer (5'-AAGGGCGTTTTTAGATTTTT-3') were prepared from the urease gene sequence according to the report of Labigne et al. [16]. PCR amplification was carried out in a total volume of 50 μL containing 2 μL of 2 mmol/L dNTPs, 1 μL containing 50 pmol of primer 1, 1 μL containing 50 pmol of primer 2 (synthesized by ABI Automatic synthesizer), 1 unit of Taq DNA polymerase (Promega), 5 μL of 10 × PCR reaction buffer, 3 mmol/L of MgCl$_2$, 2 μL of DNA template containing 0.5 ng of extracted DNA and total volume rounded to 50 μL by double distilled water. The reaction was carried out in a Perkin Elmer 9700 thermal cycler. The amplification cycle consisted of an initial denaturation of target DNA at 95°C for 5 min and then denaturation at 94°C for 1 min, primer annealing at 56°C for 1 min and extension at 72°C for 1 min. The final cycle included an extension step for 5 min at 72°C to ensure full extension of the product. Samples were amplified through 35 consecutive cycles. Negative reagent control reactions were performed with each batch of amplifications, consisting of tubes containing distilled water in place of the DNA samples. Five μL of PCR product was electrophoresed on a 1.5% agarose gel to ensure homogeneity and yield. PCR amplification resulted in a homogeneous DNA fragment of the expected size of 820 bp for ure C gene.

PCR-RFLP

The amplified products obtained by PCR were subjected to restriction endonuclease digestion for 2 hours at 37°C in 20 microliter (µl) volume, as recommended [17]. The digested samples were analyzed by agarose gel (3%, wt/volume) electrophoresis. Restriction enzyme Sau-3 (5U) and Hha I (5 U), (New England Biolabs) were used on the basis of sequence data available for this amplified product. The restriction enzyme HhaI recognized on the 820-bp *UreC* gene amplified PCR product restriction site 5'...GCG$^\downarrow$ C ...3' giving 2 fragments varying in size from 100 bps to 550 bps and showing 4 band patterns while restriction enzyme Sau3A1 recognized site 5'...$^\downarrow$ GATC..3'giving 3 fragments ranging in size from 50 bps to 600 bps having 7 bands patterns, respectively. RFLP analysis by HhaI and Sau 3A together generated eleven distinguishable digestion patterns. Small variations (<10 bps) in the size of the restriction fragments were not considered a different pattern. In case of an identical restriction pattern from antrum and body, the patient was considered to have an infection by the same *H. pylori* strain while by restriction fragments that exceeded amplified fragment size and yielded different restriction fragments, patient was considered to be infected by different *H. pylori* strains.

Statistical assessment

The statistical package for social science SPSS (Release 16, standard version, copyright © SPSS; 1989–2007) was used for data analysis. The descriptive analysis was done for demographic and clinical features. Results were presented as mean ± standard deviation for quantitative variables and number (percentage) for qualitative variables. Differences in proportion were assessed by using Pearson Chi square, Fisher exact or likelihood ratio test where appropriate. P value less than 0.05 was considered as statistically significant, all *p* values were two sided.

Results

All one hundred-twenty patients with *H. pylori* infection had positive ^{14}C-UBT. Rapid urease test was positive in 116 out of 120 (97%) and negative in 4 out of 120 (3%). Histology demonstrated *H. pylori* associated gastritis in 114 out of 120 (95%) and nonspecific gastritis in 6(5%).

Four patients negative by RUT had positive C-14 UBT and *H. pylori* positive gastritis while six patients demonstrating nonspecific gastritis had positive ^{14}C-UBT and RUT. The distribution of negative RUT ($p = 1$ and $p = 0.69$) and histology ($p = 0.600$ and $p = 0.095$) for *H. pylori* infection were not associated with age and gender.

Recurrence of H. pylori after successful eradication

One hundred-twenty patients had positive ^{14}C-UBTs on initial visit. After treatment 18 out of 120 (15%) were still positive and were excluded from the study. At 12 months, the ^{14}C-UBT confirmed recurrence in six patients. No statistically significant difference was seen for sex (Fisher's Exact Test $p = 1$) or age ($p = 0.697$). All cases of recurrence were from the local population. They were diagnosed as having non-ulcer dyspepsia (NUD) with evidence of endoscopic gastritis and mild to moderate chronic active gastritis on histology (Table 2). In the follow-up period, none of the 3(3%) duodenal ulcer patients with successful eradication had any symptoms suggesting ulcer though we did not do repeat endoscopy in these patients.

PCR-based RFLP analysis

In 103 of 120 isolates (86%), we demonstrated the same DNA fingerprint from isolates from the antrum and mid-body gastric sites, and the patterns were different in 17(14%). Six of the 102 patients had recurrence of *H. pylori* during the follow-up period after treatment. Five of these 6 patients were previously documented to have colonization by multiple *H. pylori* isolates while in one patient a single *H. pylori* isolate was present on antrum and corpus. Following recurrence, 4 out of 6 patients had colonization by multiple *H. pylori* isolates and 2 single *H. pylori* isolate on antrum and body.

Antibiotic susceptibility of H. pylori isolates

Forty-seven *H. pylori* isolates were cultured from pretreatment biopsies. *H. pylori* culture was negative from both antrum and corpus in patient having a positive ^{14}C-UBT at 12 month and follow up endoscopic with biopsies. Clarithromycin sensitivity was present in 30 out of 47 (64%) and amoxicillin in 45 out of 47 (98%), respectively (Table 2).

Table 2 Comparison of histology with diagnosis, bacterial colonization and antibiotic susceptibility

| | Diagnosis | | | H. pylori DNA fingerprint | | Clarithromycin | | | Amoxicillin | |
	Gastritis	Gastric Ulcer	Duodenal ulcer	Same on both sides	Different on both sides	Sensitive	Resistant	P	Sensitive	Resistant
Histology										
Grade 1	60(52)	0(0)	1(33)	48(47)	13(72)	12(40)	11(65)		22(49)	1(50)
Grade 2	51(44)	1(100)	2(67)	49(48)	5(28)	18(60)	5(29)		22(49)	1(50)
Grade 3	5(4)	0(0)	0(0)	5(5)	0(0)	0(0)	1(6)		1(2)	0(0)

*n (%) = number and percentage.

Comparison of antibiotic susceptibility and H. pylori DNA fingerprint at gastric site

H. pylori DNA fingerprints were different in antrum and corpus in 3(10%) out of 30 CLR sensitive strains compared to 10(59%) out of 17 CLR resistance *H. pylori* strains ($p = 0.001$).

By RFLP 18 patients had different DNA fingerprints in the antrum and corpus (Table 2). Of these 18 patients, *H. pylori* could be cultured from only 13 patients. Clarithromycin resistance was demonstrated by 10 out of 13 *H. pylori* isolates while 3 out of 13 were sensitive to CLR.

Comparison of histology with diagnosis and antibiotic susceptibility

The degree of gastric inflammation in majority of patients varied from grade 1 to 2 (Table 2). It was not significantly associated with diagnosis ($p = 0.66$) (Table 2). Grades of inflammation were equally associated with same or different *H. pylori* DNA fingerprints in antrum and corpus ($p = 0.08$) (Table 2). Eleven out of 17 (65%) *H. pylori* strains demonstrating CLR resistance were associated with grade 1 inflammation ($p = 0.06$) while grade 1 to 2 inflammation were equally associated with AMX resistance ($p = 0.957$), respectively (Table 2).

Discussion and conclusion

The results of this prospective study showed that rate of *H. pylori* recurrence after apparently successful eradication was low. Majority of our patients remained infection free at nine months and recurrence followed in about 6% at the end of one year. All the patients with recurrence had NUD while none occurred in cases with duodenal ulcer. Clarithromycin resistance was high in our *H. pylori* isolates and low for amoxicillin. Antibiotic susceptibility pattern was not found to be related to age and gender in this study. About 14% of our patients demonstrated colonization by multiple *H. pylori* strains. Clarithromycin resistance was associated with different *H. pylori* strains at different gastric sites as suggested by DNA fingerprinting. However, the technique used in this study looked at only one gene, and generated as few as 2 or 3 bands in some strains, making it a rather low resolution technique to declare a strain identical. Strains may show identical banding patterns in the RFLP sites in one gene, yet differ elsewhere. Furthermore, it is possible that in some subjects, the infection was eradicated, yet the subject was reinfected from family members with an identical or near-identical strain, which would be interpreted as recrudescence.

Most studies from developed countries reported less than 1% rate of *H. pylori* infection recurrence whereas relatively higher rates have been reported from developing countries [18]. True re-infection of *H. pylori* is defined as where tests for *H. pylori* infection stay negative for 12 months after eradication, and become positive again at a later stage. This is probably a rare event in developed countries. A study from the Netherlands [19] showed that at 6 years after successful triple therapy the recurrence rate of *H. pylori* infection was very low (0.19% per patient year). Recurrence rate is higher in developing countries. In a study from Bangladesh, recrudescence, associated with nitroimidazole-based treatment, occurred in 15 of 105 patients (13%) within the first 3 months while the annual reinfection rate was 13%, based on a total follow-up of 84.7 patient years [8]. Data from India on reinfection of *H. pylori* after eradication showed that the risk is low in Indian subjects at the end of one year. The eradication rate with the four-drug regimen was 89.1% (41/46). Four of the 5 nonresponders eradicated *H. pylori* with the second regimen. At the end of median one year follow-up (range 9–15 - months), one of the 45 patients (2.4%) who eradicated the organism developed reinfection; none of the 46 patients who were initially *H. pylori*-negative acquired new infection [9]. In Iran, 37 patients, aged 5 to 17 years, treated with triple omeprazole based regimen the reinfection rate of *H. pylori* was determined during a follow up period of 12 months. After eradication therapy of *H. pylori*, 34 patients had a negative repeat ^{13}C-UBT. Reinfection occurred in 5 (14.7%) patients [10].

The recurrence rate of 6% in our study is similar to that reported from Chile and China (4.2% /yr. and 1.08% /yr., respectively) [20,21]. It is, however, less than that reported in Korea (13%) [22] and Bangladesh (13%). This discrepancy might be explained by the fact that criteria to define eradication of infection, number of patients studied, and time of follow-up varied from one study to another [8,20-22]. Increased susceptibility of hosts to *H. pylori* infection and re-exposure to *H. pylori* are proposed to be the major requirements for re-infection of *H. pylori* [23,24]. Poor sanitation practices in the developing countries result in contamination of the environment with *H. pylori*, such as in drinking water, practice of eating uncooked vegetables; crowded living conditions thatl contribute to re-exposure to *H. pylori* infection and result in high prevalence of *H. pylori* infection [25-27]. Genetic factors may also play a role in re-infection of *H. pylori* infection after successful eradication. Susceptible individuals who have had *H. pylori* eradicated may be prone to re-infection with the bacterium when they are exposed to *H. pylori*-positive persons [28]. Self-prescription is also common in developing countries as medications are sold without prescriptions by pharmacies [29]. Most reports on antimicrobial therapy of *H.pylori* propose that antibiotic overuse selects for resistant strains as they eradicate the susceptible *H. pylori* population, and resistant survivors replace them as a resistant majority [30-33]. The resistance trait could be spread horizontally by plasmids to other bacterial population. Emergence of a resistance phenotype is a short-term phenomenon that takes 4 – 5 - years to emerge and the driving force is the indiscriminate, short-interval and frequent use of antibiotics [33-35]. Clarithromycin resistance rate was high in *H. pylori* isolates probably contributed to by use of this drug for other indications in the community and this might result in selection of stable macrolide-resistant *H.pylori* and indigenous microbiota [36]. Also, previously a low cure rate and a higher resistance to clarithromycin were observed among *H. pylori* positive patients with functional dyspepsia than that in peptic ulcer disease [37-39]. In an earlier study, we reported treatment failure was associated with younger mean age, *cagA* negativity and point mutations in *23S rRNA* gene of *H. pylori* [40]. In conclusion, in spite of having a high prevalence of *H. pylori* there is a low incidence of recurrence of *H. pylori* infection in our population once eradication has been achieved. In view of high CLR resistance, judicious use of antibiotics should follow in general.

Competing interest
The authors declare that they have no competing interests.

Authors' contributions
SA and JY conceived and designed the study, JY did the work; SA, JY, ZAB, KM, WJ and SH coordinated the study, RA did the histopathology; JY, SA and ZA analyzed the data, JY performed the statistical analysis. JY wrote the manuscript. All authors read and approved the final manuscript.

Acknowledgement
The work was supported by research grants from Aga Khan University Research Committee to SA. We are grateful to staff members at the Juma Research Laboratory, Aga Khan University for their assistance during this work.

Author details
[1]Department of Medicine, Aga Khan University, Stadium Road, Karachi 74800, Pakistan. [2]Department of Pathology, Aga Khan University, Stadium Road, Karachi 74800, Pakistan.

References
1. Anon: NIH consensus conference. *Helicobacter pylori* in peptic ulcer disease. NIH consensus development panel on helicobacter pylori in peptic ulcer disease. *JAMA* 1994, **272**:65–69.
2. Sipponen P: Gastric cancer: a long term consequence of *H. pylori* infection? *Scand J Gastroenterol* 1994, **29**:24–27.
3. Mera R, Fontham ET, Bravo LE, Bravo JC, Piazuelo MB, Camargo MC, Correa P: Long term follow up of patients treated for *helicobacter pylori* infection. *Gut* 2005, **54**:1536–1540.
4. Kyzekova J, Mour J: The effect of eradication therapy on histological changes in the gastric mucosa in patients with non-ulcer dyspepsia and *helicobacter pylori* infection. Prospective randomized intervention study. *Hepatogastroenterology* 1999, **46**:2048–2056.
5. Larkin CJ, Watson P: Gastric corpus atrophy following eradication of *helicobacter pylori*. *Eur J Gastroenterol Hepatol* 2001, **13**:377–382.
6. Niv Y: *H. pylori* recurrence after successful eradication. *World J Gastroenterol* 2008, **14**:1477–1478.
7. Yakoob J, Hu G, Fan X, Zhang Z: *Helicobacter pylori* detection in Chinese subjects: a comparison of two common DNA fingerprinting methods. *Br J Biomed Sci* 2001, **58**:239–243.
8. Hildebrand P, Bardhan P, Rossi L, Parvin S, Rahman A, Arefin MS, Hasan M, Ahmad MM, Glatz-Krieger K, Terracciano L, Bauerfeind P, Beglinger C, Gyr N, Khan AK: Recrudescence and reinfection with *helicobacter pylori* after eradication therapy in Bangladeshi adults. *Gastroenterology* 2001, **121**:792–798.
9. Bapat MR, Abraham P, Bhandarkar PV, Phadke AY, Joshi AS: Acquisition of *helicobacter pylori* infection and reinfection after its eradication are uncommon in Indian adults. *Indian J Gastroenterol* 2000, **19**:172–174.
10. Najafi M, Sobhani M, Khodadad A, Farahmand F, Motamed F: Reinfection rate after successful *helicobacter pylori* eradication in children. *Iranian J Pediatrics* 2010, **2**:58–62.
11. Jafri W, Yakoob J, Abid S, Siddiqui S, Awan S, Nizami SQ: *Helicobacter pylori* infection in children: population-based age-specific prevalence and risk factors in a developing country. *Acta Paediatr* 2010, **99**:279–282.
12. Morio O, Rioux-Leclercq N, Pagenault M, Corbinais S, Ramee MP, Gosselin M, Bretagne JF: Prospective evaluation of a new rapid urease test (pronto dry) for the diagnosis of *helicobacter pylori* infection. *Gastroenterol Clin Biol* 2004, **28**:6–7.
13. Price AB: The Sydney System: histological division. *J Gastroenterol Hepatol* 1991, **6**:209–222.
14. Rasool S, Abid S, Jafri W: Validity and cost comparison of 14 carbon urea breath test for diagnosis of *H. pylori* in dyspeptic patients. *World J Gastroenterol* 2007, **13**:925–929.
15. Van Zwet AA, Thijs C, Kooistra-Smid AM, Schirm J, Snijder JAM: Sensitivity of culture compared with that of polymerase chain reaction for detection of *Helicobacter pylori* from antral biopsy samples. *J Clin Microbiol* 1993, **31**:1918–1920.
16. Labigne A, Cussac V, Courcoux P: Shuttle cloning and nucleotide sequences of *helicobacter pylori* genes responsible for urease activity. *J Bacteriol* 1991, **173**:1920–1931.
17. Fujimoto S, Marshall B, Blaser M: PCR-based restriction fragment length polymorphism typing of *helicobacter pylori*. *J Clin Microbiol* 1994, **32**:331–334.
18. Zhang YY, Xia HH, Zhuang ZH, Zhong J: True re-infection of Helicobacter pylori after successful eradication–worldwide annual rates, risk factors and clinical implications. *Aliment Pharmacol Ther* 2009, **29**:145–160.
19. Van der Wouden EJ, Thijs JC, van Zwet AA, Kleibeuker JH: Six-year follow-up after successful triple therapy for *helicobacter pylori* infection in patients with peptic ulcer disease. *Eur J Gastroenterol Hepatol* 2000, **13**:1235–1239.
20. Rollan A, Giancaspero R, Fuster F, Acevedo C, Figueroa C, Hola K, Schulz M, Duarte I: The long-term reinfection rate and the course of duodenal ulcer disease after eradication of *helicobacter pylori* in a developing country. *Am J Gastroenterol* 2000, **95**:50–56.
21. Mitchell HM, Hu P, Chi Y, Chen MH, Li YY, Hazell SL: A low rate of reinfection following effective therapy against *helicobacter pylori* in a developing nation (china). *Gastroenterology* 1998, **114**:256–260.
22. Kim N, Lim SH, Lee KH, Jung HC, Song IS, Kim CY: *Helicobacter pylori* reinfection rate and duodenal ulcer recurrence in Korea. *J Clin Gastroenterol* 1998, **27**:321–326.
23. Xia HH, Talley NJ: Natural acquisition and spontaneous elimination of *helicobacter pylori* infection. *Am J Gastroenterol* 1997, **92**:1780–1787.
24. Xia HH, Talley NJ, Keane CT, O'Morain CA: Recurrence of *helicobacter pylori* infection after successful eradication: nature, possible causes and potential preventive strategies. *Digest Dis Sci* 1997, **42**:1821–1834.
25. Hulten K, Han SW, Enroth H, Klein PD, Opekun AR, Gilman RH, Evans DG, Engstrand L, Graham DY, El-Zaatari FA: *Helicobacter pylori* in the drinking water in Peru. *Gastroenterology* 1996, **110**:1031–1035.
26. Klein PD, Graham DY, Gaillour A, Opekun AR, Smith EO: Water source as risk factor of *helicobacter pylori* infection in Peruvian children. *Lancet* 1991, **337**:1503–1506.
27. Hopkins RJ, Vial PA, Ferreccio C, Ovalle J, Prado P, Sotomayor V, Russell RG, Wasserman SS, Morris JG Jr: Seroprevalence of *helicobacter pylori* in Chile: vegetable s may serve as one route of transmission. *J Infect Dis* 1993, **168**:222–226.
28. Azuma T, Konishi J, Tanaka Y, Hirai M, Ito S, Kato T, Kohli Y: Contribution of HLA-DQA gene to host's response against *helicobacter pylori*. *Lancet* 1994, **343**:542–543.
29. Sturm AW, van der Pol R, Smits AJ, van Hellemondt FM, Mouton SW, Jamil B, Minai AM, Sampers GH: Over-the-counter availability of antimicrobial agents, self-medication and patterns of resistance in Karachi, Pakistan. *J Antimicrob Chemother* 1997, **39**:543–547.

30. Yakoob J, Jafri W, Abid S, Jafri N, Abbas Z, Hamid S, Islam M, Anis K, Shah HA, Shaikh H: **Role of rapid urease test and histopathology in the diagnosis of** *helicobacter pylori* **infection in a developing country.** *BMC Gastroenterol* 2005, **5**:38.

31. Sharara AI, Chedid M, Araj GF, Barada KA, Mourad FH: **Prevalence of** *Helicobacter pylori* **resistance to metronidazole, clarithromycin, amoxycillin and tetracycline in Lebanon.** *Int J Antimicrob Agents* 2002, **19**:155–158.

32. Wu H, Shi XD, Wang HT, Liu JX: **Resistance of** *helicobacter pylori* **to metronidazole, tetracycline and amoxycillin.** *J Antimicrob Chemother* 2000, **46**:121–123.

33. Bennett PM: **Plasmid encoded antibiotic resistance: acquisition and transfer of antibiotic resistance genes in bacteria.** *Br J Pharmacol* 2008, **153**:S347–S357.

34. Mégraud F: **Resistance of** *helicobacter pylori* **to antibiotics.** *Aliment Pharmacol Ther* 1997, **11**(Suppl 1):43–53.

35. Aguilar GR, Ayala G, Fierros-Zárate G: *Helicobacter pylori*: **recent advances in the study of its pathogenicity and prevention.** *Salud Publica Mex* 2001, **43**:237–247.

36. Sjölund M, Tano E, Blaser MJ, Andersson DI, Engstrand L: **Persistence of resistant staphylococcus epidermidis after single course of clarithromycin.** *Emerg Infect Dis* 2005, **11**:1389–1393.

37. Broutet N, Tchamgoué S, Pereira E, Lamouliatte H, Salamon R, Mégraud F: **Risk factors for failure of** *helicobacter pylori* **therapy results of an individual data analysis of 2751 patients.** *Aliment Pharmacol Ther* 2003, **17**:99–109.

38. Graham DY: **Antibiotic resistance in** *helicobacter pylori*: **implications for therapy.** *Gastroenterology* 1998, **115**:1272–1277.

39. Houben MH, van de Beek D, Hensen EF, de Craen AJ, Rauws EA, Tytgat GN: **A systematic review of** *helicobacter pylori* **eradication therapy: the impact of antimicrobial resistance on eradication rates.** *Aliment Pharmacol Ther* 1999, **13**:1047–1055.

40. Yakoob J, Jafri W, Abbas Z, Abid S, Naz S, Khan R, Khalid A: **Risk factors associated with** *helicobacter pylori* **infection treatment failure in a high prevalence area.** *Epidemiol Infect* 2011, **139**:581–590.

Prevalence and risk factors of *Helicobacter pylori* infection in Korea: Nationwide multicenter study over 13 years

Seon Hee Lim[1†], Jin-Won Kwon[2†], Nayoung Kim[3,4*], Gwang Ha Kim[5], Jung Mook Kang[1], Min Jung Park[1], Jeong Yoon Yim[1], Heung Up Kim[6], Gwang Ho Baik[7], Geom Seog Seo[8], Jeong Eun Shin[9], Young-Eun Joo[10], Joo Sung Kim[1,4] and Hyun Chae Jung[4]

Abstract

Background: The aim of this study was to evaluate the time trend of seropositivity of *Helicobacter pylori* (*H. pylori*) over the period of 13 years in an asymptomatic Korean population, and investigate associated risk factors.

Methods: This cross-sectional nationwide multicentre study surveyed anti-*H. pylori* IgG antibodies in 19,272 health check-up subjects (aged [greater than and equal to]16 years) in 2011. Risk factors for *H. pylori* infection were investigated using logistic regression. Seropositivity in asymptomatic subjects without *H. pylori* eradication was compared between the years 1998 and 2005. Birth cohort effects were also evaluated.

Results: After exclusion of subjects with a history of *H. pylori* eradication therapy (n = 3,712, 19.3%) and gastric symptoms (n = 4,764, 24.7%), the seroprevalence of *H. pylori* infection was 54.4% in 10,796 subjects. This was significantly lower than the seroprevalence of 59.6% in 2005 and that of 66.9% in 1998, and this decrease of seropositivity of *H. pylori* became widespread across all ages and in most areas of the country. This decreasing trend could be explained by cohort analysis. All younger birth cohorts had a lower seroprevalence of *H. pylori* than older birth cohorts at the same age. Decreased seroprevalence within the same birth cohorts also accounted for this phenomenon. Clinical risk factors of *H. pylori* infection were higher cholesterol level ([greater than and equal to] 240 mg/dl) (OR = 1.33; 95% CI = 1.14-1.54), male gender, older age, low income, and residence in a rural area.

Conclusions: A decreasing trend of *H. pylori* seroprevalence due to a birth cohort effect requires further studies on its related human host factors as well as socio-economic and hygienic factors. In addition, the relationship between *H. pylori* infection and high cholesterol level needs more investigation regarding underlying pathogenesis.

Keywords: Helicobacter pylori, Seroprevalence, Epidemiology, Cohort

Background

Helicobacter pylori (*H. pylori*), a cause of peptic ulcer disease, gastric adenocarcinoma, and low-grade gastric mucosa associated lymphoid tissue (MALT) lymphoma [1] has been falling due to improved sanitation and better living conditions [2,3]. However, its prevalence is reported to be still high, especially in Asia including

* Correspondence: nayoungkim49@empal.com
†Equal contributors
3Department of Internal Medicine, Seoul National University Bundang Hospital, Seongnam, Korea
4Department of Internal Medicine and Liver Research Institute, Seoul National University College of Medicine, Seoul, Korea

South Korea. From the public health perspective, observation of prevalence trends and confirmation of risk factors for *H. pylori* infection are important to establish health policies to prevent *H. pylori* related diseases.

There are many studies regarding the prevalence and risk factors of *H. pylori* infection, and older age was commonly considered as the main risk factor [4,5]. One study mentioned that adults have a continuous risk of *H. pylori* infection, resulting in increased seroprevalence during lifetime as a function of age [6]. However, this does not mean that young people have a higher seroprevalence when they get older, showing that cross sectional presentation does not necessarily give an accurate picture of lifetime trends. Also, there are limited studies on lifetime trends for *H. pylori* seroprevalence [7,8].

In South Korea, previous study also indicated a decreasing pattern of *H. pylori* infection during a time period between 1998 and 2005 [9]. As Korea is in a dynamic state of progression from a developing country into a developed country, it may be valuable to evaluate the seroprevalence of *H. pylori* in Korea. In accordance with this point of view, the aim of this study was to investigate the trends of seropositivity of *H. pylori* in asymptomatic Korean subjects over 16 years of age together with cohort effects between the years 1998 and 2011, and to find factors related to *H. pylori* infection.

Methods
Study population
This is a cross-sectional nationwide multicentre study of adult subjects aged 16 years or older who visited healthcare centers for routine health check-up between January and December 2011 in South Korea. The subjects were enrolled prospectively in 2011 under a predefined protocol. The institutions participating in this study were healthcare centers located in Seoul and in the seven provinces of South Korea.

Informed consent was obtained from each subject. All subjects were invited to answer the questionnaire which was the same as previous study's [9] under the supervision of a well-trained interviewer. The questionnaire included information regarding demographic data (i.e. age, sex, and residence), socioeconomic data (i.e. monthly income and education level), medical history (such as *H. pylori* eradication therapy, history of gastric operation, and family history of gastric cancer (GC)), and upper gastrointestinal (GI) symptoms (such as indigestion, bloating, epigastric soreness, regurgitation, or heartburn), that persisted for at least one month within the last 3 years.

Subjects were categorized into 3 education levels: low (middle school graduate or less), middle (high school graduate or university dropout), and high (university graduate or graduate of a postgraduate course). Monthly family income was classed as 3 groups: low household income (< US $ 3,000 per month), middle income (US $ 3,000 to 10,000 per month), and high income (> US $ 10,000 per month).

Clinical and laboratory evaluations
Anthropometric measurements (weight and height) were done by trained nurses using a standardized protocol.

Blood samples were obtained from the antecubital vein in the morning after overnight fasting, and serum samples were separated after centrifugation. Serum cholesterol, triglyceride, and fasting glucose were measured by an automatic analyser, Alisei® (Seac, Pomezia, Italy). To compare these results according to seropositivity of *H. Pylori*, we

categorized the level of total cholesterol (TC) as normal (≤240 mg/dl) and abnormal (>240 mg/dl), trigryceride (TG) as ≤150 mg/dl and >150 mg/dl, and fasting glucose as ≤100 mg/dl and >100 mg/dl, respectively.

Anti-*H. pylori* IgG was measured using *H. pylori*-EIA-Well in Healthcare System Gangnam Center and Genedia *H. pylori* ELISA at the remaining centers using the same kits as those in the previous studies [9,10]. Genedia *H. pylori* ELISA, developed from Korean *H. pylori* strains showed a sensitivity of 97.8% and a specificity of 92% [11]. *H. pylori*-EIA-Well showed a sensitivity of 95.6% and a specificity of 97.8% when Genedia *H. pylori* ELISA was used as the gold standard [9].

Statistical analysis
Evaluation of risk factors of each group according to eradication of H. pylori
Demographic and clinical information were summarized by descriptive statistics. To investigate risk factors for *H. pylori* seropositivity and influential factors having a history of *H. pylori* eradication, multivariable logistic regression was used. A significance level of $p < 0.05$ was used for all analyses.

Comparison of trends of seroprevalence of H. pylori in 1998, 2005, and 2011
Trends of seroprevalence of *H. pylori* were compared using the published data of 1998 [10] and 2005 [9]. For this comparison, study subjects in each time period were restricted to asymptomatic subjects without a history of *H. pylori* eradication and gastric operation. For statistical comparison of trends of seroprevalence of *H. pylori* in 1998, 2005, and 2011, the Cochrane-Armitage trend test, which is a modified Pearson chi-square test to examine the association between a binary outcome and a variable with multiple categories with order, was conducted.

Analysis of cohort effects
In addition, the seroprevalence of *H. pylori* by birth cohort group was also drawn. To examine birth cohort effects, we created synthetic cohorts from the successive cross-sectional data of 1998, 2005, and 2011. For this analysis, relevant raw data in 1998 and 2005 were obtained from the authors and reconstructed for the analysis of birth cohort. Data from 1998 was considered to be those in 1999 because the successive cross-sectional data should span with same interval. The interval of three cross-sectional data was 6 years. The aggregate birth cohort from 1930 to 1972 was restructured into 8 groups using the standard approach for cohort analysis [12]. In detail, a birth cohort was obtained by subtracting age from year (i.e. Birth cohort of 1974.5 (birth cohort of 1972–77) = Year of 1998 – Age of 24.5 (22–27 years old)). For example, people aged 22–27 years in 1998 (considered as data in 1999), those

aged 28–33 years in 2005, and those aged 34–39 years in 2011 were considered to be in the same birth cohort, born between 1972 and 1977. Using this approach for other age groups in each year, eight birth cohorts (1972–77, 1966–71, 1960–65, 1954–59, 1948–53, 1942–47,1936-41,1930-35) had three estimates of *H. pylori* seroprevalence at 6 year intervals for 12 years.

Ethics statement
The protocol of this study was approved by the main Institutional Review Board of Seoul National University Hospital (IRB No. H-1011-038-339).

Results
Seroprevalence and eradication history of *H. pylori* in total subjects
The seroprevalence of *H. pylori* was 52.8% (8,216/15,560) after exclusion of *H. pylori* eradicated history in 19,272 eligible subjects and 54.4% (5,882/10,796) after exclusion of symptomatic subjects (Figure 1).

The demographics and clinical characteristics by group are presented in Table 1.

Among the 19,272 subjects, 19.3% reported a history of eradication therapy for *H. pylori* infection. By logistic regression modeling, the influencing factors for having a history of eradication therapy for *H. pylori* infection were male, older age, higher income, living in Seoul (Capital area), the presence of GI symptom and GC family history (Table 2).

Risk factors for *H. pylori* infection in asymptomatic subjects without a history of *H. pylori* eradication
The risk factors for *H. pylori* infection in asymptomatic subjects without a history of *H. pylori* eradication were

significantly associated with gender, age, geographic area, economic status, education level, and cholesterol level (Table 3). Seropositivity of *H. pylori* was significantly lower in females than in males (OR = 0.79, 95% CI = 0.71-0.87). By age, seroprevalence increased in a nearly linear fashion from 20 to 59 years of age. However, the prevalence remained steady from 60 years of age. Regarding residence, when compared with Seoul, other provinces except for Gyeonggi and Kangwon had a higher risks of *H. pylori* seropositivity. Subjects with high income and high education level had a lower likelihoods of having *H. pylori* seropositivity. Subjects with a higher TC level (≥240 mg/dl) had a 30% higher likelihood of having *H. pylori* seropositivity compared with subjects with a lower TC (<240 mg/dl) (OR = 1.33, 95% CI = 1.14-1.54) after adjustments for BMI, age, and income level. However, blood glucose level and TG level did not affect the seropositivity of *H. pylori* infection after adjustment for other variables. Family history of GC and BMI level did not affect the seropositivity of *H. pylori*.

Comparison of seroprevalence of *H. pylori* among 2011, 2005, and 1998 in asymptomatic subjects without a history of *H. pylori* eradication
Comparison of seroprevalence of *H. pylori* from 1998, 2005 and 2011 was performed, and the data from 1998 and 2005 were investigated by the Korean *H. pylori* Study Group [10] and our group [9], respectively. The overall seroprevalence of *H. pylori* infection was 54.4% (95% CI: 53.5-55.4%) in 2011 which is significantly decreased from 66.9 % (95% CI: 65.4-68.6%) in 1998, and 59.6 % (95% CI: 58.5-60.7%) in 2005 (p < 0.001) (Panel A of Figure 2). There was a statistically significant reduction between 1998 and 2005, and between 2005 and 2011.

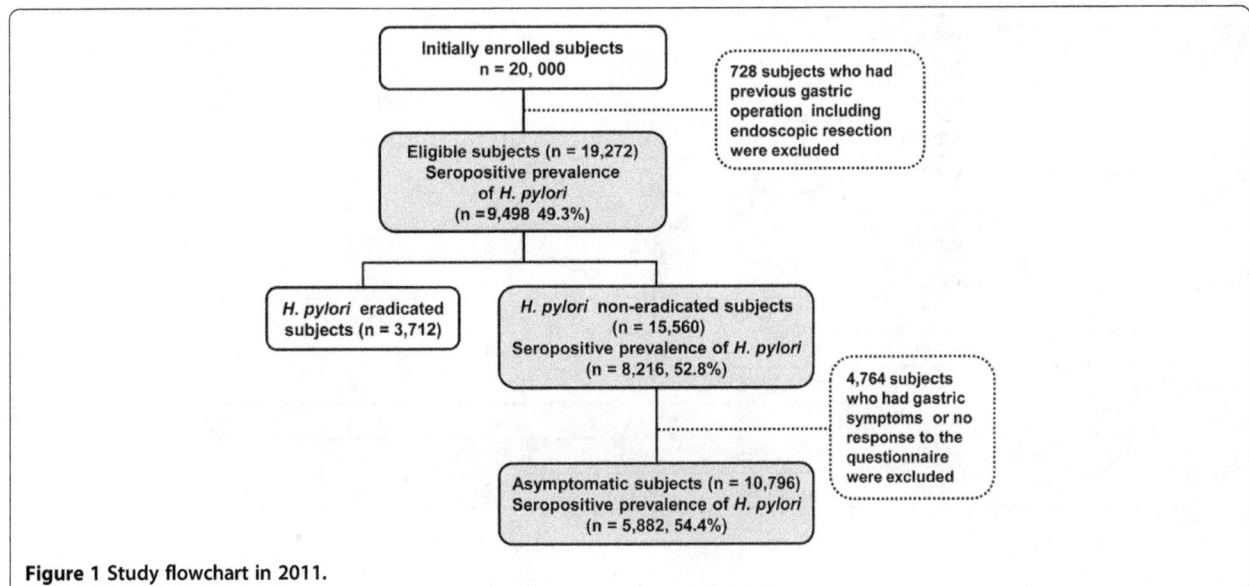

Figure 1 Study flowchart in 2011.

Table 1 Baseline characteristics of subjects

		Subjects without GI operation history		Subjects without history of *H. pylori* eradication		Asymptomatic subjects without history of *H. pylori* eradication	
		n	(%)	n	(%)	n	(%)
Total		19,272	(100.0)	15,560	(100.0)	10,796	(100.0)
Sex	Male	10,557	(54.8)	8,311	(53.4)	6,085	(56.4)
	Female	8,715	(45.2)	7,249	(46.6)	4,711	(43.6)
	Subtotal	19,272	(100.0)	15,560	(100.0)	10,796	(100.0)
Age (years)	16-19	34	(0.2)	33	(0.2)	17	(0.2)
	20-29	798	(4.1)	777	(5.0)	421	(3.9)
	30-39	2,853	(14.8)	2,607	(16.8)	1,659	(15.4)
	40-49	5,087	(26.4)	4,198	(27.0)	2,913	(27.0)
	50-59	6,176	(32.0)	4,709	(30.3)	3,403	(31.5)
	60-69	3,358	(17.4)	2,493	(16.0)	1,840	(17.0)
	≥70	966	(5.0)	743	(4.8)	543	(5.0)
	Subtotal	19,272	(100.0)	15,560	(100.0)	10,796	(100.0)
Geographic area	Seoul	10,755	(55.8)	8,515	(54.8)	5,829	(54.0)
	Gyeonggi	3,025	(15.7)	2,403	(15.5)	1,683	(15.6)
	Chungcheong	863	(4.5)	740	(4.8)	536	(5.0)
	Kyungsang	1,630	(8.5)	1,313	(8.4)	914	(8.5)
	Cholla	1,807	(9.4)	1,553	(10.0)	1,194	(11.1)
	Kangwon	588	(3.1)	466	(3.0)	331	(3.1)
	Jeju	589	(3.1)	555	(3.6)	299	(2.8)
	Subtotal[*]	19,257	(100.0)	15,545	(100.0)	10,786	(100.0)
Household income[**]	low	2,114	(12.5)	1,838	(13.5)	1,247	(13.2)
	medium	11,049	(65.2)	8,843	(65.1)	6,197	(65.6)
	high	3,781	(22.3)	2,910	(21.4)	2,005	(21.2)
	Subtotal[*]	16,944	(100.0)	13,591	(100.0)	9,449	(100.0)
Education level[***]	low	1,743	(9.5)	1,458	(9.9)	984	(9.7)
	medium	3,667	(20.0)	3,004	(20.4)	1,981	(19.4)
	high	12,928	(70.5)	10,250	(69.7)	7,223	(70.9)
	Subtotal[*]	18,338	(100.0)	14,712	(100.0)	10,188	(100.0)
Body mass index (kg/m^2)	<18.5	840	(4.4)	736	(4.8)	412	(3.9)
	18.5 - <23.0	7,696	(40.6)	6,245	(40.7)	4,237	(39.8)
	23.0 - <25.0	4,818	(25.4)	3,821	(24.9)	2,759	(25.9)
	≥25.0	5,625	(29.6)	4,530	(29.5)	3,249	(30.5)
	Subtotal[*]	18,979	(100.0)	15,332	(100.0)	10,657	(100.0)
Cholesterol (mg/dl)	<240	16,671	(90.5)	13,417	(90.4)	9,228	(90.1)
	≥240	1,755	(9.5)	1,428	(9.6)	1,013	(9.9)
	Subtotal[*]	18,426	(100.0)	14,845	(100.0)	10,241	(100.0)
TG (mg/dl)	<150	14,651	(79.7)	11,873	(80.1)	8,118	(79.4)
	≥150	3,736	(20.3)	2,941	(19.9)	2,102	(20.6)
	Subtotal*	18,387	(100.0)	14,814	(100.0)	10,220	(100.0)
Glucose (mg/dl)	<100	12,999	(70.7)	10,667	(72.0)	7,206	(70.5)
	100 - <126	4,438	(24.1)	3,399	(22.9)	2,459	(24.1)
	≥126	955	(5.2)	747	(5.0)	555	(5.4)
	Subtotal*	18,392	(100.0)	14,813	(100.0)	10,220	(100.0)

Table 1 Baseline characteristics of subjects (Continued)

Family history of gastric cancer	No	16,470	(86.6)	13,418	(87.5)	9,473	(88.2)
	Yes	2,556	(13.4)	1,910	(12.5)	1,270	(11.8)
	Subtotal*	19,026	(100.0)	15,328	(100.0)	10,743	(100.0)
GI symptoms	No	13,121	(68.8)	10,796	(70.3)		
	Yes	5,954	(31.2)	4,568	(29.7)		
	Subtotal*	19,075	(100.0)	15,364	(100.0)		

*Subjects with missing values were excluded.
**Household income was classified as low (less than US $ 3,000), medium (US $ 3,000 to 10,000), or high (more than US $ 10,000).
***Education level was classified as low (middle school graduates or less), middle (high school graduates or university dropouts), or high (university graduates or graduates of a postgraduate course).
GI gastrointestinal.

According to geographic area, the seroprevalence showed a significant downward trend in most of areas over time except in Kyungsang and Kangwon. (Panel B of Figure 2).

The seroprevalence of *H. pylori* and 95% CI at intervals of 10 years of age in 1998, 2005, and 2011 were plotted in Panel C of Figure 2. The seroprevalence of *H. pylori* was decreased in the all age groups over time with statistical significance from 1998 to 2011. A steep decreasing pattern was observed for subjects under 40 years of age between 1998 and 2005. However, when the time period was

Table 2 Multivariate analysis of factors affecting *H. pylori* eradication therapy

		Total	Subjects with history of *H. pylori* eradication		Odds ratio	95% CI	
			n	%			
Total		19,272	3,712	19.3			
Sex	Male	10,557	2,246	21.3	Ref		
	Female	8,715	1,466	16.8	0.77	0.71	0.84
Age (years)	16-19	34	1	2.9	2.27	0.28	18.21
	20-29	798	21	2.6	Ref		
	30-39	2,853	246	8.6	4.22	2.44	7.31
	40-49	5,087	889	17.5	9.32	5.44	15.94
	50-59	6,176	1,467	23.8	14.33	8.39	24.48
	60-69	3,358	865	25.8	16.91	9.87	28.97
	≥70	966	223	23.1	16.73	9.58	29.20
Geographic area	Seoul	10,755	2,240	20.8	Ref		
	Gyeonggi	3,025	622	20.6	0.97	0.87	1.08
	Chungcheong	863	123	14.3	0.76	0.61	0.94
	Kyungsang	1,630	317	19.4	0.85	0.74	0.99
	Cholla	1,807	254	14.1	0.68	0.58	0.80
	Kangwon	588	122	20.7	1.30	1.04	1.64
	Jeju	589	34	5.8	0.27	0.19	0.39
Household income*	Low	2,114	276	13.1	0.70	0.58	0.83
	Medium	11,049	2,206	20.0	0.96	0.87	1.05
	High	3,781	871	23.0	Ref		
Education level**	Low	1,743	285	16.4	0.70	0.59	0.84
	Medium	3,667	663	18.1	0.87	0.78	0.97
	High	12,928	2,678	20.7	Ref		
GI symptoms	No	13,121	2,325	17.7	Ref		
	Yes	5,954	1,386	23.3	1.60	1.47	1.73
Family history of gastric cancer	No	16,470	3,052	18.5	Ref		
	Yes	2,556	646	25.3	1.34	1.21	1.49

*, **, GI, same as those of Table 1.
CI confidence Interval, Ref reference.
Total subject number of multivariable logistic regression was 16,770.

Table 3 Risk factors for *H. pylori* seropositivity in asymptomatic subjects without a history of *H. pylori* eradication and gastric operation (Multivariable logistic regression)

		Total	*H. pylori* Seropositivity				
			N	%	Odds ratio	95% CI	
Total		10,796	5,882	54.5			
Sex	Male	6,085	3,472	57.1	Ref		
	Female	4,711	2,410	51.2	0.79	0.71	0.87
Age (years)	16-19	17	2	11.8	0.55	0.11	2.68
	20-29	421	111	26.4	Ref		
	30-39	1,659	698	42.1	1.55	1.18	2.04
	40-49	2,913	1,531	52.6	2.39	1.83	3.11
	50-59	3,403	2,088	61.4	3.52	2.70	4.60
	60-69	1,840	1,134	61.6	3.57	2.70	4.71
	≥70	543	318	58.6	3.11	2.24	4.31
Geographic area	Seoul	5,829	2,917	50.0	Ref		
	Gyeonggi	1,683	898	53.4	1.07	0.95	1.21
	Chungcheong	536	297	55.4	1.29	1.05	1.58
	Kyungsang	914	595	65.1	1.29	1.06	1.57
	Cholla	1,194	790	66.2	1.66	1.41	1.96
	Kangwon	331	200	60.4	1.19	0.92	1.54
	Jeju	299	176	58.9	1.36	1.05	1.77
Household Income*	Low	1,247	785	63.0	1.21	1.00	1.45
	Medium	6,197	3,416	55.1	1.07	0.96	1.19
	High	2,005	1,042	52.0	Ref		
Education**	Low	984	629	63.9	1.01	0.84	1.23
	Medium	1,981	1,165	58.8	1.13	1.00	1.28
	High	7,223	3,779	52.3	Ref		
Body Mass Index (kg/m^2)	<18.5	412	180	43.7	1.03	0.81	1.31
	18.5 - <23.0	4,237	2,224	52.5	Ref		
	23.0 - <25.0	2,759	1,565	56.7	0.98	0.88	1.10
	≥25	3,249	1,830	56.3	0.95	0.84	1.06
Cholesterol (mg/dl)	<240	9,228	4,882	52.9	Ref		
	≥240	1,013	624	61.6	1.33	1.14	1.54
Triglyceride (mg/dl)	<150	8,118	4,316	53.2	Ref		
	≥150	2,102	1,179	56.1	0.98	0.87	1.10
Glucose (mg/dl)	<100	7,206	3,786	52.5	Ref		
	100 – <126	2,459	1,378	56.0	0.93	0.84	1.04
	≥126	555	328	59.1	0.98	0.80	1.19
Family history of gastric cancer	No	9,473	5,152	54.4	Ref		
	Yes	1,270	700	55.1	0.96	0.84	1.09

*, **, GI, CI, Ref, same as those of Table 2.
Total subject number of multivariable logistic regression was 8,688.

extended to 2011, the declining trend was more prominent in older age groups, resulting in an overall decrease for all age groups.

The birth cohort effects

To observe lifetime trends, the seroprevalence of *H. pylori* of categorized birth cohorts against age were plotted as shown in Figure 3. Each line connects the values for the same cohort-group in different age groups. For example, a line first represents a birth cohort of 1972–77 in all graphs. At the same age of 28–33 years (mean 30.5 years old), a younger birth cohort of 1972–77 had a lower seroprevalence of *H. pylori* when compared with a older birth cohort of 1966–71. Likewise, all younger birth cohorts at the same age had a lower seroprevalence of *H. pylori* compared with older birth cohorts. Within

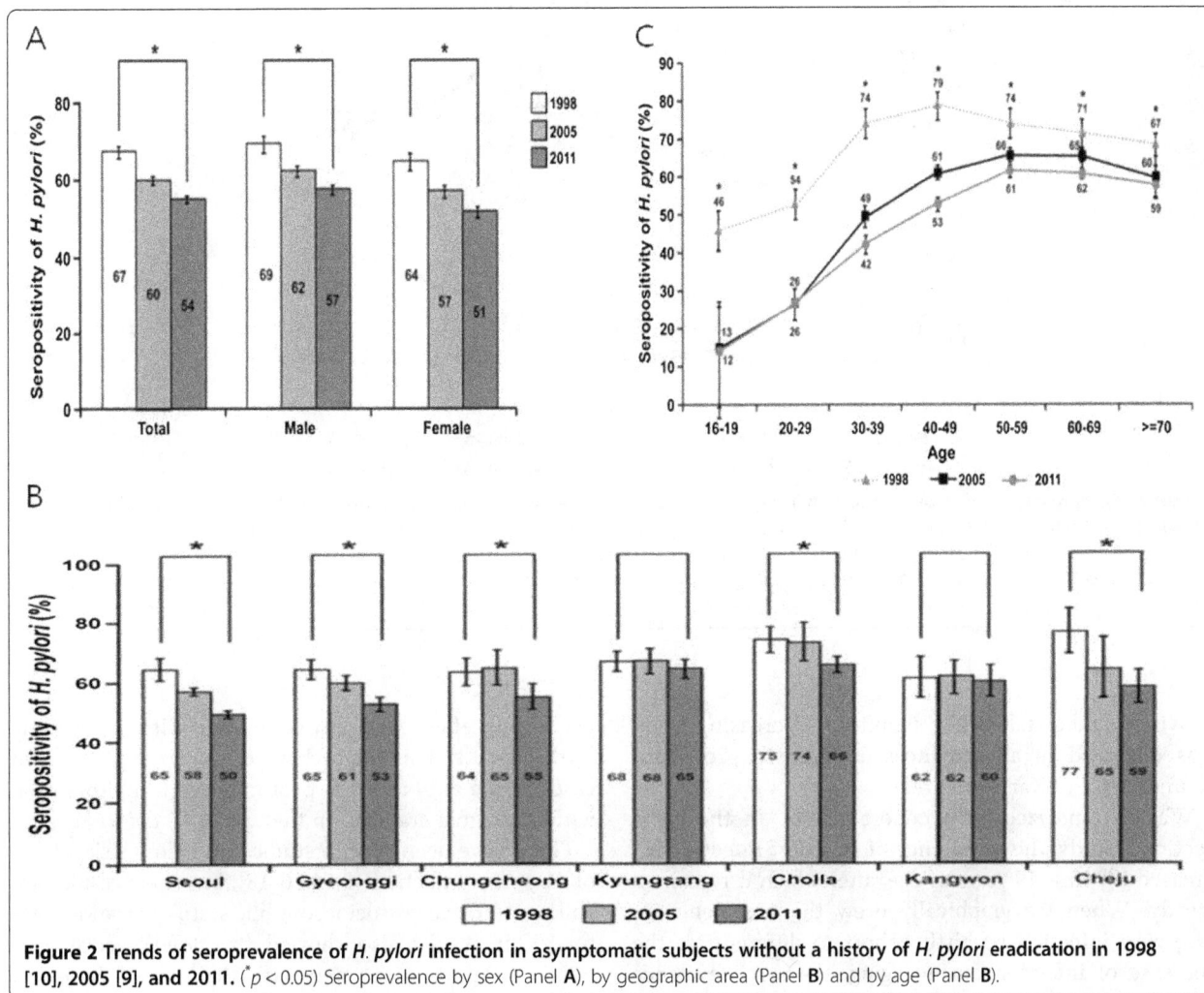

Figure 2 Trends of seroprevalence of *H. pylori* infection in asymptomatic subjects without a history of *H. pylori* eradication in 1998 [10], 2005 [9], and 2011. ($^*p$ < 0.05) Seroprevalence by sex (Panel **A**), by geographic area (Panel **B**) and by age (Panel **B**).

the same birth cohort, most birth cohorts had decreasing pattern of seropositivity of *H. pylori* except for a birth cohort of 1972–1977. This birth cohort showed a decreasing pattern from 22–27 to 28–33 years of age, but it showed a very slight increase (from 41% to 43%) from 28–33 to 34–39 years of age.

Discussion

The decreasing trend (from 66.9% to 54.4%) of seroprevalence of *H. pylori* over 13 years was explained by birth cohort analysis, and a relationship between *H. pylori* infection and high cholesterol level was found in this large cohort.

A drop in the seroprevalence of *H. pylori* infection has been observed in previous studies [2,3,13]. This trend was most often explained by a combination of various factors including rapid economic growth, improved sanitation, and widespread use of antibiotics and proton pump inhibitors [2,3]. Similarly, the overall seroprevalence of *H. pylori* significantly decreased in the last survey of the Korean population in 2005 [9] compared with

that in 1998 [10], but the declining trend was different depending on the age groups and areas. Although the drop in *H. pylori* infection was bigger in younger age groups of subjects 40 years old or less for seven years from 1998 to 2005, the difference of seroprevalence in older groups during same periods was smaller, as shown in the upper two lines of figure 2C. In addition, regarding areas, only subjects who lived in Seoul (capital) and Gyeonggi province which surrounds the capital, showed a clear declining trend during the same periods, but not in all districts in previous study [9]. Furthermore, subjects who lived in Chungcheong province showed a slight increase between 1998 and 2005.

However, when we extended the time period to 2011 in this study, this decreasing trend was more prominent for all ages over 13 years. Similarly, a Japanese study of seropositivity trends of *H. pylori* over a period of 10 years from 1992 to 2002–2006 also found declining trends of seropositivity for all age groups [13]. Regarding province, there was no increasing pattern in any

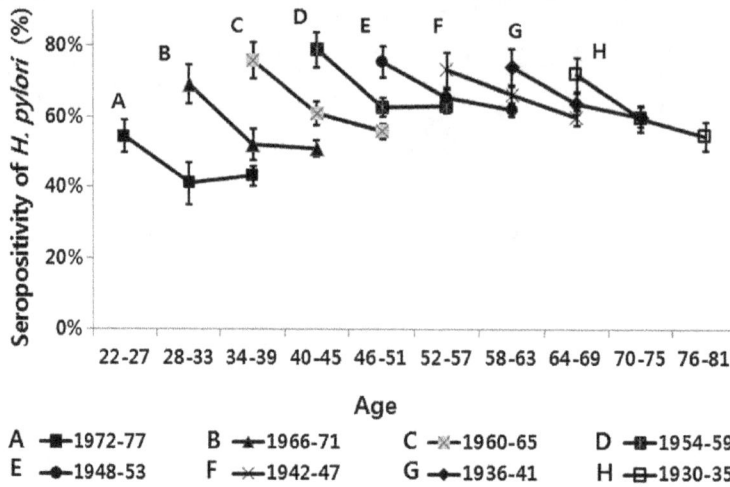

Figure 3 Seroprevalence of *H. pylori* infection in asymptomatic subjects without a history of *H. pylori* eradication in birth cohort against age. Each line connects the values for the same cohort-group in different age group. For example, the first line shows the seroprevalence of *H. pylori* in a birth cohort of 1972–77 for ages of 22–39 years, and the second line shows the seroprevalence of *H. pylori* in a birth cohort of 1966–71 for ages of 28–45 years. All younger birth cohorts at the same age have a lower seroprevalence of *H. pylori* than older birth cohorts.

province, and a statistically significant decreasing trend was observed in all provinces except two provinces, Kyungsang and Kangwon areas.

We also analyzed birth cohort effects. In the cross sectional study, the prevalence of *H. pylori* infection increased till 40 – 49 years of age, after which it remained steady. When we graphically drew the prevalence in *H. pylori* infection by birth cohort to differentiate the increase of infection during aging, the seroprevalence was lower in younger birth cohort (i.e. people who were born later) than the older birth cohort (people who were born earlier) at the same age, showing a clear cohort effect in subjects up to 40–45 years of age. This phenomenon could be explained by continuous influx of younger birth cohorts [7]. A similar birth cohort effect for *H. pylori* infection was observed in Western studies [2,3,7,8]. In addition, *H. pylori* infection in adults is mostly acquired by the age of 15 years [7,8]. One study which followed children (1–3 years old) for 21 years indicated that the annual seroconversion rate had a highest risk at the age of 4–5 years, and newly acquired *H. pylori* infections mostly occurred by the age of 10 years [14]. However, there is a doubt whether only a birth cohort effect could explain this pattern. That is, one study in Canada mentioned that an increasing pattern of *H. pylori* infection with advancing age may be due to the continuous risk of infection in adults rather than cohort effects [6]. The decrease of *H. pylori* seroprevalence with advancing age within the same birth cohort in our study strongly suggests that aging is not likely to raise risk of *H. pylori* infection. There was a

decreasing effect with advancing age within the same birth cohorts. This might have occurred as a result of cases taking antibiotics or proton pump inhibitors even without formal eradication therapy of *H. pylori* [15].

There have been several studies regarding risk factors of *H. pylori* infection [9,14,16-18], but their results are still unclear, except socioeconomic status as the risk factors. Our results also showed that lower social economic status is associated with the risk of *H. pylori* infection in a cross sectional analysis. Furthermore, subjects with lower social economic status had a lower likelihood of taking *H. pylori* eradication therapy in the present study. Interestingly, our study showed a relationship between cholesterol level and seropositivity of *H. pylori*. Subjects who had a TC level of ≥240 mg/dl were 1.3 times more likely to be seropositive for *H. pylori*. In frequency analysis, higher levels of TG and glucose as well as TC were also associated with *H. pylori* infection, but after adjusting for demographic variables, clinical information, and socioeconomic status(i.e. age, BMI, income and etc.), only TC among metabolic parameters was related to *H. pylori* infection. So far, the results regarding the relationship between lipid parameters such as TC, TG and low-density lipoprotein cholesterol (LDL-C) levels and *H. pylori* seropositivity have not been consistent. Some studies [19-21] reported no relationship, but several studies reported higher atherogenic lipid parameter levels in *H. pylori* seropositive subjects in comparison with seronegative ones [22-24] as seen in the present study. Our study results could be convincing for demonstrating the effect of *H. pylori* infection on atherosclerotic disease because the positive relationship between TC and *H. pylori* seropositivity was persistent even after adjustment for BMI and age in a large cohort. The mechanism of how *H. pylori* infection modifies the serum lipid profiles is still not clear, but a plausible explanation is that systemic inflammatory response to the bacterium induces changes in lipid and lipoprotein metabolism [25]. That is, chronic *H. pylori* infection has been postulated to shift the lipid profile toward an atherogenic direction *via* the action of proinflammatory cytokines, such as interleukins 1 and 6, interferon-alpha, and tumor necrosis factor-alpha. These cytokines are capable of affecting lipid metabolism in various ways, including activation of adipose tissue lipoprotein lipase, stimulation of hepatic fatty acid synthesis, influencing lipolysis and the increasing hepatic HMG-CoA reductase activity [26,27]. Thus, *H. pylori* infection could play a role in the atherosclerotic process and may be a reliable indicator for the assessment of cardiovascular disease risk.

There are several limitations which should be acknowledged in this study. First, the relationship between *H. pylori* infection and its risk factors in the cross sectional study could not be proven conclusively. However, this is an unavoidable limitation in the cross sectional study. Second, we compared the time trends of seroprevalence of *H. pylori* using two previous studies [9,10]. However, the responsible author (N.K.) did play main role in these previous studies, and the population in 2011 study was restricted to have comparability of *H. pylori* seroprevalence. In other words, the subjects in 2011 study were restricted to asymptomatic people without a history of *H. pylori* eradication and GI operation. Moreover, this study was carried out nationwide, so our findings represent a national trend, not a local phenomenon. Nonetheless, the study subjects in 1998 involved a relatively lower population from Seoul and Gyeonggi, (capital city and its near city) compared with the population in 2005 and 2011. Generally people in capital cities have higher socioeconomic conditions than those living in other areas. It may account for much higher seroprevalence in 1998 compared with 2005/2011. However, the change of seroprevalence by the strata (e.g. age, sex, region, etc.) over time periods may indicate that our overall result is not much influenced by a different proportion of subjects from provinces. Third, for the generation of synthetic cohort, cross-sectional data should have the same interval. However, our data did not have the same interval as the previous data. This is the reason why we considered the data from 1998 as equivalent to those from 1999. This intentional modification could have caused bias, but we think that the bias may be negligible because *H.pylori* seroprevalence was not changed much by one-year.

Conclusion

In conclusion, we confirmed that the seropositivity of *H. pylori* declined across all age groups from 1998 to 2011 using nationwide data, an effect which originated from birth cohort effects and continuous risk reduction of *H. pylori* infection during one's life time. In addition, we found that high TC level as well as lower social economic status had a relationship with *H. pylori* infection. These results may suggest the importance of management of *H. pylori* infection in younger age and the effect of *H. pylori* infection on atherosclerosis.

Abbreviations
GC: Gastric cancer; GI: Gastrointestinal; H. pylori: Helicobacter pylori; TG: Triglyceride; TC: Total cholesterol.

Competing interests
All authors declare that they have no conflict of interest.

Authors' contributions
SHL carried out the acquisition of data, analysis and interpretation of data, and drafting of the manuscript; JK carried out statistical analysis, interpretation of data, and drafting of the manuscript; NK carried out study concept and design, critical revision of the manuscript for important intellectual content and study supervision as a corresponder; GHK participated in acquisition of the data of southeastern part of Korea; JMK participated in design of the study and acquisition of data; MJP participated in acquisition of data; JYY participated in acquisition of data and study concept; HUK participated in acquisition of the data of southernmost part of Korea; GHB participated in acquisition of the data of northeastern part of Korea; GSS participated in acquisition of the data of western part of Korea; JES participated in acquisition of the data of middle upcountry of Korea; YEJ participated in acquisition of the data of southwestern part of Korea ;JSK participated in technical or material support and study supervision ;HCJ participated in study supervision and provided general support. All authors read and approved the final manuscript.

Acknowledgments
This work was supported by the National Research Foundation of Korea (NRF) grant for the Global Core Research Center (GCRC) funded by the Korea government (MSIP) (No. 2011-0030001).

Author details
[1]Seoul National University Hospital, Healthcare System Gangnam Center, Healthcare Research Institute, Seoul, Korea. [2]College of Pharmacy, Kyungpook National University, Daegu, Korea. [3]Department of Internal Medicine, Seoul National University Bundang Hospital, Seongnam, Korea. [4]Department of Internal Medicine and Liver Research Institute, Seoul National University College of Medicine, Seoul, Korea. [5]Department of Internal Medicine, Pusan National University School of Medicine, Busan, Korea. [6]Department of Internal Medicine, School of Medicine, Jeju National University, Jeju, Korea. [7]Department of Internal Medicine, Hallym University College of Medicine, Chuncheon, Korea. [8]Department of Internal Medicine, Wonkwang University Hospital, Iksan, Korea. [9]Department of Internal medicine, Dankook University College of Medicine, Chonan, Korea. [10]Department of Internal Medicine, Chonnam National University Medical School, Gwangju, Korea.

References
1. Egan BJ, Holmes K, O'Connor HJ, O'Morain CA: **Helicobacter pylori gastritis, the unifying concept for gastric diseases.** *Helicobacter* 2007, 12(Suppl 2):39–44.
2. Parsonnet J: **The incidence of Helicobacter pylori infection.** *Aliment Pharmacol Ther* 1995, 9(Suppl 2):45–51.
3. Roosendaal R, Kuipers EJ, Buitenwerf J, Meuwissen SG, van Kamp GJ, Vandenbroucke-Grauls CM: **Helicobacter pylori and the birth cohort effect:**

evidence of a continuous decrease of infection rates in childhood. *Am J Gastroenterol* 1997, **92:**1480–1482.

4. Taylor DN, Blaser MJ: **The epidemiology of Helicobacter pylori infection.** *Epidemiol Rev* 1991, **13:**42–59.

5. Graham DY, Malaty HM, Evans DG, Evans DJ Jr, Klein PD, Adam E: **Epidemiology of Helicobacter pylori in an asymptomatic population in the United States. Effect of age, race, and socioeconomic status.** *Gastroenterology* 1991, **100:**1495–1501.

6. van Zanten SJ V, Pollak PT, Best LM, Bezanson GS, Marrie T: **Increasing prevalence of Helicobacter pylori infection with age: continuous risk of infection in adults rather than cohort effect.** *J Infect Dis* 1994, **169:**434–437.

7. Banatvala N, Mayo K, Megraud F, Jennings R, Deeks JJ, Feldman RA: **The cohort effect and Helicobacter pylori.** *J Infect Dis* 1993, **168:**219–221.

8. Kosunen TU, Aromaa A, Knekt P, Salomaa A, Rautelin H, Lohi P, Heinonen OP: **Helicobacter antibodies in 1973 and 1994 in the adult population of Vammala, Finland.** *Epidemiol Infect* 1997, **119:**29–34.

9. Yim JY, Kim N, Choi SH, Kim YS, Cho KR, Kim SS, Seo KS, Kim HU, Baik GH, Sin CS, Cho SH, Oh BH: **Seroprevalence of Helicobacter pylori in South Korea.** *Helicobacter* 2007, **12:**333–340.

10. Kim JH, Kim HY, Kim N, Kim SW, Kim JG, Kim JJ, Roe IH SJK, Sim JG, Ahn H, Yoon BC, Lee SW, Lee YC, Chung IS, Jung HY, Hong WS, Choi KW: **Seroepidemiological study of Helicobacter pylori infection in asymptomatic people in South Korea.** *J Gastroenterol Hepatol* 2001, **16:**969–975.

11. Kim SY, Ahn JS, Ha YJ, Doh HJ, Jang MH, Chung SI, Park HJ: **Serodiagnosis of Helicobacter pylori infection in Korean patients using enzyme-linked immunosorbent assay.** *J Immunoassay* 1998, **19:**251–270.

12. Kwon JW, Song YM, Sung J, Sohn Y, Cho SI: **Varying patterns of BMI increase in sex and birth cohorts of Korean adults.** *Obesity (Silver Spring)* 2007, **15:**277–282.

13. Shiota S, Murakami K, Fujioka T, Yamaoka Y: **Population-based strategies for Helicobacter pylori-associated disease management: a Japanese perspective.** *Expert Rev Gastroenterol Hepatol* 2010, **4:**149–156.

14. Malaty HM, El-Kasabany A, Graham DY, Miller CC, Reddy SG, Srinivasan SR, Yamaoka Y, Berenson GS: **Age at acquisition of Helicobacter pylori infection: a follow-up study from infancy to adulthood.** *Lancet* 2002, **359:**931–935.

15. Kim N, Lim SH, Lee KH, Kim JM, Cho SI, Jung HC, Song IS: **Seroconversion of Helicobacter pylori in Korean male employees.** *Scand J Gastroenterol* 2005, **40:**1021–1027.

16. Perez-Perez GI, Rothenbacher D, Brenner H: **Epidemiology of Helicobacter pylori infection.** *Helicobacter* 2004, **9**(Suppl 1):1–6.

17. The EUROGAST Study Group: **Epidemiology of, and risk factors for, Helicobacter pylori infection among 3194 asymptomatic subjects in 17 populations.** *Gut* 1993, **34:**1672–1676.

18. Moayyedi P, Axon AT, Feltbower R, Duffett S, Crocombe W, Braunholtz D, Richards IDG, Dowell AC, Forman D: **Relation of adult lifestyle and socioeconomic factors to the prevalence of Helicobacter pylori infection.** *Int J Epidemiol* 2002, **31:**624–631.

19. Danesh J, Peto R: **Risk factors for coronary heart disease and infection with Helicobacter pylori: meta-analysis of 18 studies.** *BMJ* 1998, **316:**1130–1132.

20. Oshima T, Ozono R, Yano Y, Oishi Y, Teragawa H, Higashi Y, Yoshizumi M, Kambe M: **Association of Helicobacter pylori infection with systemic inflammation and endothelial dysfunction in healthy male subjects.** *J Am Coll Cardiol* 2005, **45:**1219–1222.

21. Paximadas S, Pagoni ST, Kosmidis M, Tsarouchas X, Christou M, Chatziantonakis N, Papachilleos P: **The lipid profile in adults with negative or positive antibody Helicobacter pylori [abstract].** *Atherosclerosis supplement* 2005, **6:**74.

22. Kucukazman M, Yavuz B, Sacikara M, Asilturk Z, Ata N, Ertugrul DT, Yalcin AA, Yenigum EC, Kizilca G, Okten H, Akin KO, Nazligul Y: **The relationship between updated Sydney System score and LDL cholesterol levels in patients infected with Helicobacter pylori.** *Dig Dis Sci* 2009, **54:**604–607.

23. Laurila A, Bloigu A, Nayha S, Hassi H, Leinonen M, Saikku P: **Association of Helicobacter pylori infection with elevated serum lipids.** *Atherosclerosis* 1999, **142:**207–210.

24. Majka J, Rog T, Konturek PC, Konturek SJ, Bielanski W, Kowalsky M, Szczudlik A: **Influence of chronic Helicobacter pylori infection on ischemic cerebral stroke risk factors.** *Med Sci Moni* 2002, **8:**CR675–CR684.

25. Gallin JI, Kaye D, O'Leary WM: **Serum lipids in infection.** *N Engl J Med* 1969, **281:**1081–1086.

26. Grunfeld C, Gulli R, Moser AH, Gavin LA, Feingold KR: **Effect of tumor necrosis factor administration in vivo on lipoprotein lipase activity in various tissues of the rat.** *J Lipid Res* 1989, **30:**579–585.

27. Memon RA, Grunfeld C, Moser AH, Feingold KR: **Tumor necrosis factor mediates the effects of endotoxin on cholesterol and triglyceride metabolism in mice.** *Endocrinology* 1993, **132:**2246–2253.

16

Gene expression analysis of a *Helicobacter pylori*-infected and high-salt diet-treated mouse gastric tumor model: identification of CD177 as a novel prognostic factor in patients with gastric cancer

Takeshi Toyoda[1,2†], Tetsuya Tsukamoto[3*†], Masami Yamamoto[4], Hisayo Ban[2], Noriko Saito[2], Shinji Takasu[1], Liang Shi[5], Ayumi Saito[6], Seiji Ito[7], Yoshitaka Yamamura[7], Akiyoshi Nishikawa[8], Kumiko Ogawa[1], Takuji Tanaka[9] and Masae Tatematsu[10]

Abstract

Background: *Helicobacter pylori* (*H. pylori*) infection and excessive salt intake are known as important risk factors for stomach cancer in humans. However, interactions of these two factors with gene expression profiles during gastric carcinogenesis remain unclear. In the present study, we investigated the global gene expression associated with stomach carcinogenesis and prognosis of human gastric cancer using a mouse model.

Methods: To find candidate genes involved in stomach carcinogenesis, we firstly constructed a carcinogen-induced mouse gastric tumor model combined with *H. pylori* infection and high-salt diet. C57BL/6J mice were given *N*-methyl-*N*-nitrosourea in their drinking water and sacrificed after 40 weeks. Animals of a combination group were inoculated with *H. pylori* and fed a high-salt diet. Gene expression profiles in glandular stomach of the mice were investigated by oligonucleotide microarray. Second, we examined an availability of the candidate gene as prognostic factor for human patients. Immunohistochemical analysis of CD177, one of the up-regulated genes, was performed in human advanced gastric cancer specimens to evaluate the association with prognosis.

Results: The multiplicity of gastric tumor in carcinogen-treated mice was significantly increased by combination of *H. pylori* infection and high-salt diet. In the microarray analysis, 35 and 31 more than two-fold up-regulated and down-regulated genes, respectively, were detected in the *H. pylori*-infection and high-salt diet combined group compared with the other groups. Quantitative RT-PCR confirmed significant over-expression of two candidate genes including *Cd177* and *Reg3g*. On immunohistochemical analysis of CD177 in human advanced gastric cancer specimens, over-expression was evident in 33 (60.0%) of 55 cases, significantly correlating with a favorable prognosis ($P = 0.0294$). Multivariate analysis including clinicopathological factors as covariates revealed high expression of CD177 to be an independent prognostic factor for overall survival.

(Continued on next page)

* Correspondence: ttsukamt@fujita-hu.ac.jp
†Equal contributors
[3]Department of Pathology, Fujita Health University School of Medicine, Toyoake, Japan
Full list of author information is available at the end of the article

(Continued from previous page)

Conclusions: These results suggest that our mouse model combined with *H. pylori* infection and high-salt diet is useful for gene expression profiling in gastric carcinogenesis, providing evidence that CD177 is a novel prognostic factor for stomach cancer. This is the first report showing a prognostic correlation between CD177 expression and solid tumor behavior.

Keywords: Cd177, Gastric cancer, *Helicobacter pylori*, Microarray, Salt

Background

Stomach cancer is the fourth most common cancer and second leading cause of cancer-related death worldwide [1]. *Helicobacter pylori* (*H. pylori*) is now recognized as a major risk factor for chronic gastritis and stomach cancer development [2]. In addition, environmental and host factors have also been shown to influence gastric carcinogenesis, and salt (sodium chloride, NaCl) and salty food are of particular importance, based on evidence from a number of epidemiological and experimental studies [3-6]. Thus, combined exposure to *H. pylori* infection and excessive salt intake appears to be very important for the development and progression of gastric tumors, although the detailed mechanisms, especially in terms of gene expression profiles, remain to be clarified.

High throughput microarray technology provides a powerful tool for comprehensive gene analysis, already applied to assess gene expression patterns in both human samples and animal models of gastric disorders [7-16]. Although many researchers have focused on gene expression in *H. pylori*-treated gastric cell lines [17-19], results in cell culture do not necessarily correlate with expression of specific genes in the *in vivo* microenvironment featuring host immune responses and stromal-epithelial interactions in cancers. Carcinogen-treated Mongolian gerbils have been used as a useful animal model of *H. pylori*-associated gastric carcinogenesis [20-24], and we previously reported that a synergistic interaction between *H. pylori* infection and high-salt intake accelerates chronic inflammation and tumor development in the stomachs of these animals [25,26]. Unfortunately, there is little information available for the gerbil genome, hampering genetic and molecular analysis. Therefore, attention has focused on mouse models [12,13], and establishment of a mouse model for stomach cancer featuring salt and *H. pylori* exposure is needed for investigations targeting genes involved in gastric carcinogenesis.

Previous microarray studies using rodent models did not distinguish and characterize expression profiles based on the interaction of *H. pylori* infection and salt intake. In the present study, we examined gene expression in the gastric mucosa in a *H. pylori*-infected and high-salt diet-treated mouse gastric tumor model by oligonucleotide microarray and found two candidate up-regulated genes including *Cd177* and *Reg3g*. We also investigated the

expression of CD177 in human advanced gastric cancers by immunohistochemistry, and obtained evidence as a potential prognostic factor for stomach carcinogenesis.

Methods

Inoculation with *H. pylori*

H. pylori was prepared by the same method as described previously [27,28]. Briefly, *H. pylori* (Sydney strain 1) was inoculated on Brucella agar plates (Becton Dickinson, Cockeysville, MD, USA) containing 7% (v/v) heat-inactivated fetal bovine serum (FBS) and incubated at 37°C under microaerophilic conditions at high humidity for 2 days. Then, bacteria grown on the plates were introduced into Brucella broth (Becton Dickinson) supplemented with 7% (v/v) FBS and incubated under the same conditions for 24-h. After 24-h fasting, animals were intra-gastrically inoculated *H. pylori* (1.0×10^8 colony-forming units). Before inoculation, the broth cultures of *H. pylori* were checked under a phase-contrast microscope for bacterial shape and mobility.

Animals and experimental protocol

Fifty-six specific pathogen-free male, 5- or 6-week-old C57BL/6J mice (CLEA Japan, Tokyo, Japan) were used in this study. All animals were housed in plastic cages on hardwood-chip bedding in an air-conditioned biohazard room with a 12-h light/12-h dark cycle, and allowed free access to food and water throughout. The experimental design was approved by the Animal Care Committee of the Aichi Cancer Center Research Institute, and the animals were cared for in accordance with institutional guidelines as well as the Guidelines for Proper Conduct of Animal Experiments (Science Council of Japan, June 1st, 2006).

The experimental design is illustrated in Figure 1A. The mice were divided into 4 groups (Groups A-D); 21, 5, 15, and 15 mice were assigned to A, B, C, and D groups, respectively, at the commencement of the experiment. Animals of Groups B and D were inoculated with *H. pylori* intra-gastrically on alternate weeks (total 7 times), while mice of the other groups were inoculated with Brucella broth alone. All mice were given *N*-methyl-*N*-nitrosourea (MNU, Sigma Chemical, St Louis, MO, USA) in their drinking water at the concentration of 120 ppm on alternate weeks (total exposure was 5 weeks). For this purpose

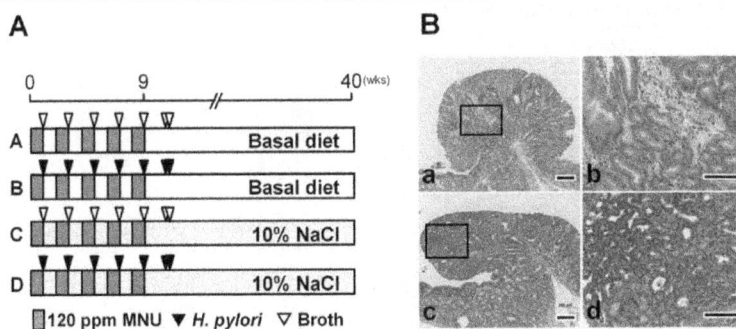

Figure 1 Experimental design and histopathological findings. A: Experimental design. Five- to six-week-old male C57BL/6J mice were inoculated with *H. pylori* SS1 strain (Groups B and D) or Brucella broth (Groups A and C). All animals were administered 120 ppm MNU in their drinking water on alternate weeks (total exposure, 5 weeks). Mice of Groups C and D were given basal diet (CE-2) containing 10% NaCl. **B**: Histopathological findings for MNU-induced mice gastric tumors. (a and b) Gastric adenoma in the pyloric region of an MNU-treated and *H. pylori*-infected mouse (Group B). (c and d) Gastric adenocarcinoma observed in Group B. Note the high cell density and cellular and structural atypia. Bar = 200 (a and c) or 100 μm (b and d).

MNU was freshly dissolved in distilled water three times per week. Mice of Groups C and D received CE-2 diets (basal sodium content of 0.36%; CLEA Japan) containing 10% NaCl. During the exposure period, one animal of Group B, one of Group C and six of Group D died or became moribund and they were excluded from the experiment. At 40 weeks, the remained animals were subjected to deep anesthesia and laparotomy with excision of the stomach.

Histological evaluation

For histological examination, the stomachs were fixed in 10% neutral-buffered formalin for 24-h, sliced along the longitudinal axis into strips of equal width, and embedded in paraffin. Four-μm thick sections were prepared and stained with hematoxylin and eosin (H&E) for histological observation. Tumors were classified into adenoma and adenocarcinoma based on cellular and morphological atypia and invasive growth to submucosa as we reported previously [21].

RNA preparation and oligonucleotide microarray analysis

Total RNA was extracted from the whole gastric mucosa including both tumor and peripheral tissue using an RNeasy Plus Mini Kit (Qiagen, Hilden, Germany) and its quality checked with a microchip electrophoresis system (i-chip SV1210; Hitachi Chemical, Tokyo, Japan). High-quality samples were selected, and pooled for each group to avoid individual difference for oligonucleotide microarray assessment (Group A, n = 3; B, n = 4; C, n = 6; D, n = 7). The CodeLink Mouse Whole Genome Bioarray (Applied Microarrays, Tempe, AZ, USA) containing 35,587 probe sets per chip was used to analyze gene expression profiles. Hybridization, processing, and scanning were performed by Filgen, Inc. (Nagoya, Japan), scan data images being analyzed using a software

package (Microarray Data Analysis Tool, Filgen). Complete-linkage hierarchical clustering was also examined on the four groups using a qualified probe subset (Filgen).

Quantitative real-time RT-PCR of expression profiles in mice stomach

Relative quantitative real-time RT-PCR was performed using a StepOne Real-Time PCR System (Applied Biosystems, Foster City, CA, USA) with the mouse-specific glyceraldehyde-3-phosphate dehydrogenase (*Gapdh*) gene as an internal control. After DNase treatment, first strand cDNAs were synthesized from total RNA using a Super-Script VILO cDNA Synthesis Kit (Invitrogen, Carlsbad, CA, USA). The PCR was accomplished basically following the manufacturer's instructions using a QuantiTect SYBR Green PCR Kit (Qiagen). The primer sequences for each gene are listed in Table 1. Specificity of the PCR reactions was confirmed using a melt curve program provided with the StepOne software and electrophoresis of the PCR samples in 3% agarose gels. The expression levels of mRNAs were normalized to the mRNA level of *Gapdh* and compared with the control mice (Group A) by the $\Delta\Delta CT$ method.

Patients and tumor specimens

A total of 55 cases of primary advanced gastric cancer, surgically resected at Aichi Cancer Center Hospital (Nagoya, Japan) between 1995 and 2002, were investigated after obtaining informed consent. The study was approved by the ethics committee of Aichi Cancer Center. The patients were all male and the mean age and median follow-up period were 58.6 ± 10.2 years and 83 weeks, respectively. None had received preoperative chemotherapy or radiotherapy. Carcinomas with adjacent mucosa tissue were fixed and embedded in paraffin, and sectioned for staining

Table 1 Primer sequences for relative quantitative real-time RT-PCR

Gene	Sequences	Product length	Accession no.
Gapdh	5'-AACGGATTTGGCCGTATTG-3'	140	NM_008084
	5'-TTGCCGTGAGTGGAGTCATA-3'		
Cd177	5'-AGGGGTGCCACTCACTGTTA-3'	128	NM_026862
	5'-CCGATTGTTTTGGAGTCACC-3		
Reg3g	5'-GTATGGATTGGGCTCCATGA-3'	106	NM_011260
	5'-GATTCGTCTCCCAGTTGATG-3'		
Muc13	5'-CCTAATCCCTACGCAAACCA-3'	124	NM_010739
	5'-TCTGCCCATTTCTCCTTGTC-3'		

Gapdh glyceraldehyde-3-phosphate dehydrogenase, Reg3g regenerating islet-derived protein 3 gamma, Muc13 mucin 13.

with H&E. Classification of tumor staging and diagnosis of advanced cases were made according to the Japanese Classification of Gastric Carcinomas [29]. The cancers had invaded the muscularis propria (T2 for TNM classification), the subserosa (T3), or the serosa and the peritoneal cavity (T4a), sometimes involving adjacent organs (T4b).

Immunohistochemistry using human gastric cancer tissue

We examined expression of CD177, for which a commercial primary antibody was available, in human gastric cancer tissues by immunohistochemistry. After inhibition of endogenous peroxidase activity by immersion in 3% hydrogen peroxide/methanol solution, antigen retrieval was carried out with 10 mM citrate buffer (pH 6.0) in a microwave oven for 10 min at 98°C. Then, sections were incubated with a mouse monoclonal anti-CD177 antibody (clone 4C4, diluted 1:100, Abnova, Taipei, Taiwan). Staining for CD177 was performed using a Vectastain Elite ABC Kit (Vector Laboratories, Burlingame, CA, USA) and binding visualized with 0.05% 3,3'-diaminobenzidine. The results of CD177 immunostaining in neoplastic cells were classified into four degrees; grade 0 (none, 0-10% of positive cells), grade 1 (weak, 10-30%), grade 2 (moderate, 30-60%), and grade 3 (strong, over 60%) based on proportion of stained cells, and cases showing moderate to strong staining were considered as positive.

Statistical analysis

The Chi-square test with Bonferroni correction was used to assess incidences of gastric tumor. Quantitative values including multiplicity of tumor and relative expression of mRNA were represented as means ± SD or SE, and differences between means were statistically analyzed by ANOVA or the Kruskal-Wallis test followed by the Tukey test for multiple comparisons. Overall survival was estimated using the Kaplan-Meier method and the log-rank test for comparisons. Correlations between CD177 expression and clinicopathological factors were analyzed by ANOVA or Chi-square test. Multivariate analysis was performed to examine whether CD177 over-expression was an independent prognostic factor using the Cox proportional-hazards regression model. P values of < 0.05 were considered to be statistically significant.

Results

Incidences and multiplicities of gastric tumors

The effective number of mice and the observed incidences and multiplicities of gastric tumors are summarized in Table 2. Tumors developed in the gastric mucosa of all MNU-treated groups (Groups A-D) (Figure 1B). In high-salt diet-treated groups (Groups C and D), the incidence of gastric tumor in Group D (*H. pylori*-infected; 100%) was significantly higher than that in Group C (non-infected; 50.0%) ($P < 0.05$). In basal diet groups (Groups A

Table 2 Incidence and multiplicity of gastric tumors in MNU-treated mice

Group	Effective number	Treatment	Incidence (%)			Multiplicity (no. of tumor/mouse)		
			Adenoma	Carcinoma	Total tumor	Adenoma	Carcinoma	Total tumor
A	21	MNU	3(14.3)	13(61.9)	13(61.9)	0.1 ± 0.4[a]	0.8 ± 0.7	0.9 ± 0.8
B	4	MNU + H. pylori	4(100)[b]	4(100)	4(100)	1.5 ± 0.6	1.8 ± 1.0	3.3 ± 1.0[c]
C	14	MNU + 10% NaCl	2(14.3)	6(42.9)	7(50.0)	0.2 ± 0.6	0.8 ± 1.0	1.0 ± 1.2
D	9	MNU + H. pylori + 10% NaCl	4(44.4)	8(88.8)	9(100)[d]	0.4 ± 0.5[e]	2.1 ±1.4[d]	2.6 ± 1.1[d]

Values for multiplicity are expressed as means ± SD. Incidences were generally assessed by Chi-square test, followed by pairwise analysis with Bonferroni correction. Multiplicities were generally analyzed by ANOVA, followed by the Tukey test for multiple comparison. [a]$P < 0.01$ vs. Group B, [b]$P < 0.01$ vs. Group A, [c]$P < 0.05$ vs. Group A, [d]$P < 0.05$ vs. Group C, [e]$P < 0.05$ vs. Group B.

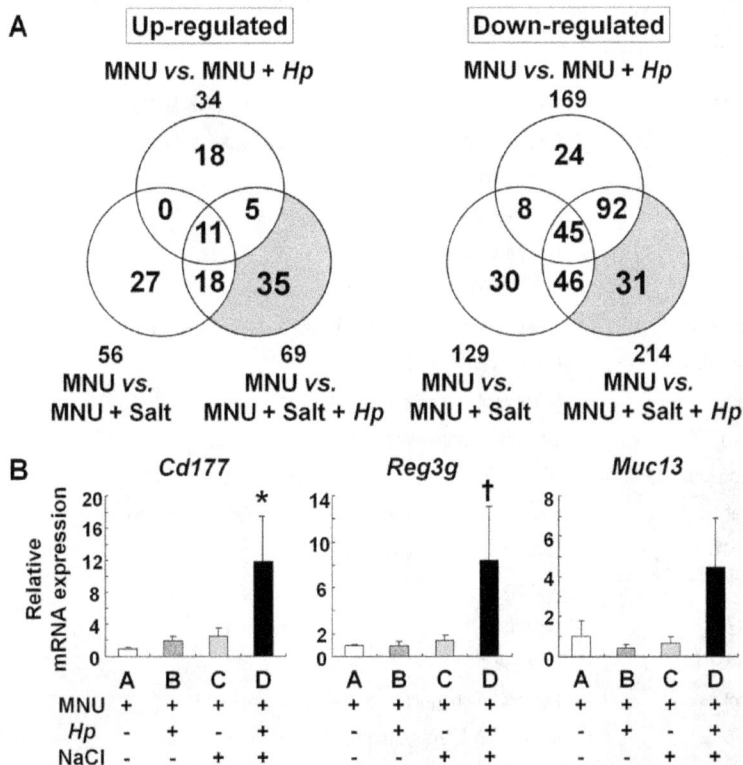

Figure 2 Global gene analysis in the glandular stomach of MNU-treated mice using oligonucleotide microarray. A: Number of genes up- or down-regulated more than two-fold in the stomach of MNU-treated mice. In Venn's diagram, the circles indicate up- (left) or down-regulated (right) genes in the stomach of MNU-treated mice with *H. pylori* infection, high-salt diet or their combination. The shaded area represents the up- or down-regulated genes more than two-fold only by the combination. **B**: Quantitative real-time RT-PCR analysis of three selected up-regulated genes (*Cd177*, *Reg3g*, and *Muc13*) in the stomachs of MNU-treated mice. Expression levels of the genes in each sample were normalized by *Gapdh* as internal control using ΔΔCT method. Relative expression levels were represented as the X-fold change relative to Group A (fixed as 1.0). Statistical analysis was performed by the Kruskal-Wallis test for general analysis and Tukey test for multiple comparison. Bars, SE; *, $P < 0.01$ *vs.* Group A and < 0.05 *vs.* Group C; †, $P < 0.01$ *vs.* Group C.

and B), the incidence was also increased by *H. pylori*-infection (Group A, 61.9% and Group B, 100%), albeit without statistical significance. The multiplicities of total tumors in both *H. pylori*-infected groups (Group B, 3.3 ± 1.0 tumors/mouse and Group D, 2.6 ± 1.1) were markedly higher than those in non-infected groups (Group A, 0.9 ± 0.8 and Group C, 1.0 ± 1.2) ($P < 0.05$). The multiplicity of gastric adenocarcinoma in Group D (2.1 ± 1.4) was slightly higher than that in Group B (1.8 ± 1.0) and significantly increased over the Group C value (0.8 ± 1.0) ($P < 0.05$). In contrast, the multiplicities of adenomas in Groups A and D (0.1 ± 0.4 and 0.4 ± 0.5, respectively) were significantly lower than in Group B (1.5 ± 0.6) ($P < 0.05$ and 0.01).

Gene expression profiling in the glandular stomachs by oligonucleotide microarray

With oligonucleotide microarrays, compared with the non-infected and basal diet-treated group (Group A), 34 genes were up-regulated and 169 were down-regulated

more than two-fold in *H. pylori*-infected mice (Group B), 56 up-regulated and 129 down-regulated in high-salt diet-treated mice (Group C), and 69 up-regulated and 214 down-regulated in the combined group (Group D) (Figure 2A). Taken together, as shown in Table 3, we found that 35 genes were up-regulated and 31 genes were down-regulated more than two-fold only by the combination of *H. pylori* infection and high-salt diet. In addition, hierarchical clustering analysis was performed on the four groups with a total of 303 qualified probes using the complete-linkage clustering algorithm (Figure 3). Thirty-one probes including *Cd177*, *Reg3g* and *Muc13* were confirmed to be within a cluster of probes up-regulated only in Group D. Subsequent analysis in the present study was focused on these genes, because it was considered that the genes in which expression was altered only in the combined group might be associated with gastric carcinogenesis and progression in humans.

The entire results of this microarray analysis have been submitted and are readily retrievable from the

Table 3 Regulated genes by combination of *H. pylori* infection and high-salt diet in mouse gastric mucosa

Accession no.	Symbol	Genes/proteins	Fold changes
Up-regulated genes			
XM_357640	Igk-V8	Immunoglobulin kappa chain variable 8 (V8)	14.4
XM_001472541	Ighg	Immunoglobulin heavy chain (gamma polypeptide)	9.2
NM_026862	Cd177	CD177 antigen	7.3
NM_011260	Reg3g	Regenerating islet-derived 3 gamma	6.1
NM_023137	Ubd	Ubiquitin D	4.3
XM_144817	Igk-V34	Immunoglobulin kappa chain variable 34 (V34)	4.1
NM_007675	Ceacam10	Carcinoembryonic antigen-related cell adhesion molecule 10	3.7
NM_183322	Khdc1a	KH domain containing 1A	3.3
NM_011475	Sprr2i	Small proline-rich protein 2I	3.2
NM_175165	Tprg	Transformation related protein 63 regulated	3.2
NM_175406	Atp6v0d2	ATPase, H+ transporting, lysosomal V0 subunit D2	3.0
NM_009703	Araf	v-raf murine sarcoma 3611 viral oncogene homolog	2.6
NM_026822	Lce1b	Late cornified envelope 1B	2.5
NM_016958	Krt14	Keratin 14	2.5
NM_212487	Krt78	Keratin 78	2.4
NM_009807	Casp1	Caspase 1	2.4
NM_146037	Kcnk13	Potassium channel, subfamily K, member 13	2.4
NM_019450	Il1f6	Interleukin 1 family, member 6	2.3
NM_008827	Pgf	Placental growth factor	2.3
XM_893506	Klk12	Kallikrein related-peptidase 12	2.3
NM_016887	Cldn7	Claudin 7	2.3
NM_029360	Tm4sf5	Transmembrane 4 superfamily member 5	2.2
NM_172301	Ccnb1	Cyclin B1	2.2
NM_010739	Muc13	Mucin 13, epithelial transmembrane	2.2
NM_011165	Prl4a1	Prolactin family 4, subfamily a, member 1	2.2
NM_010162	Ext1	Exostoses (multiple) 1	2.2
NM_011704	Vnn1	Vanin 1	2.1
NM_011082	Pigr	Polymeric immunoglobulin receptor	2.1
NM_007769	Dmbt1	Deleted in malignant brain tumors 1	2.1
NM_022984	Retn	Resistin	2.1
NM_173037	Tmco 7	Transmembrane and coiled-coil domain 7	2.1
NM_009100	Rptn	Repetin	2.1
NM_007630	Ccnb2	Cyclin B2	2.1
NM_001081060	Slc9a3	Solute carrier family 9 (sodium/hydrogen exchanger), member 3	2.0
NM_146588	Olfr1030	Olfactory receptor 1030	2.0
Down-regulated genes			
NM_008753	Oaz1	Ornithine decarboxylase antizyme 1	0.31
NM_027126	Hfe2	Hemochromatosis type 2 (juvenile) (human homolog)	0.33
NM_053206	Magee2	Melanoma antigen, family E, 2	0.33
NM_010924	Nnmt	Nicotinamide N-methyltransferase	0.41
NM_026260	Tctn3	Tectonic family member 3	0.41
NM_181039	Lphn1	Latrophilin 1	0.43
NM_008312	Htr2c	5-hydroxytryptamine (serotonin) receptor 2C	0.43

Table 3 Regulated genes by combination of _H. pylori_ infection and high-salt diet in mouse gastric mucosa _(Continued)_

NM_146667	Olfr740	Olfactory receptor 740	0.44
NM_007550	Blm	Bloom syndrome homolog (human)	0.44
NM_011243	Rarb	Retinoic acid receptor, beta	0.44
NM_184052	Igf1	Insulin-like growth factor 1	0.45
NM_013893	Reg3d	Regenerating islet-derived 3 delta	0.46
NM_008645	Mug1	Murinoglobulin 1	0.46
NM_029550	Keg1	Kidney expressed gene 1	0.46
NM_019388	Cd86	CD86 antigen	0.46
NM_011316	Saa4	Serum amyloid A 4	0.47
NM_007811	Cyp26a1	Cytochrome P450, family 26, subfamily a, polypeptide 1	0.47
NM_011538	Tbx6	T-box 6	0.48
NM_011086	Pip5k3	Phosphatidylinositol-3-phospate/phosphatidylinositol 5-kinase, type III	0.48
NM_133723	Asph	Aspartate-beta-hydroxylase	0.48
NM_001081390	Palld	Palladin, cytoskeletal associated protein	0.48
NM_007858	Diap1	Diaphanous homolog 1 (Drosophila)	0.48
NM_053271	Rims2	Regulating synaptic membrane exocytosis 2	0.48
NM_153163	Cadps2	Ca2+–dependent activator protein for secretion 2	0.49
NM_007541	Bglap1	Bone gamma carboxyglutamate protein 1	0.49
NM_031871	Ghdc	GH3 domain containing	0.49
NM_025545	Aptx	Aprataxin	0.49
NM_177322	Agtr1a	Angiotensin II receptor, type 1a	0.49
NM_026872	Ubap2	Ubiquitin-associated protein 2	0.49
NM_028045	Erv3	Endogenous retroviral sequence 3	0.49
NM_011641	Trp63	Transformation related protein 63	0.49

public database NCBI Gene Expression Omnibus (GEO) with the accession number GSE29444 (sample number: GSM728857-60).

Quantitative real-time RT-PCR analysis of gene expression profiles in MNU-treated mouse stomachs

Relative quantitative real-time RT-PCR analysis of three selected up-regulated genes (_Cd177_, _Reg3g_, and _Muc13_) in _H. pylori_-infected and high-salt diet-treated mice confirmed increased expression of _Cd177_ and _Reg3g_, as shown in Figure 2B, with significant differences. Although expression level of _Muc13_ in Group D was higher than all other groups, there was no statistical significance among them ($P = 0.0712$ _vs._ Group C).

Immunohistochemical expression of CD177 in human advanced gastric cancers and correlation with clinicopathological factors

On immunohistochemical analysis of human gastric cancer tissues, CD177 was observed not only in the membranes and cytoplasms of infiltrated neutrophils, but also in gastric cancer cells of both well- and poorly-differentiated

adenocarcinomas (Figure 4A). Cancer cells of signet-ring cell type (2 cases) were negative for CD177. Among 55 gastric cancer cases, moderate to strong expression of CD177 was observed in 33 (60.0%) (Table 4).

The follow-up period of the patients ranged from 9 to 606 weeks (median = 83 weeks). Five-year survival rates for CD177-positive and negative were 39.4% and 18.2%, respectively. From the Kaplan-Meier survival curve analysis, CD177-positive expression was associated with better overall survival ($P = 0.0294$, log-rank test) (Figure 4B). There was no statistically significant correlation of CD177 expression with age, histological classification, depth of invasion, and lymph node metastasis (Table 4).

Multivariate analysis for overall survival of human gastric cancer cases

Using the Cox proportional hazards model, multivariate analysis of clinicopathological variables, including the patient age, tumor histological classification, invasion depth, lymph node metastasis, and CD177 expression (Table 5), revealed the last to be an independent factor for overall survival ($P = 0.0323$). Patient age and low

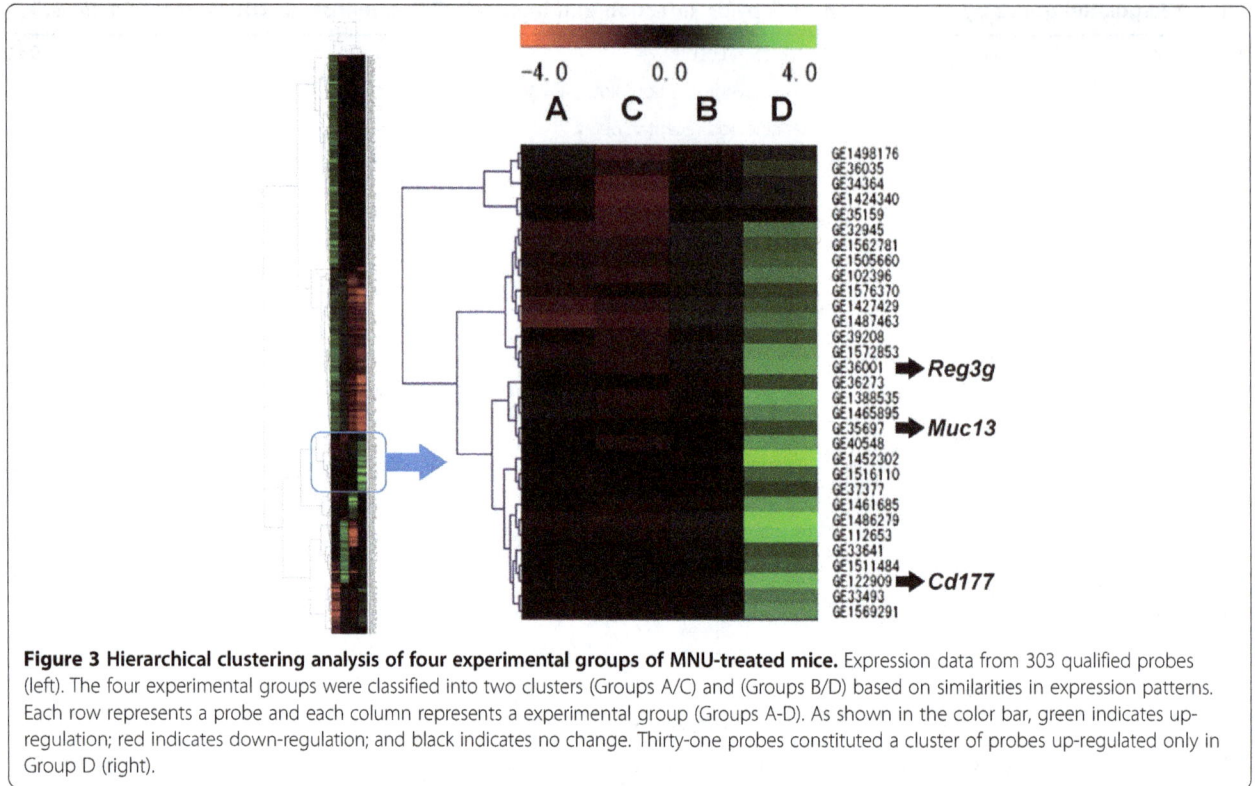

Figure 3 Hierarchical clustering analysis of four experimental groups of MNU-treated mice. Expression data from 303 qualified probes (left). The four experimental groups were classified into two clusters (Groups A/C) and (Groups B/D) based on similarities in expression patterns. Each row represents a probe and each column represents a experimental group (Groups A-D). As shown in the color bar, green indicates up-regulation; red indicates down-regulation; and black indicates no change. Thirty-one probes constituted a cluster of probes up-regulated only in Group D (right).

differentiation of adenocarcinoma were also associated with poor overall survival (P = 0.0439 and 0.0017, respectively). Tumor invasion depth and lymph node metastasis were not independent factors of gastric cancer cases in the present study (P > 0.05).

Discussion

In the present study, we demonstrated that the mouse model combined with *H. pylori* infection and high-salt diet is a useful tool to investigate the detailed mechanisms both of development and progression of gastric

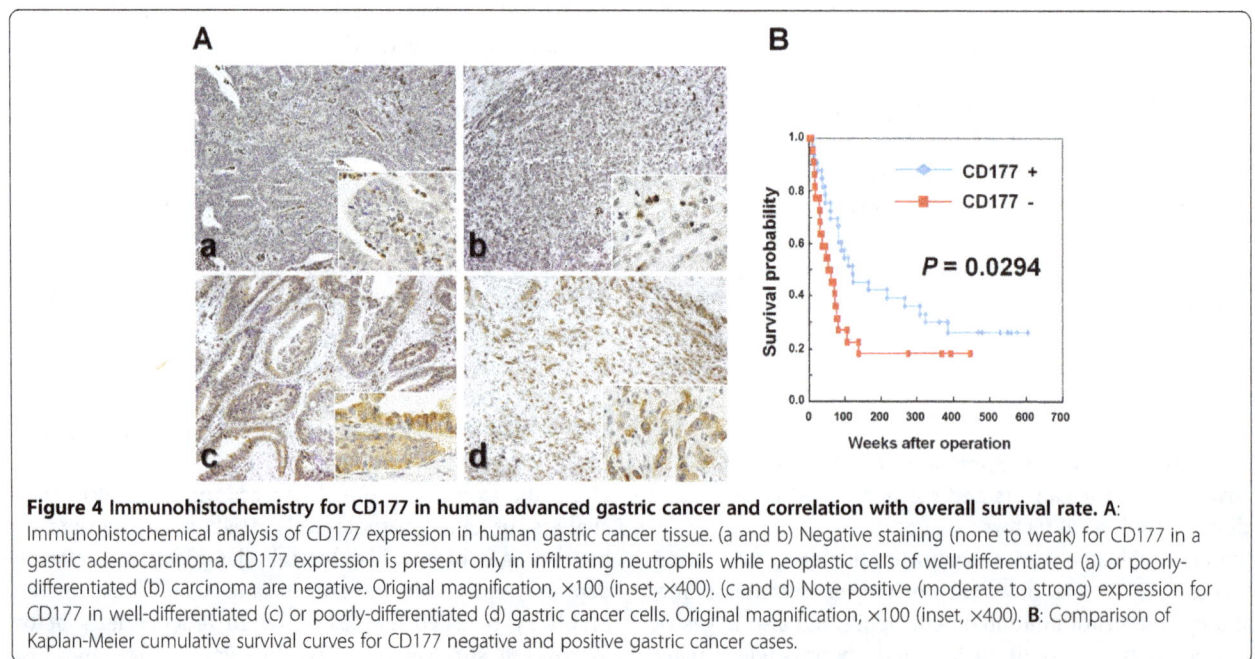

Figure 4 Immunohistochemistry for CD177 in human advanced gastric cancer and correlation with overall survival rate. A: Immunohistochemical analysis of CD177 expression in human gastric cancer tissue. (a and b) Negative staining (none to weak) for CD177 in a gastric adenocarcinoma. CD177 expression is present only in infiltrating neutrophils while neoplastic cells of well-differentiated (a) or poorly-differentiated (b) carcinoma are negative. Original magnification, ×100 (inset, ×400). (c and d) Note positive (moderate to strong) expression for CD177 in well-differentiated (c) or poorly-differentiated (d) gastric cancer cells. Original magnification, ×100 (inset, ×400). **B:** Comparison of Kaplan-Meier cumulative survival curves for CD177 negative and positive gastric cancer cases.

Table 4 CD177 expression in gastric carcinomas and its correlation with clinicopathological factors

	Case no.	CD177 Over-expression				P value‡
		Positive		Negative		
		Strong	Moderate	Weak	None	
Gastric adenocarcinomas	55	18	15	17	5	
Age						
Years (means ± SD)		55.3 ± 10.4	60.2 ± 8.13	59.8 ± 11.0	60.4 ± 13.0	0.5039
Histological classification						
Well/moderately-differentiated type*	21	6	9	4	2	0.1904
Poorly-differentiated/Signet-ring cell type**	34	12	6	13	3	
Depth of invasion†						
T1-3	27	5	10	10	2	0.2011
T4	26	11	5	7	3	
Lymph node metastasis						
N0	6	1	2	2	1	0.7869
N1-3	49	17	13	15	4	

* Lauren's intestinal type, ** Lauren's diffuse type, † Case number was reduced to fifty-three because the depth of invasion was not classified in two cases,
‡ ANOVA and Chi-square test were performed for age and other factors, respectively.

neoplasms. A number of rodent models of gastric cancer have been developed under various conditions, including *H. pylori* or *H. felis* infection, exposure to chemical carcinogens, and genetic modification [21,30]. Since *H. pylori* is known as a most closely-associated risk factor in man, animal models with infection of the bacterium, such as that utilizing Mongolian gerbils, are considered to be particularly important to mimic the background of human gastric carcinogenesis. On the other hand, there is a consensus that gastric cancer is a multifactorial disease [31]. Epidemiological studies and animal experiments have demonstrated that development of stomach cancer is also associated with many other factors including salt intake, alcohol drinking and cigarette, containing a wide variety of chemical carcinogen. In the present study, we attempted to mimic the gastric environment of human high-risk group exposed to combination of *H. pylori* infection, salt intake, and carcinogen.

As might be expected, there are both advantages and disadvantages of *Helicobacter*-infected mouse models. Instability of *cag* pathogenicity islands (PAI), a particularly important virulence factor of *H. pylori*, has been reported in the mouse model using SS1 strain [32]. Multiplicity of gastric tumors is difficult to examine in the gerbil model, because almost all of the stomach tumors in gerbils show invasive growth into the lamina propria or muscle layer. In the present study, our results demonstrated that *H. pylori* infection increased not only incidence but also multiplicity of gastric tumors in MNU-treated mice. Thus, the mouse model presented here has advantages in respect to investigate the multiplicity and tissue sampling for gene expression analysis.

In this study, we focused on the genes in which the expression was regulated only in *H. pylori*-infection and high-salt diet combined mice, which are expected to reflect the background of human high-risk group, to explore examples which might be associated with tumor progression. The two up-regulated genes selected, *Cd177* and *Reg3g* could be confirmed to exhibit significant over-expression by relative quantitative RT-PCR. Expression level of *Muc13* showed a tendency for increase with combination of *H. pylori* and salt, although this was not statistically significant. *Muc13* is a recently identified gene encoding transmembrane mucin that is expressed in the stomach to large intestine [33]. Shimamura et al. have reported that overexpression of *Muc13* is associated with differentiation towards the intestinal (differentiated) type of human gastric cancer [34]. In addition, the combined expression of

Table 5 Multivariate analysis of prognostic factos in patients with gastric cancer using Cox proportional hazard model

Factors	Hazard ratio	95% CI	P value
CD177 expression (negative)	2.07	1.063-4.021	0.0323
Age (year)	1.04	1.001-1.071	0.0439
Histological type (poorly-differentiated)	4.06	1.695-9.742	0.0017
Depth of invasion (high grade)	1.64	0.790-3.410	0.1838
Lymph node metastasis (positive)	3.40	0.773-14.92	0.1055

MUC13 with other metaplasia biomarkers is shown to be a prognostic indicator in several types of gastric cancer [35]. In the present study, all gastric tumors observed in MNU-treated mice were histologically of differentiated type. The REG protein family is also known to be associated with gastric cancer development and *Reg1α* and *Reg4* have been suggested as prognostic markers for advanced stomach cancers in man [36]. The present results indicate the possibility that *Reg3g* is also involved with progression of stomach tumor.

Immunohistochemical analysis of CD177 in advanced gastric cancer specimens showed expression to be significantly correlated with a good prognosis and survival rate after surgery. Importantly, multivariate analysis with clinicopathological factors as covariates further revealed high expression to be an independent prognostic factor for overall survival, as along with patient's age and histological classification. To our knowledge, the present study is the first to provide evidence that high expression of CD177 is associated with favorable prognosis in advanced gastric cancer.

CD177 is a member of the leukocyte antigen 6 (Ly-6) gene superfamily, encoding two neutrophil-associated proteins, NB1 and PRV-1 [37,38]. The NB1 glycoprotein is typically expressed on a subpopulation of neutrophils, located at plasma membranes and secondary granules. Recent studies have demonstrated that CD177 is overexpressed in neutrophils from 95% of patients with polycythemia vera and in half of patients with essential thrombocythemia [37]. Gonda et al. have reported a microarray analysis that *Cd177* expression in whole gastric tissue of *H. felis*-infected mice with mucosal dysplasia is reduced by folic acid supplementation [39]. Because they compared stage-matched groups to detect up- or down-regulated genes only by treatment of folic acid, it is unclear if *Cd177* expression is associated with gastritis or dysplasia. In our microarray results, there were no significant differences in expression of *Ela2*, which is a neutrophil-specific gene [40], and histological degrees of neutrophil infiltration were almost same among *H. pylori*-infected groups (data not shown). Therefore, the up-regulation of *Cd177* observed in this study was considered to be caused not by increased infiltration of neutrophils into the gastric mucosa but by a change of gene expression in tumor cells. NB1 is similar in structure to urokinase-type plasminogen activator receptor (uPAR), which is known to be associated with cell adhesion and migration [37]. Thus, there is a possibility that CD177 also acts as a regulator of adhesion and migration of neoplastic cells in gastric tumor. Further studies are needed to clarify the association between CD177 expression in gastric epithelial cells and tumor progression.

Conclusions

We demonstrated that the mouse model combined with *H. pylori* infection and high-salt diet is suitable for investigation of global gene expression associated with gastric tumor development and progression. Furthermore, our results suggest that CD177 expression might be associated with a favorable prognosis of gastric adenocarcinomas in man.

Abbreviations

FBS: Fetal bovine serum; *Gapdh*: Glyceraldehyde-3-phosphate dehydrogenase; H&E: Hematoxylin and eosin; *H. pylori*: Helicobacter pylori; Ly-6: Leukocyte antigen 6; MNU: N-methyl-N-nitrosourea; *Muc13*: Mucin 13; PAI: Pathogenicity islands; *Reg3g*: Regenerating islet-derived 3 gamma; RT-PCR: Reverse transcription-polymerase chain reaction; uPAR: Urokinase-type plasminogen activator receptor.

Competing interests

The authors declare that they have no competing interests.

Authors' contributions

TTo and TTs designed the study under the supervision of AN, KO, TTa and MT. MY, HB, NS, ST, LS and AS participated in the animal handling and procedures. Clinical sample collection and suggestions were provided by SI and YY. Sample analysis and evaluation were performed by TTo, TTs and MY. All authors read and approved the final manuscript.

Acknowledgements

This study was supported by Grant-in Aid for the Third-term Comprehensive 10-year Strategy for Cancer Control from the Ministry of Health, Labour and Welfare, Japan, Grant-in-Aid for the Cancer Research from the Ministry of Health, Labour and Welfare, Japan, and Grant-in-Aid for Young Scientists B (20790318 and 22700935) from the Ministry of Education, Culture, Sports, Science and Technology, Japan.

Author details

[1]Division of Pathology, National Institute of Health Sciences, Tokyo, Japan. [2]Division of Oncological Pathology, Aichi Cancer Center Research Institute, Nagoya, Japan. [3]Department of Pathology, Fujita Health University School of Medicine, Toyoake, Japan. [4]Faculty of Veterinary Medicine, Nippon Veterinary and Life Science University, Tokyo, Japan. [5]Chemicals Safety Department, Mitsui Chemicals Inc, Mobara, Japan. [6]Department of Pathology and Matrix Biology, Mie University Graduate School of Medicine, Tsu, Japan. [7]Department of Gastroenterological Surgery, Aichi Cancer Center Hospital, Nagoya, Japan. [8]Biological Safety Research Center, National Institute of Health Sciences, Tokyo, Japan. [9]The Tohkai Cytopathology Institute: Cancer Research and Prevention, Gifu, Japan. [10]Japan Bioassay Research Center, Hadano, Japan.

References

1. Jemal A, Bray F, Center MM, Ferlay J, Ward E, Forman D: **Global cancer statistics.** *CA Cancer J Clin* 2011, **61:**69–90.
2. Uemura N, Okamoto S, Yamamoto S, Matsumura N, Yamaguchi S, Yamakido M, Taniyama K, Sasaki N, Schlemper RJ: **Helicobacter pylori infection and the development of gastric cancer.** *N Engl J Med* 2001, **345:**784–789.
3. Kono S, Hirohata T: **Nutrition and stomach cancer.** *Cancer Causes Control* 1996, **7:**41–55.
4. Tsugane S: **Salt, salted food intake, and risk of gastric cancer: epidemiologic evidence.** *Cancer Sci* 2005, **96:**1–6.
5. Joossens JV, Hill MJ, Elliott P, Stamler R, Lesaffre E, Dyer A, Nichols R, Kesteloot H: **Dietary salt, nitrate and stomach cancer mortality in 24 countries. European cancer prevention (ECP) and the INTERSALT cooperative research group.** *Int J Epidemiol* 1996, **25:**494–504.
6. Nozaki K, Shimizu N, Inada K, Tsukamoto T, Inoue M, Kumagai T, Sugiyama A, Mizoshita T, Kaminishi M, Tatematsu M: **Synergistic promoting effects of Helicobacter pylori infection and high-salt diet on gastric carcinogenesis in Mongolian gerbils.** *Jpn J Cancer Res* 2002, **93:**1083–1089.
7. Abe M, Yamashita S, Kuramoto T, Hirayama Y, Tsukamoto T, Ohta T, Tatematsu M, Ohki M, Takato T, Sugimura T, *et al*: **Global expression analysis of N-methyl-N'-nitro-N-nitrosoguanidine-induced rat stomach**

carcinomas using oligonucleotide microarrays. *Carcinogenesis* 2003, **24**:861–867.

8. Hasegawa S, Furukawa Y, Li M, Satoh S, Kato T, Watanabe T, Katagiri T, Tsunoda T, Yamaoka Y, Nakamura Y: Genome-wide analysis of gene expression in intestinal-type gastric cancers using a complementary DNA microarray representing 23,040 genes. *Cancer Res* 2002, **62**:7012–7017.

9. Boussioutas A, Li H, Liu J, Waring P, Lade S, Holloway AJ, Taupin D, Gorringe K, Haviv I, Desmond PV, *et al*: Distinctive patterns of gene expression in premalignant gastric mucosa and gastric cancer. *Cancer Res* 2003, **63**:2569–2577.

10. El-Rifai W, Frierson HF Jr, Harper JC, Powell SM, Knuutila S: Expression profiling of gastric adenocarcinoma using cDNA array. *Int J Cancer* 2001, **92**:832–838.

11. Hofman VJ, Moreilhon C, Brest PD, Lassalle S, Le Brigand K, Sicard D, Raymond J, Lamarque D, Hebuterne XA, Mari B, *et al*: Gene expression profiling in human gastric mucosa infected with Helicobacter pylori. *Mod Pathol* 2007, **20**:974–989.

12. Kobayashi M, Lee H, Schaffer L, Gilmartin TJ, Head SR, Takaishi S, Wang TC, Nakayama J, Fukuda M: A distinctive set of genes is upregulated during the inflammation-carcinoma sequence in mouse stomach infected by Helicobacter felis. *J Histochem Cytochem* 2007, **55**:263–274.

13. Takaishi S, Wang TC: Gene expression profiling in a mouse model of Helicobacter-induced gastric cancer. *Cancer Sci* 2007, **98**:284–293.

14. Hippo Y, Taniguchi H, Tsutsumi S, Machida N, Chong JM, Fukayama M, Kodama T, Aburatani H: Global gene expression analysis of gastric cancer by oligonucleotide microarrays. *Cancer Res* 2002, **62**:233–240.

15. Huff JL, Hansen LM, Solnick JV: Gastric transcription profile of Helicobacter pylori infection in the rhesus macaque. *Infect Immun* 2004, **72**:5216–5226.

16. Vivas JR, Regnault B, Michel V, Bussiere FI, Ave P, Huerre M, Labigne A, DE MM, Touati E: Interferon gamma-signature transcript profiling and IL-23 upregulation in response to Helicobacter pylori infection. *Int J Immunopathol Pharmacol* 2008, **21**:515–526.

17. Maeda S, Otsuka M, Hirata Y, Mitsuno Y, Yoshida H, Shiratori Y, Masuho Y, Muramatsu M, Seki N, Omata M: cDNA microarray analysis of Helicobacter pylori-mediated alteration of gene expression in gastric cancer cells. *Biochem Biophys Res Commun* 2001, **284**:443–449.

18. Marcos NT, Magalhaes A, Ferreira B, Oliveira MJ, Carvalho AS, Mendes N, Gilmartin T, Head SR, Figueiredo C, David L, *et al*: Helicobacter pylori induces beta3GnT5 in human gastric cell lines, modulating expression of the SabA ligand sialyl-Lewis x. *J Clin Invest* 2008, **118**:2325–2336.

19. Mills JC, Syder AJ, Hong CV, Guruge JL, Raaii F, Gordon JI: A molecular profile of the mouse gastric parietal cell with and without exposure to Helicobacter pylori. *Proc Natl Acad Sci USA* 2001, **98**:13687–13692.

20. Tatematsu M, Nozaki K, Tsukamoto T: Helicobacter pylori infection and gastric carcinogenesis in animal models. *Gastric Cancer* 2003, **6**:1–7.

21. Tsukamoto T, Mizoshita T, Tatematsu M: Animal models of stomach carcinogenesis. *Toxicol Pathol* 2007, **35**:636–648.

22. Toyoda T, Tsukamoto T, Takasu S, Hirano N, Ban H, Shi L, Kumagai T, Tanaka T, Tatematsu M: Pitavastatin fails to lower serum lipid levels or inhibit gastric carcinogenesis in Helicobacter pylori-infected rodent models. *Cancer Prev Res* 2009, **2**:751–758.

23. Toyoda T, Tsukamoto T, Takasu S, Shi L, Hirano N, Ban H, Kumagai T, Tatematsu M: Anti-inflammatory effects of caffeic acid phenethyl ester (CAPE), a nuclear factor-kappaB inhibitor, on Helicobacter pylori-induced gastritis in Mongolian gerbils. *Int J Cancer* 2009, **125**:1786–1795.

24. Magari H, Shimizu Y, Inada K, Enomoto S, Tomeki T, Yanaoka K, Tamai H, Arii K, Nakata H, Oka M, *et al*: Inhibitory effect of etodolac, a selective cyclooxygenase-2 inhibitor, on stomach carcinogenesis in Helicobacter pylori-infected Mongolian gerbils. *Biochem Biophys Res Commun* 2005, **334**:606–612.

25. Toyoda T, Tsukamoto T, Hirano N, Mizoshita T, Kato S, Takasu S, Ban H, Tatematsu M: Synergistic upregulation of inducible nitric oxide synthase and cyclooxygenase-2 in gastric mucosa of Mongolian gerbils by a high-salt diet and Helicobacter pylori infection. *Histol Histopathol* 2008, **23**:593–599.

26. Kato S, Tsukamoto T, Mizoshita T, Tanaka H, Kumagai T, Ota H, Katsuyama T, Asaka M, Tatematsu M: High salt diets dose-dependently promote gastric chemical carcinogenesis in Helicobacter pylori-infected Mongolian gerbils associated with a shift in mucin production from glandular to surface mucous cells. *Int J Cancer* 2006, **119**:1558–1566.

27. Shimizu N, Inada KI, Tsukamoto T, Nakanishi H, Ikehara Y, Yoshikawa A, Kaminishi M, Kuramoto S, Tatematsu M: New animal model of glandular stomach carcinogenesis in Mongolian gerbils infected with Helicobacter pylori and treated with a chemical carcinogen. *J Gastroenterol* 1999, **34**(Suppl. 11):61–66.

28. Takasu S, Tsukamoto T, Cao XY, Toyoda T, Hirata A, Ban H, Yamamoto M, Sakai H, Yanai T, Masegi T, *et al*: Roles of cyclooxygenase-2 and microsomal prostaglandin E synthase-1 expression and beta-catenin activation in gastric carcinogenesis in N-methyl-N-nitrosourea-treated K19-C2mE transgenic mice. *Cancer Sci* 2008, **99**:2356–2364.

29. Japanese Gastric Cancer Association: Japanese Classification of Gastric Carcinoma - 2nd English Edition. *Gastric Cancer* 1998, **1**:10–24.

30. Oshima H, Oguma K, Du YC, Oshima M: Prostaglandin E2, Wnt, and BMP in gastric tumor mouse models. *Cancer Sci* 2009, **100**:1779–1785.

31. Fock KM, Talley N, Moayyedi P, Hunt R, Azuma T, Sugano K, Xiao SD, Lam SK, Goh KL, Chiba T, *et al*: Asia-Pacific consensus guidelines on gastric cancer prevention. *J Gastroenterol Hepatol* 2008, **23**:351–365.

32. Thompson LJ, Danon SJ, Wilson JE, O'Rourke JL, Salama NR, Falkow S, Mitchell H, Lee A: Chronic Helicobacter pylori infection with Sydney strain 1 and a newly identified mouse-adapted strain (Sydney strain 2000) in C57BL/6 and BALB/c mice. *Infect Immun* 2004, **72**:4668–4679.

33. Williams SJ, Wreschner DH, Tran M, Eyre HJ, Sutherland GR, McGuckin MA: Muc13, a novel human cell surface mucin expressed by epithelial and hemopoietic cells. *J Biol Chem* 2001, **276**:18327–18336.

34. Shimamura T, Ito H, Shibahara J, Watanabe A, Hippo Y, Taniguchi H, Chen Y, Kashima T, Ohtomo T, Tanioka F, *et al*: Overexpression of MUC13 is associated with intestinal-type gastric cancer. *Cancer Sci* 2005, **96**:265–273.

35. Suh YS, Lee HJ, Jung EJ, Kim MA, Nam KT, Goldenring JR, Yang HK, Kim WH: The combined expression of metaplasia biomarkers predicts the prognosis of gastric cancer. *Ann Surg Oncol* 2012, **19**:1240–1249.

36. Yamagishi H, Fukui H, Sekikawa A, Kono T, Fujii S, Ichikawa K, Tomita S, Imura J, Hiraishi H, Chiba T, *et al*: Expression profile of REG family proteins REG Ialpha and REG IV in advanced gastric cancer: comparison with mucin phenotype and prognostic markers. *Mod Pathol* 2009, **22**:906–913.

37. Stroncek DF, Caruccio L, Bettinotti M: CD177: A member of the Ly-6 gene superfamily involved with neutrophil proliferation and polycythemia vera. *J Transl Med* 2004, **2**:8.

38. Kissel K, Santoso S, Hofmann C, Stroncek D, Bux J: Molecular basis of the neutrophil glycoprotein NB1 (CD177) involved in the pathogenesis of immune neutropenias and transfusion reactions. *Eur J Immunol* 2001, **31**:1301–1309.

39. Gonda TA, Kim YI, Salas MC, Gamble MV, Shibata W, Muthupalani S, Sohn KJ, Abrams JA, Fox JG, Wang TC, *et al*: Folic acid increases global DNA methylation and reduces inflammation to prevent Helicobacter-associated gastric cancer in mice. *Gastroenterology* 2012, **142**:824–833.

40. Sturrock A, Franklin KF, Wu S, Hoidal JR: Characterization and localization of the genes for mouse proteinase-3 (Prtn3) and neutrophil elastase (Ela2). *Cytogenet Cell Genet* 1998, **83**:104–108.

17

Gastric bacterial Flora in patients Harbouring *Helicobacter pylori* with or without chronic dyspepsia: analysis with matrix-assisted laser desorption ionization time-of-flight mass spectroscopy

Verima Pereira[1], Philip Abraham[1*], Sivaramaiah Nallapeta[2] and Anjali Shetty[3]

Abstract

Background: The gastric microbiota has recently been implicated in the causation of organic/structural gastroduodenal diseases (gastric and duodenal ulcers, gastric cancer) in patients with *Helicobacter pylori* (H. pylori) infection. We aimed to ascertain, in patients harbouring *H. pylori*, the role of the gastric microbiota in the causation of symptoms (chronic dyspepsia) in the absence of organic disease.

Methods: Seventy-four gastric biopsy samples obtained at endoscopy from patients with ($n = 21$) or without ($n = 53$) chronic dyspepsia, and that tested positive by the bedside rapid urease test for *H. pylori* infection, were cultured for detection of *H. pylori* and non-*H. pylori* organisms. The cultured organisms were identified by matrix-assisted laser desorption ionization time-of-flight mass spectroscopy (MALDI-TOF MS).

Results: A total of 106 non-*H. pylori* isolates were obtained from 74 patients' samples. This included 33 isolates (median 2, range 1–2 per patient) from dyspeptic and 73 (median 2, range 1–2 per patient) from non-dyspeptic patients. These were identified from the Bruker Biotyper 2 database as Staphylococcus spp., Streptococcus spp., Lactobacillus spp., Micrococcus spp., Enterococcus spp., Pseudomonas spp., Escherichia spp., Klebsiella spp. and Bacillus spp., Staphylococcus and Lactobacillus were identified significantly more commonly in dyspeptics and Streptococcus, Pseudomonas, *Escherichia coli* and *Klebsiella pneumoniae* in non-dyspeptics. All identified organisms belonged to the phyla Firmicutes and Proteobacteria.

Conclusions: There is a qualitative difference in the gastric microbial spectrum between patients harbouring *H. pylori* with and without chronic dyspepsia. Whether these organisms have an independent role in the development or prevention of dyspepsia or act in concurrence with *H. pylori* needs study.

Keywords: Gastric microbiome, Gastric microbiota, *Helicobacter pylori* pathogenicity, MALDI-TOF

* Correspondence: dr_pabraham@hindujahospital.com
[1]Division of Gastroenterology, P D Hinduja Hospital, V S Marg, Mahim, Mumbai 400016, India
Full list of author information is available at the end of the article

Background

Traditionally, the human stomach has been viewed as an inhospitable environment for microorganisms mainly because of its acidic lumen [1]. With the discovery of *Helicobacter pylori (H. pylori)* and other gastric Helico-bacters, and subsequent insight into the mechanisms by which these organisms adapt to the gastric environment, the stomach is no longer considered sterile and the adaptative mechanisms of local organisms are becoming clearer [2].

Bacterial counts in the human stomach were tradition-ally believed to range from 0 to 10^3 cfu/g [3]; these figures were based on studies with organisms that can be cultured and identified by standard biochemical techniques. More advanced techniques have brought to light one fact: the normal stomach is host to many more organisms than have been identified by standard culture techniques. Studies found colonisation by a complex microbiota be-longing mainly to the Proteobacteria, Firmicutes, Acti-nobacteria and Fusobacterium phyla, which was clearly different from the microbiota described in the mouth and oesophagus [4]. A high prevalence of non-*H. pylori* bacteria has been found, the majority of which were Streptococcus and Staphylococcus [5, 6].

H. pylori infects up to 50% of the world's population [3]. It has been implicated in the causation of various gastroduodenal (duodenal ulcers, MALT lymphoma, gastric cancer) as well as extraintestinal (e.g., refractory an-aemia, idiopathic thrombocytopenic purpura) diseases [7]. Why only a small fraction of those infected will pro-gress to disease development has been the subject of ex-tensive investigation. Several pathogenic factors have been identified within the organism that enable colonisation and progression to disease [3]. Recent attention has also focused on host factors [6–8], with increasing interest in the role of the gastric microbiota particularly in the caus-ation of gastric cancer, in the presence of *H. pylori* infec-tion [9–14]. The role of the human gut microbiota in health and disease in general has been reviewed in detail recently [15].

More common than the development of organic disease is the development of symptoms (chronic dyspepsia) in patients with *H. pylori* infection even in the absence of organic disease (so-called functional dyspepsia). Although the role of *H. pylori* infection in functional dyspepsia is still being debated, eradication of the infection with anti-bacterial therapy has been shown to provide symptom re-lief more than with placebo [16]. It is not clear whether the relief is due to eradication of this infection or of any concurrent gastric bacterial population [17]. In support of an important role for non-*H. pylori* bacteria in the caus-ation of disease is the finding in a longitudinal study that treatment for *H. pylori* decreased the occurrence of gastric cancer even in those in whom the organism could not be eradicated [18].

A qualitative difference in the gastric microbiota in per-sons infected with *H. pylori* has been mentioned [8, 9]; which of the two (*H. pylori* and non-*H. pylori* bacteria) influenced the other is not clear. Little is known about the gastric microbiota in patients with *H. pylori* infection with dyspepsia in the absence of organic disease.

Finally, there is information on the gastric microflora in the West [4, 10, 12–14], but reports on the gastric microbiota in developing countries are few [8]. The gastric microbiota of Indian subjects has not been studied by ad-vanced techniques. Why is this important? We expect it to be different in developing countries from what has been reported from the more hygienic environs of the West. Besides, in the context of *H. pylori* infection, it is worth noting that while antibody to this infection is rather wide-spread in a country like India [19], the incidence of gastric cancer is not as high as would then be expected [20]; the reasons for this are only speculative [21].

Our primary aim was therefore to characterise the culturable gastric microbiota in patients with *H. pylori* infection with or without chronic dyspepsia in the absence of organic disease. Simultaneously we wished to determine if there is any qualitative difference in the Indian gastric microbiota as compared to that described from the West, in the presence of *H. pylori* infection. For these purposes, we used matrix-assisted laser desorption ionization time-of-flight mass spectrometry (MALDI-TOF MS) for bacter-ial identification [22]. A higher accuracy is obtained with this technique compared with the phenotypic methods reported before [23].

Methods
Subjects

During an 11-month period (September 2013 – August 2014), 74 consecutive patients (40 men, 34 women) under-going upper gastrointestinal endoscopy for indications de-cided by their treating physician, who had not received any antibiotic for three months prior or acid-suppression ther-apy for four weeks prior, and who consented to obtaining endoscopic gastric biopsy for the purpose of the study, were enrolled. Patients who had comorbid illness (e.g., renal failure, chronic NSAID use) or obvious organic disease on endoscopy (ulcers, cancer) that can cause dyspepsia were excluded.

With diligent sterile precautions and after flushing the endoscope working channel with sterile normal saline, two sets each of mucosal biopsy samples were taken using single-use forceps, from the gastric antrum and body. One set was placed in a commercial urea-based strip (Halifax Research Laboratory, Kolkata) for the bed-side rapid urease test (RUT) for *H. pylori* infection. The second set was transported in ice packs at 4 °C to the cul-ture laboratory within an hour of collection, using sterile 0.9% saline as transport medium. Samples that yielded positive results on RUT were taken for *H. pylori* culture and further examinations. Tissue was not taken for histologic examination.

The institution's Ethics Committee reviewed and approved the study protocol (reference number 760-PA-13 dated August 22, 2013) and informed written consent was obtained from each patient.

The 74 patients were divided into two groups, namely, those with chronic dyspepsia (greater than six months' duration) as the indication for endoscopy (dyspeptics; $n = 21$; median age 48, range 21 to 66 years) and those whose indications for endoscopy were other than dyspepsia (non-dyspeptics; $n = 53$; median age 47, range 22 to 79 years). As mentioned earlier, those with organic disease that can cause dyspepsia were excluded. The dyspeptics group thus had functional dyspepsia, as defined by the Rome III criteria [24]. The non-dyspeptic group included patients with the following indications: dysphagia, anaemia suspected to be due to gastrointestinal blood loss, search for primary cancer, and screening for varices in portal hypertension.

Tissue culture

The selected samples were dispersed using a homogeniser. Each homogenate was inoculated into sterile tryptic soy broth and the samples were plated on non-selective Brucella blood agar and Mueller Hinton agar plates supplemented with 5% human blood, starch and human serum. They were then incubated at 37 °C under microaerophilic, aerobic and anaerobic conditions for 5 to 7 days.

Small translucent colonies were selected for Giemsa's staining and tested for urease, catalase and oxidase activity. Curved rods resembling *Helicobacter* that were positive for all the three enzyme activity tests were identified as *H. pylori*.

The non-*H. pylori* colonies were subjected to Gram staining and colony characteristics study (size, shape, colour, margins, opacity, elevation), and to MALDI-TOF MS for identification.

Identification by MALDI-TOF MS

The method we used was similar to that used by Hu et al. [23] Appropriately 5–10 mg of colony was scraped and suspended in 300 µL deionized water in an Eppendorf tube and mixed; 900 µL ethanol was added to it and further mixed. The sample was then centrifuged at 12000 rpm for 2 min. The supernatant was decanted and centrifuged again and the ethanol was pipetted off without disturbing the bacterial pellet, which was then dried for 2–3 min. Fifty µL formic acid (70% in water) was added to the dry pellet and mixed, and 50 µL acetonitrile was then added. After centrifugation again at 12000 rpm for 2 min, 1 µL of the supernatant containing the bacterial extract was

transferred on to the 96-well steel plate and dried. One µL of matrix solution containing saturated solution of cyano-4-hydroxycinnamic acid in 50% acetonitrile + 2.5% trifluoroacetic acid was added and allowed to air dry at room temperature.

Measurement was done with Microflex LT mass spectrometer (Bruker Daltonics; Germany) equipped with a 200 Hz smartbeam laser. The parameter settings were as follows: delay 320 ns; ion source (i) 20 kV; ion source (ii) 18.5 kV, lens voltage 8.5 kV; and mass range 2–15 kDa. Each run was validated with an *Escherichia coli (E. coli)* control sample where the presence of 10 specific proteins ensured that the spectrometer was set properly. Raw spectra of the strains were analysed by MALDI Biotyper 2.0 software (Bruker Daltonics; Germany) using the default settings.

A list of peaks up to 100 was generated. The threshold for peak acceptance was a signal-to-noise (S/N) ratio of 3. After alignment, peaks with a mass-to-charge (m/z) ratio difference of less than 200 ppm were considered to be identical. The peak lists generated were used for matches against the reference library, by directly using the integrated pattern-matching algorithm of the software. All parameters were the same regardless of the bacteria analysed [3] and a score was attributed to each identification.

Statistical analysis

Fisher's exact test was used to compare the frequency of micro-organisms in dyspeptic patients and non-dyspeptic patients.

Results

The ATCC culture of *E. coli* (positive control) was correctly identified with a score of > 2. The yields on both plates (Brucella blood agar and Mueller Hinton agar) were identical for the types of organisms, as identified on MALDI-TOF.

From the 74 biopsy samples, 106 isolates were obtained. These included 33 isolates (median 2, range 1 to 2 per patient) from dyspeptic and 73 (median 2, range 1–2 per patient) from non-dyspeptic patients; there was no difference in the isolation rates between the two groups.

The 106 isolates included 32 of Staphylococcus spp., 29 of Streptococcus spp., 18 of Lactobacillus spp., 11 of *Klebsiella pneumoniae*, 8 of *Escherichia coli*, 5 of *Pseudomonas mosselii*, and one each of Micrococcus, *Enterococcus faecium* and Bacillus (Fig. 1). All the organisms identified belonged to the phyla Firmicutes and Proteobacteria. The Staphylococcus species identified included *Staph. aureus*, *Staph. equorum*, *Staph. haemolyticus*, *Staph. auricularis*, *Staph. hominis*, *Staph. warneri* and *Staph. xylosus*. The Streptococcus species identified included *Strep. salivarius*, *Strep. oralis*, *Strep. sanguinis*, *Strep. gordonii* and *Strep. parasanguinis*. The Lactobacillus species included *L. brevis*

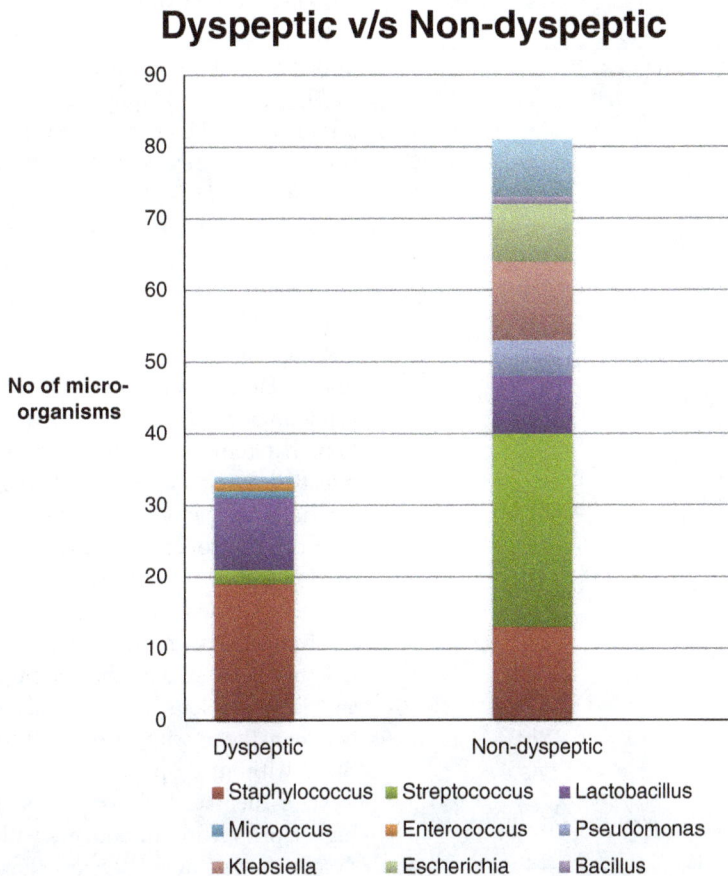

Fig. 1 Genera isolated in the two groups (dyspeptics and non-dyspeptics) with *H. pylori* infection

and *L. paracasei. Micrococcus luteus, Enterococcus faecium, Pseudomonas mosselii, Escherichia coli, Klebsiella pneumonia,* and Bacillus spp. were the others identified.

Staphylococcus spp. and Lactobacillus spp. were significantly more commonly identified in dyspeptics; Streptococcus spp., *Pseudomonas mosselii, Escherichia coli* and *Klebsiella pneumoniae* were more common in non-dyspeptics (Tables 1 and 2).

The MALDI-TOF spectra of the four commonest identified species are shown in Fig. 2.

Discussion

We describe a qualitative difference in the bacterial spectrum in subjects with *H. pylori* infection who do and do not have chronic dyspepsia. The former excluded patients who had obvious organic gastroduodenal or systemic disease that could cause dyspepsia, and met the Rome III criteria for functional dyspepsia [24]. No subgroup analysis (as epigastric pain syndrome and postprandial distress syndrome) was done. We excluded patients who had recently received antibiotic or acid-suppression therapy; none of our patients was on long-term NSAID use. Subsequent to the initiation of our study, the Rome

IV diagnostic criteria for functional dyspepsia were introduced [25]. These differ importantly from the Rome III criteria by defining a severity threshold for identifying symptom as 'bothersome' and by providing a cut-off for symptom frequency.

Table 1 Genera isolated in the two groups (dyspeptics and non-dyspeptics) with *H. pylori* infection

Genera	Dyspeptic (*n* = 21) No. (%)	Non-dyspeptic (*n* = 53) No. (%)	*p* value
Staphylococcus	19 (90.5)	13 (24.5)	0.00
Streptococcus	2 (9.5)	27 (50.9)	0.0011
Lactobacillus	10 (47.6)	8 (15)	0.0060
Micrococcus	1 (4.8)	0 (0)	0.2837
Enterococcus	1 (4.8)	0 (0)	0.2837
Pseudomonas	0 (0)	5 (9.4)	0.0625
Escherichia	0 (0)	8 (15)	0.007
Klebsiella	0 (0)	11 (20.8)	0.0009
Bacillus	0 (0)	1 (1.9)	1
Total No.	33	73	

Total of 106 species were identified from 74 samples

Table 2 Species isolated in the two groups (dyspeptics and non-dyspeptics) with *H. pylori* infection

Micro-organisms	Dyspeptic (*n* = 21)	Non-dyspeptic (*n* = 53)
Staphylococcus aureus	8 (38.1%)	5 (9.4%)
Staphylococcus equorum	1 (4.8%)	0
Staphylococcus haemolyticus	3 (14.3%)	2 (3.8%)
Staphylococcus auricularis	1 (4.8%)	0
Staphylococcus hominis	2 (9.5%)	3 (5.7%)
Staphylococcus warneri	4 (19.1%)	0
Staphylococcus xylosus	0	3 (5.7%)
Streptococcus salivarius	0	11 (20.8%)
Streptococcus oralis	1 (4.8%)	4 (7.6%)
Streptococcus sanguinis	0	8 (15.1%)
Streptococcus gordonii	1 (4.8%)	0
Streptococcus parasanguinis	0	4 (7.6%)
Lactobacillus brevis	5 (23.8%)	8 (15.1%)
Lactobacillus paracasei	5 (23.8%)	0
Micrococcus luteus	1 (4.8%)	0
Enterococcus faecium	1 (4.8%)	0
Pseudomonas mosselii	0	5 (9.4%)
Escherichia coli	0	8 (15.1%)
Klebsiella pneumoniae	0	11 (20.8%)
Bacillus spp	0	1 (1.9%)
Total No.	33	73

Since it would be unethical to perform endoscopies and obtain biopsies in persons without gastroduodenal indications (truly healthy individuals), our comparator group was a diseased-control group that had patients with the infection but without dyspepsia even if they had other structural disease.

Studies from the West have explored the gastric microbiota in the absence and presence of *H. pylori* infection [11]; several studies have also explored the role of the gastric microbiota in the development of structural disease, particularly gastric cancer, in the presence of *H. pylori* infection [10–14]. We attempted to address the issue of why some individuals with *H. pylori* infection develop chronic dyspepsia and others do not, a clinical scenario that is much more common in this infection than the development of structural disease.

We found Staphylococcus spp., Streptococcus spp. and Lactobacillus spp. as the most frequently identified organisms in the samples we studied. The species we isolated on cuture belonged to the phyla Firmicutes and Proteobacteria; Bik et al [4] and others from the West [12–14] reported (on 16 s rRNA sequencing) the presence of Proteobacteria, Firmicutes, Actinobacteria, Bacteroidetes and Fusobacteria phyla in the stomach of those with *H. pylori* infection. Interestingly, the flora in *H. pylori*-positive

patients with chronic dyspepsia in our study was dominated by Staphylococcus and Lactobacillus (in that order of prevalence); those without dyspepsia showed dominance by Streptococcus, Staphylococcus and Klebsiella. There was a significant difference in the organisms in the two groups, with Staphylococcus and Lactobacillus more commonly identified in dyspeptics and Streptococcus, Pseudomonas, *Escherichia coli* and *Klebsiella pneumoniae* more common in non-dyspeptics. Lactobacillus is one of the species that has been incriminated in the progression to gastric cancer in *H. pylori*-positive individuals [26].

A role for *H. pylori* in the causation of gastroduodenal disease (acid-peptic diseases, low-grade MALT lymphoma, carcinoma) has been established [27, 28]. However, a question that remains is why only some individuals with this infection develop disease while the majority do not. *H. pylori* virulence factors have been extensively studied in this regard [3]; factors such as the host diet have also been studied, but a clear answer has not been forthcoming. A role for host environment factors (gastric microbiome) has recently received extensive attention [8, 10, 23]. However, we are not aware of studies that attempted to differentiate the gastric microbiota in individuals with *H. pylori* infection, between those with chronic (functional) dyspepsia and those without dyspepsia.

An earlier study by Hu et al [23] had shown that a higher proportion of patients with non-ulcer (functional) dyspepsia had non-*H. pylori* flora as compared to those with gastric ulcer [23], suggesting a role for these concurrent organisms in the causation of symptoms. They, however, did not specify any qualitative difference. They observed an overall high prevalence of Streptococcus, Neisseria, Rothia and Staphylococcus in their patients with *H. pylori* infection; we observed a high prevalence of Staphylococcus spp. and Lactobacillus spp. in chronic dyspeptics and Streptococcus spp., Pseudomonas, *Escherichia coli* and *Klebsiella pneumoniae* in non-dyspeptics. Of these, Staphylococcus and Klebsiella are urease-producing organisms.

We suggest a possibility that some or all of these organisms play a role (bacteria-bacteria, bacteria-host, or bacteria-host-bacteria) in the causation of symptoms in *H. pylori* infection. What the range of interactions among human-associated microbes might be is not clear, nor how this may influence host health or disease [29]. Maldonado-Contreras et al [8] have suggested various mechanisms of interactions between *H. pylori* and non-*H. pylori* organisms in the stomach. The interactions of *H. pylori* with the other bacteria detected in the stomach may be influenced by host response [3, 5, 6, 8, 30–32]. It is likely that *H. pylori* creates special niches that allow the survival and colonisation of bacteria in the stomach [33].

It is well known that colonisation by *H. pylori* leads to changes in the gastric milieu, including raising the pH

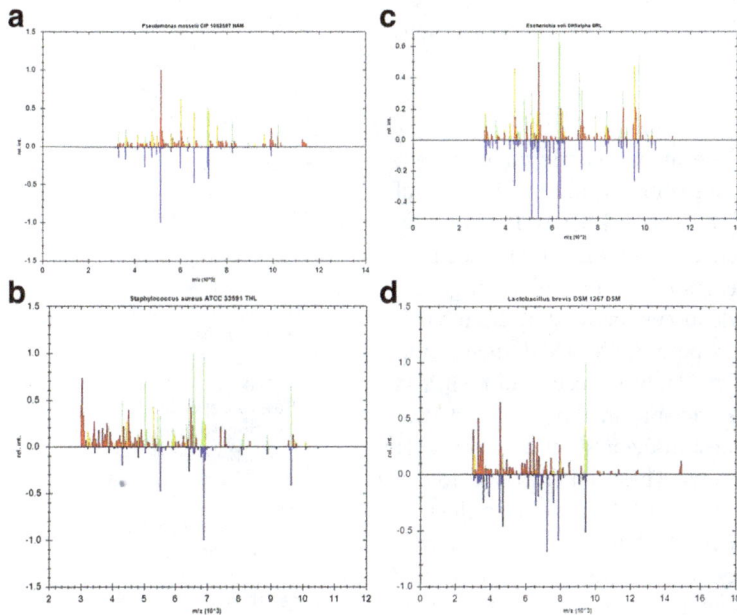

Fig. 2 MALDI-TOF MS spectra of 4 commonest organisms isolated (**a** *Pseudomonas mosselii;* **b** *Staphylococcus aureus;* **c** *Escherichia coli;* **d** *Lactobacillus brevis*)

to > 4, which facilitates colonisation by other bacteria [34]. Multiple non-*H. pylori* organisms have been isolated from the stomach in patients with hypochlorhydria [35]. It could be that the spectrum we obtained was influenced by concomitant *H. pylori* infection. But, if it was, we would expect the influence to be similar in both our study groups, namely, dyspeptics and non-dyspeptics.

On the other hand, Bik et al. [4], who used a metagenomic approach, found no influence of *H. pylori* on the diversity of gastric microbiota. They also showed that there is no difference in the microbiota isolated from the gastric antrum and corpus, which justifies our decision to pool samples from these two regions. The relationship between *H. pylori* and the gastric microbiota is thus still controversial [33].

We also describe, probably for the first time, the culturable gastric flora in an Indian population, as identified using MALDI-TOF MS, a technique that identifies organisms more reliably than the standard culture techniques (morphology and biochemical tests) [36]. The organisms we identified in *H. pylori*-positive individuals may not reflect the spectrum in the general (asymptomatic) Indian population, and so cannot be compared with studies from the healthy population in the West.

Our study had limitations. We used culture (and MALDI-TOF MS) as the identifying technique; this identifies only viable microflora. Metagenomics is a high-end technique that will increase the yield of the microflora by also identifying DNA from dead organisms. Which of these is a more faithful representation of the functional microflora is not clear [26]. Importantly, we did not study the gastric

histology in our subjects, and so cannot comment on the presence or absence of inflammation and atrophy, common accompaniments of *H. pylori* infection. This could be a major confounder: the gastric environment, including the pH and the presence of inflammation, can obviously influence the microbial spectrum. Besides, the presence of inflammation and/or atrophy may be an indicator of the virulence of the *H. pylori* strains in these patients, a factor we did not study; the latter could contribute to the development of symptoms in addition to possibly influencing the concomitant microflora. We also had no information on the smoker status of our patients. Finally, we did not explore the potential pathogenicity of bacterial types we isolated. Although some of the organisms we isolated are known to be pathogens in other sites and clinical situations, we do not know yet about their pathogenic ability in the gastric environs.

Information regarding the contribution of the concurrent gastrointestinal microbiome to the development of disease is still in its infancy. Future studies are needed to elucidate whether and to what extent *H. pylori* infection perturbs the established microbiota, and how the concomitant microbiota influence development of symptoms and disease. Such studies should factor in the limitations in our study, in order to get a clearer understanding. Increasing evidence supports the hypothesis that although *H. pylori* is the most relevant, it may not be the only local bacterial culprit leading to gastric diseases. There may be a role for non-*H. pylori* components of the gastric microbiota in both gastric and extragastric diseases. Conversely, some components of the gastric microbiota have been shown to exert antibacterial and probiotic properties, which may be exploited for the prevention and treatment of gastric diseases [37].

Conclusions

The changes that take place in the gastric environment during *H. pylori* infection are complex and involve several factors. A combination of these would determine not only the composition of the gastric microbiota but also the progress toward different diseases [32]. Our finding of gastric flora dominated by Staphylococcus followed by Lactobacillus in patients with *H. pylori*-positive chronic dyspepsia and by Streptococcus followed by Staphylococcus and Klebsiella (along with gram-negative bacteria) in those without dyspepsia adds an area of interest in the interaction of bacteria in the causation of symptoms. These findings add to the now-popular belief that individual bacteria identified in individual gut disease may not be lone players but may be influenced in their pathogenicity by the community they live in. Although this is an attractive proposition, it is too early to state whether manipulating the concomitant microflora will offer an alternative approach to preventing or managing these diseases or symptoms.

Acknowledgements
We thank the doctors of the Division of Gastroenterology and nurses in the Endoscopy Suite of P D Hinduja Hospital for kindly providing us the biopsy samples. We also thank the staff of the Division of Microbiology for their co-operation and support. We are grateful to the National Education Society for the intramural funding for this project.

Funding
This work was supported by an intramural grant from the National Education Society of P D Hinduja Hospital, Mahim, Mumbai 400016, India. The funding agency had no role in the design of the study and collection, analysis, and interpretation of data and in writing the manuscript.

Authors' contributions
PA conceived and designed the work. VP collected the data. VP, SN and AS analysed the data. VP and PA interpreted the data and drafted the article. All authors critically revised the article and approved the final manuscript.

Consent for publication
Not applicable.

Competing interests
The authors declare that they have no competing interests

Author details
¹Division of Gastroenterology, P D Hinduja Hospital, V S Marg, Mahim, Mumbai 400016, India. ²Bruker Daltonics, Bangalore, India. ³Division of Microbiology, P D Hinduja Hospital, Mumbai, India.

References
1. Von Rosenvinge EC, O'May GA, Macfarlane S, Macfarlane GT, Shirtliff ME. Microbial biofilms and gastrointestinal diseases. Pathog Dis. 2013;67(1):25–38.
2. Merrell DS, Goodrich ML, Otto G, Lucy S, Falkow S, Tompkins LS. pH-regulated gene expression of the gastric pathogen helicobacter pylori. Infect Immun. 2003;71(6):3529–39.
3. Sheh A, Fox JG. The role of the gastrointestinal microbiome in helicobacter pylori pathogenesis. Gut Microbes. 2013 Jan 19;4(6):505–31.
4. Bik EM, Eckburg PB, Gill SR, Nelson KE, Purdom EA, Francois F, et al. Molecular analysis of the bacterial microbiota in the human stomach. Proc Natl Acad Sci U S A. 2006 Jan 17;103(3):732–7.
5. Yang I, Nell S, Suerbaum S. Survival in hostile territory: the microbiota of the stomach. FEMS Microbiol Rev. 2013;37(5):736–61.
6. Zilberstein B, Quintanilha AG, MAA S, Pajecki D, Moura EG, PRA A, et al. Digestive tract microbiota in healthy volunteers. Clinics (Sao Paulo). 2007 Feb;62(1):47–54.
7. Malfertheiner P, Megraud F, O'Morain CA, Gisbert JP, Kuipers EJ, Axon AT, et al. Management of *Helicobacter pylori* infection – the Maastricht V/Florence consensus report. Gut. 2017 Jan;66(1):6–30.
8. Maldonado-Contreras A, Goldfarb KC, Godoy-Vitorino F, Karaoz U, Contreras M, Blaser MJ, et al. Structure of the human gastric bacterial community in relation to helicobacter pylori status. ISME J. 2011 Apr;5(4):574–9.
9. Coker OO, Dai Z, Nie Y, Zhao G, Cao L, Nakatsu G, et al. Mucosal microbiome dysbiosis in gastric carcinogenesis. Gut 2017 Aug 1; 2017–314281 (Epub ahead of print).
10. Abreu MT, Peek RM Jr. Gastrointestinal malignancy and the microbiome. Gastroenterology. 2014 May;146(6):1534–46.
11. Khosravi Y, Dieye Y, Poh B. Culturable bacterial microbiota of the stomach of helicobacter pylori positive and negative gastric disease patients. Sci World. 2014;2014:610421.
12. Li TH, Qin Y, Sham PC, Lau KS, Chu K-M, Leung WK. Alterations in gastric microbiota after H. Pylori eradication and in different histological stages of gastric carcinogenesis. Sci Rep. 2017;7:44935.
13. Yu G, Torres J, Hu N, Medrano-Guzman R, Herrera-Goepfert R, Humphrys MS, et al. Molecular characterization of the human stomach microbiota in gastric cancer patients. Front Cell Infect Microbiol. 2017;7:302 (online).
14. Sohn S-H, Kim N, Jo HJ, Kim J, Park JH, Nam RH, et al. Analysis of gastric body microbiota by pyrosequencing: possible role of bacteria other than *Helicobacter pylori* in the gastric carcinogenesis. J Cancer Prev. 2017 Jun 30; 22(2):115–25.
15. Wang B, Yao M, Lv L, Ling Z, Li L. The human microbiota in health and disease. Engineering. 2017 Feb 1;3(1):71–82.
16. Suzuki H, Moayyedi P. Helicobacter pylori infection in functional dyspepsia. Nat Rev Gastroenterol Hepatol. 2013;10:168–74.
17. Holtmann G, Talley NJ. Functional dyspepsia. Curr Opin Gastroenterol. 2015 Nov;31(6):492–8.
18. Ma JL, Zhang L, Brown LM, Li JY, Shen L, Pan KF, et al. Fifteen-year effects of *Helicobacter pylori*, garlic, and vitamin treatments on gastric cancer incidence and mortality. J Natl Cancer Inst. 2012;104(6):488–92.
19. Tewari R, Nijhawan V, Mishra M, Cleary JM, Salopal T, Martínez-Lorenzana G, et al. Prevalence of helicobacter pylori, cytomegalovirus, and chlamydia pneumoniae immunoglobulin seropositivity in coronary artery disease patients and normal individuals in north Indian population. Med J Armed Forces India. 1998;68(1):53–7.
20. Ghoshal UC, Chaturvedi R, Correa P. The enigma of helicobacter pylori infection and gastric cancer. Indian J Gastroenterol. 2010;29(3):95–100.
21. Misra V, Pandey R, Misra SP, Dwivedi M. Helicobacter pylori and gastric cancer: Indian enigma. World J Gastroenterol. 2014;20(6):1503–9.
22. Clark AE, Kaleta EJ, Arora A, Wolk DM. Matrix-assisted laser desorption ionization - time of flight mass spectrometry: a fundamental shift in the routine practice of clinical microbiology. Clin Microbiol Rev. 2013 Jul 3;26(3): 547–603.
23. Hu Y, He L-H, Xiao D, Liu G-D, Gu Y-X, Tao X-X, et al. Bacterial flora concurrent with helicobacter pylori in the stomach of patients with upper gastrointestinal diseases. World J Gastroenterol. 2012 Mar 21;18(11):1257–61.
24. Tack J, Talley NJ, Camilleri M, Hollmann G, Hu P, Malagelada JR, et al. Functional gastroduodenal disorders. Gastroenterology. 2006;130:1466–79.
25. Stanghellini V, Chan FKL, Hasler WL, Malagelada JR, Suzuki H, Tack J, Talley NJ. Gastroduodenal disorders. Gastroenterology. 2016;150:1380–92.
26. Noto JM, Peek RM Jr. The gastric microbiome, its interaction with *Helicobacter pylori*, and its potential role in the progression to stomach cancer. PLoS Pathog. 2017;13(10):e1006573.

27. Linz B, Balloux F, Moodley Y, Manica A, Liu H, Roumagnac P, et al. An African origin for the intimate association between humans and helicobacter pylori. Nature. 2007 Feb 22;445(7130):915–8.

28. Kusters JG, van Vliet AHM, Kuipers EJ. Pathogenesis of helicobacter pylori infection. Clin Microbiol Rev. 2006 Jul;19(3):449–90.

29. Faust K, Sathirapongsasuti JF, Izard J, Segata N, Gevers D, Raes J, Huttenhower C. Microbial co-occurrence relationships in the human microbiome. PLoS Comput Biol. 2012;8(7):e1002606.

30. Wen Y, Marcus EA, Matrubutham U, Gleeson MA, Scott DR, Sachs G. Acid-adaptive genes of helicobacter pylori. Infect Immun. 2003 Oct;71(10):5921–39.

31. Moyat M, Velin D. Immune Responses to helicobacter pylori infection. World J Gastroenterol. 2014 May 21;20(19):5583–93.

32. Yarandi SS, Hebbar G, Sauer CG, Cole CR, Ziegler TR. Diverse roles of leptin in the gastrointestinal tract: modulation of motility, absorption, growth, and inflammation. Nutrition. 2011 Mar;27(3):269–75.

33. Nardone G, Compare D. The human gastric microbiota: is it time to rethink the pathogenesis of stomach diseases? United Eur Gastroenterol J. 2015;3(3):255–60.

34. Human CP. Gastric carcinogenesis: a multistep and multifactorial process – first American Cancer Society award lecture on cancer epidemiology and prevention. Cancer Res. 1992 Dec 15;52(24):6735–40.

35. Williams C, KE MC. Proton pump inhibitors and bacterial overgrowth. Aliment Pharmacol Ther. 2006 Jan 1;23(1):3–10.

36. Calderaro A, Arcangeletti M-C, Rodighiero I, Buttrini M, Gorrini C, Motta F, et al. Matrix-assisted laser desorption/ionization time-of- flight (MALDI-TOF) mass spectrometry applied to virus identification. Sci Rep. 2014 Jan;4:6803.

37. Ianiro G, Molina-Infante J, Gasbarrini A. Gastric microbiota. Helicobacter. 2015;20:68–71.

18

Dietary habits and *Helicobacter pylori* infection: a cross sectional study at a Lebanese hospital

Shafika Assaad[1], Rawan Chaaban[2], Fida Tannous[3] and Christy Costanian[4]* (ID)

Abstract

Background: To examine the association between dietary habits and *Helicobacter pylori* (*H. pylori*) infection among patients at a tertiary healthcare center in Lebanon.

Methods: This cross-sectional study was conducted on 294 patients in 2016, at a hospital in Northern Lebanon. Participants were interviewed using a structured questionnaire to collect information on socio-demographic and lifestyle characteristics; dietary habits were ascertained via a short food frequency questionnaire (FFQ). *H. pylori* status (positive vs. negative) was determined after upper GI endoscopy where gastric biopsy specimens from the antrum, body, and fundus region were collected and then sent for pathology analysis. Multivariable logistic regression was conducted to identify the association between socio-demographic, lifestyle, dietary and other health-related variables with H pylori infection.

Results: The prevalence of *H. pylori* infection was found to be 52.4% in this sample. Results of the multivariable analysis showed that *H. pylori* infection risk was higher among participants with a university education or above (OR = 2.74; CI = 1.17–6.44), those with a history of peptic ulcers (OR = 3.80; CI = 1.80–8.01), gastric adenocarcinoma (OR = 3.99; CI = 1.35–11.83) and vitamin D level below normal (OR = 29.14; CI = 11.77–72.13). In contrast, hyperglycemia was protective against *H. pylori* (OR = 0.18; CI = 0.03–0.89). No relationship between dietary habits and *H. pylori* infection was found in the adjusted analysis.

Conclusions: Socio-demographic and clinical variables are found to be associated with *H. pylori*, but not with dietary factors. Further studies are needed to investigate the effect of diet on *H. pylori* risk.

Keywords: Dietary habits, *Helicobacter pylori*, Socio-demographic factors, Lebanon

Background

Helicobacter pylori (*H. pylori*) infection is one of the most prevalent chronic gastric infections, affecting more than 50% of the world population [1–3][1]. The microorganism is the first formally recognized bacterial carcinogen, leading to the development of various upper gastro-intestinal disorders including gastritis, gastroduodenal ulcer diseases and gastric cancer [4]. The latter was established to be the second leading cause of cancer-related death worldwide [5, 6]. Epidemiological studies have demonstrated that *H. pylori* infection is most prevalent in developing countries and among populations with low socioeconomic background [2, 7, 8]. In addition to income and education level, living standards such as sanitation and hygiene, crowding index, and source of drinking water have been shown to be risk factors of *H. pylori* [3, 8, 9]. Major variations in prevalence rates were observed among different ethnic groups, suggesting a possible genetic susceptibility [2, 3, 8–10]. Lifestyle factors are also believed to contribute to *H. pylori* infection development. Studies on the association of smoking and alcohol consumption with the infection show conflicting results. While some have found that smoking was associated with an increased risk for *H. pylori*, and that alcohol consumption had no effect on it [11–13], others have concluded that both smoking and

---
* Correspondence: chc01@yorku.ca
[4]School of Kinesiology and Health Science, York University, Toronto, ON M3J1P3, Canada

alcohol consumption had a protective effect against the infection [14, 15].

Previous studies worldwide have investigated the relationship between dietary patterns and *H. pylori*, with many being published over 20 years ago. Some studies have found that salty, pickled, fermented, or smoked foods increased the risk of *H. pylori* infection [16–18], while another found no association between *H. pylori* and pickled food [19]. Also, high intake of fruits, vegetables or of antioxidants were found to be protective factors infection in some studies [17, 19]. Moreover, Eslami et al. [20] reported that lower consumption of raw vegetables was significantly associated with higher risk of *H. pylori* infection in a group of Iranian students. A recent case-control study of patients with peptic ulcer ($n = 190$) and control group ($n = 125$) in Pune, India, found that meat consumption (OR = 2.35, 95% CI = 1.30–4.23) as well as the consumption of restaurant food increased the risk for *H. pylori* infection, while chili peppers intake was protective against it (OR = 0.20, 95% CI = 0.10–0.37) [11].

Research has also been conducted in the Middle East and North Africa (MENA) region on the association between *H. pylori* and diet [21, 22], however no conclusive evidence on this relationship exists yet. Studies on the prevalence of *H. pylori* infection in Lebanon are scarce [23–25]. In addition, risk factors for *H. pylori* infection, especially lifestyle and dietary factors, have not been comprehensively investigated in in this context. Given the high prevalence of modifiable cardio-metabolic risk factors in the MENA region, and Lebanon in particular, and given the high burden of this infection in developing countries, a study investigating the role of dietary habits in *H. pylori* infection is warranted. This study aims to examine the association between dietary habits and *H. pylori* infection among adult patients undergoing endoscopic examination at a tertiary health care center in Lebanon.

Methods

Study design and participants

This cross sectional study was conducted between March 2016 and December 2016, at Centre Hospitalier du Nord-Zgharta, a major tertiary care hospital in the North region of Lebanon. Study participants aged 18 years or above were recruited at the gastroenterological unit as they were being referred for endoscopic examination of the upper gastrointestinal (GI) tract (gastroscopy) to obtain a biopsy. A retrospective chart review was conducted to determine study eligibility. Only patients with gastrointestinal (dyspeptic) symptoms, mainly epigastric pain and gastritis and who were undergoing gastroscopy were included in the study. Patients were excluded if they had a history of *H. pylori* eradication therapy, a history of antibiotic, antacid,

H_2 blocker, proton pump inhibitors (PPI), bismuth compound, or nonsteroidal anti-inflammatory drug (NSAID) use during the previous 4 weeks, or had a previous diagnosis of other inflammatory diseases, such as coeliac disease, inflammatory bowel disease or allergies, or had gastric perforation or hemorrhage, or a history of abdominal surgery. Based on these eligibility criteria, a total of 294 participants were consecutively recruited for this study. Informed consent of the participants was obtained and all completed questionnaires were anonymous and confidential. Approval to conduct the present study was granted by the administration of the participating hospital. This study protocol was reviewed and approved by the institutional review board at the Lebanese University.

Data collection and measures

A structured questionnaire was administered by one trained interviewer during face-to-face interviews prior to the endoscopic examination. The questionnaire was composed of five sections: socio-demographic characteristics that included age, sex, educational level, marital status, occupation and monthly income; lifestyle characteristics gathering information on cigarette and arguileh smoking statuses and frequencies, alcohol consumption, stress, total number of hours slept and frequency and intensity of physical activity; dietary habits and a short food frequency questionnaire (FFQ). The FFQ was adapted from a validated questionnaire used by Yassibas et al. [26], and assessed the frequency of consuming 13 types of food (milk, yogurt, salty cheese, red meat, salami or ham, sausages, hot dogs, hamburgers, chicken, fish, green vegetables, tuberous vegetables, and grains). Frequency was assessed through selecting one of five categories ("less than once per month or none", "1-2 times a month", "1–2 times a week", "3-4 times a week" and "every day"); the last three frequency categories were combined into "once or more per week" for the statistical analysis. Questions on dietary habits were also adapted such as type of drinking water during childhood, coffee consumption, chili pepper consumption, eating rate, food temperature, salt status of dishes, and consumption of food from outside the house.

A clinical section also collected information on history of digestive diseases including gastroenteritis, peptic ulcer, esophagitis and hepatitis; and gastric cancer types and stages. Family history of cancer was also reported. Medical records of patients were also retrieved and reviewed. Information was obtained on biochemical measurements including glycemia level (above normal> 1.2 g/L), HDL (below normal< 0.45 g/L), LDL (above normal> 1.6 g/L), total cholesterol (above normal > 2.1 g/L), triglyceride (above normal> 1.5 g/L), iron level (below normal < 50 µg/L) and vitamin D level (below normal< 20 nanog/L) via medical chart abstraction. These variables were recoded as binary (normal level versus not) based on widely known cut off levels for each parameter. Systolic and diastolic blood pressures and anthropometrics including height and weight were also collected from patients' records. Hypertension was defined as having a systolic blood pressure above 140 mmHg or a diastolic pressure above 90 mmHg. Body mass index was calculated by dividing the weight (kilograms) by the square of height (meters) and was classified into four categories: underweight (< 18. 5), normal weight (18.5–24.9), overweight (25.0–29.9) and obese (≥30.0).

Outcome assessment

Identification of the microorganism was done according to standard procedures.

H. pylori status (positive vs. negative) was determined after upper GI endoscopy where gastric biopsy specimens from the antrum, body, and fundus region were collected in a plate containing formalin buffer. These samples were then sent to the pathology laboratory and examined by a pathologist. Contamination detection was performed with hematoxylin and eosin (H&E) [27]. Semi-quantitative method of scoring according to the Updated Sydney Classification System was undertaken.

Statistical analysis

All eligible questionnaires were coded. Student's *t* -tests was conducted to examine differences in continuous variables including age, duration of smoking, duration of drinking alcohol, and number of coffee cups consumed per day between cases and non-cases. Chi-square analyses were used to compare frequency distributions of categorical variables with the two groups of *H. pylori* infection. Univariate logistic regression was performed to evaluate the crude association between dietary factors and *H. pylori* status. Next, multivariable backward regression analysis was employed to examine the association of risk factors controlling for potential confounders *H. pylori* infection was the dependent variable in all regression models. Odds ratio (OR) and 95% confidence interval (CI) were calculated. Sample size calculations were performed assuming the following parameters: alpha error = 0.05, power = 80%, expected effect size: odds ratio (OR) = 1.4, proportion of people with the outcome (*H. pylori*) = 0.50, thereby yielding a required sample size of at least 200 participants. A two tailed *p*-value of <.05 was considered as statistically significant. All statistical analyses were performed using the Statistical Package for Social Sciences (version 22.0, SPSS, Inc).

Results

The total number of study participants was 294. The mean age of the sample was 40.55 years (SD ± 14.11), with a proportion of females larger than males (63.3% vs 36.7%). The prevalence of *H. pylori* infection was found to be 52. 4% in this sample. Tables 1, 2, 3, 4, 5, and 6 show the differences in terms of characteristics between *H. pylori* positive and *H. pylori* negative subjects *H. pylori* infection was significantly lower among hyperglycemic subjects ($p = 0.006$) and those with vitamin D levels below normal ($p < 0.001$) (Table 2). Lifestyle and dietary factors were similar between *H. pylori* positive and *H. pylori* negative subjects, except for frequency of milk consumption with *H. pylori* being more prevalent among subjects who consumed milk 1–2 times per month and once or more per week in comparison to those who consumed milk less than once per month ($p = 0.030$) (Tables 3 and 4). Table 5 shows that *H. pylori* was more prevalent among subjects with peptic ulcer ($p < 0.001$); subjects with history of hepatitis C were less likely to be *H. pylori* positive ($p = 0.022$). *H. pylori* infection was more common among subjects with gastric adenocarcinoma ($p = 0.005$) (Table 6). Table 6 highlights results of the bivariate and multivariable logistic analyses. Hyperglycemia (OR = 0.26; CI = 0.08–0.83), vitamin D deficiency (OR = 24.57; CI = 10.78–56.03), consuming milk 1–2 times per month (OR = 2.23; CI = 1.21–4.10), history of peptic ulcer or gastric (OR = 4.20; CI = 2.23–7.90; OR = 3.58; CI = 1.40 = 9.15, respectively), and a history of hepatitis C (OR = 0.19; CI = 0.04 = 0.92) were associated with *H. pylori* infection at the bivariate level. After adjustment for significant variables at the univariate levels and potential predictors as indicated by the literature, the risk of *H. pylori* infection was significantly higher among participants with a university education or above (OR = 2.74; CI = 1.17–6.44) versus those with a lower education level. Patients who reported a vitamin D deficiency were more likely to be *H. pylori* positive than those with normal vitamin D levels (OR = 29.14; CI = 11.77–72.13). Subjects with a history of peptic ulcers were almost 4 times more likely to be *H. pylori* positive (OR = 3.80; CI = 1.80–8.01). Patients with gastric adenocarcinoma (OR = 3.99; CI = 1.35–11.83) were also at a 4 times increased odds of reporting *H. pylori* infection. In contrast, subjects with hyperglycemia were more than 5 times less likely to be *H. pylori* positive (OR = 0.18; CI = 0.03–0.89).

Discussion

Prevalence of *H. pylori* infection in this study was found to be 52.4%. The risk of having the infection was significantly higher among subjects with an educational level of university or higher, with normal glycemic levels, and those with vitamin D levels below normal, after adjusting for other confounders. No association between *H. pylori* status and dietary habits was detected. Findings of this study might help clinicians make better informed decisions on treatment options based on their patients' dietary and lifestyle habits.

Table 1 Percent distribution of socio-demographic characteristics of participants

	Overall $n = 294$	H. pylori (−) $n = 140$	H. pylori (+) $n = 154$	p-value
Age (mean ± SD, years)	40.55 ± 14.11	41.04 ± 14.37	40.10 ± 13.90	0.570
Sex				
Males	108 (36.7)	48 (44.4)	60 (55.6)	0.358
Females	186 (63.3)	93 (50.0)	93 (50.0)	
Marital status				
Non married	90 (30.6)	42 (46.7)	48 (53.3)	0.768
Married	204 (69.4)	99 (48.5)	105 (51.5)	
Education				
Middle	55 (18.7)	31 (56.4)	24 (43.6)	0.379
Secondary	73 (24.8)	33 (45.2)	40 (54.8)	
University and higher	166 (56.5)	77 (46.4)	89 (53.6)	
Income (per month)				
< 660 USD	121 (41.2)	54 (44.6)	67 (55.4)	0.339
≥ 660 USD	173 (58.8)	87 (50.3)	86 (49.7)	
Employment status				
Unemployed	110 (37.4)	49 (44.5)	61 (55.5)	0.365
Employed	184 (62.6)	92 (50.0)	92 (50.0)	

Our estimate of *H. pylori* infection is comparable to the prevalence of 52% reported among the general Lebanese adult population by Naja et al. [28]. This rate is lower than that found in other countries of the MENA region including Egypt, Libya, Saudi Arabia, Iran, Oman, United Arab Emirates, and Turkey where the prevalence of *H. pylori* ranged between 70% and 94% [10, 15, 29]. The only exception was a study conducted in Gaza, Palestine where *H. pylori* prevalence was found to be 48. 3% [30]. Compared to other studies among symptomatic patients with dyspepsia or other GI symptoms conducted in this region, a review article by Khedmat et al [29] showed that studies in all countries had a higher prevalence ranging from around 70% up to 100%, except for one conducted in Jordan on 250 patients undergoing a biopsy on a specimen of the gastric antrum, reporting a prevalence of 44%. Other developing countries in Asia had prevalence rates similar to those reported in this study [10]. On the other hand, prevalence of *H. pylori* infection in Lebanon is still higher than the rates reported in developed countries including Canada, USA, Australia and Western European countries with rates that range from around 11% in Sweden to 48.8% among older adults in Germany [10].

Subjects with university degree or higher had almost three times increased risk for *H. pylori* infection (OR = 2. 74; CI = 1.17–6.44). The literature is inconsistent on the association between education level and H pylori, with some studies showing no association while others reporting a higher risk for *H. pylori* among subjects with lower education level. Naja et al. in a cross-sectional study

conducted in Lebanon on 308 participants reported no association between education level and *H. pylori* [28]. In addition, a prospective study conducted on 516 asymptomatic subjects showed no association between *H. pylori* infection and educational level in Pakistan [31]. Similarly, Fani et al [32] and Aguemon et al. [33] reported no relationship between *H. pylori* infection and education. In contrast, a cross-sectional study on 19,272 subjects aged 16 years or older in South Korea, reported that those with high education level and high income were less likely to be *H. pylori* seropositive [34]. Also, prevalence of *H. pylori* infection in Vietnamese migrant women was lower (55. 7%) than that of national Korean females (71.4%). Migrant workers in large cities of Northern China were also tested for *H. pylori* infection and had a low rate of infection (41. 5%). Indigenous populations in Northwestern Ontario in Canada, had a lower prevalence than expected (37.9%) [35] . On the other hand, this result might be due to variations in study design, ethnicities of the sample, the designated tests used to estimate prevalence, symptomatic versus cross-sectional volunteer patients, or use of suppressive medications among studies. More research is needed to investigate whether this result is due to chance or to other unknown confounding factors.

High glycemia was negatively associated with *H. pylori* risk (OR = 0.18; 95% CI = 0.03–0.89). The relationship between diabetes mellitus and *H. pylori* infection is not well established in the literature. A meta-analysis of 11 studies including 513 patients with diabetes mellitus has shown that *H. pylori* negative status was significantly associated with lower glycosylated hemoglobin (HbA1c)

Table 2 Percent distribution of medical conditions among participants

	Overall n = 294	H. pylori (−) n = 140	H. pylori (+) n = 154	p-value
Body Mass Index (kg/m²)				0.083
Underweight (< 18.5)	12 (4.1)	7 (58.3)	5 (41.7)	
Normal weight (18.5–24.9)	145 (49.3)	79 (54.5)	66 (45.5)	
Overweight (25.0–29.9)	78 (26.5)	33 (42.3)	45 (57.7)	
Obese (≥ 30)	59 (20.1)	22 (37.3)	37 (62.7)	
Hypertension				0.527
No	162 (55.1)	75 (46.3)	87 (53.7)	
Yes	132 (44.9)	66 (50.0)	66 (50.0)	
Glycemia				**0.006**
Normal (≤1.2 g/L)	278 (94.6)	128 (46.0)	150 (54.0)	
Above normal (> 1.2 g/L)	16 (5.4)	13 (81.3)	3 (18.8)	
Total Cholesterol				0.092
Normal (≤2.1 g/L)	239 (81.3)	109 (45.6)	130 (54.4)	
Above normal (> 2.1 g/L)	55 (18.7)	32 (58.2)	23 (41.8)	
Triglycerides				0.103
Normal (≤1.5 g/L)	183 (62.2)	81 (44.3)	102 (55.7)	
Above normal (> 1.5 g/L)	111 (37.8)	60 (54.1)	51 (45.9)	
HDL				0.789
Normal (≥0.45 g/L)	140 (47.6)	66 (47.1)	74 (52.9)	
Below normal (< 0.45 g/L)	154 (52.4)	75 (48.7)	79 (51.3)	
LDL				0.971
Normal (≤1.6 g/L)	265 (90.1)	127 (47.9)	138 (52.1)	
Above normal (> 1.6 g/L)	29 (9.9)	14 (48.3)	15 (51.7)	
Iron level				0.830
Normal (≥50 µg/L)	233 (79.3)	111 (47.6)	122 (52.4)	
Below normal (< 50 µg/L)	61 (20.7)	30 (49.2)	31 (50.8)	
Vitamin D level				**< 0.001**
Normal (≥20 nanog/L)	201 (68.4)	134 (66.7)	67 (33.3)	
Below normal (< 20 nanog/L)	93 (31.6)	7 (7.5)	86 (92.5)	
Family history of cancer				
No	151 (51.4)	71 (50.4)	70 (49.6)	0.740
Yes	143 (48.6)	80 (52.3)	73 (47.7)	

Bolded data are significant

levels (WMD = 0.43, 95%CI: 0.07–0.79), and a meta-analysis of 6 studies including 325 type 2 diabetic patients has shown the infection to be associated with higher fasting plasma glucose (WMD = 1.20, 95% CI: 0.17–2.23) [36]. However, eradication of *H. pylori* has not shown to improve HbA1c or glucose levels after a period of 3 months or 6 months [36–38]. On the other hand, a study conducted in Lebanon to examine the relationship between metabolic syndrome and insulin resistance with *H. pylori* found that hyperglycemia was not significantly associated with the infection [28]. In addition, Jafarzadeh et al. reported *H. pylori* seropositivity rates that were similar between participants with type 2 diabetes (76%) and healthy subjects (75%) in Rafsanjan, Iran [39]. Results from the Netherlands were also similar [40]. Interestingly, the eradication of *H. pylori* in a case-control study showed a significant increase in the incidence of obesity, hypercholesterolemia and hypertriglyceridemia after 1 year of the treatment [41]. In a review of the evidence regarding the association between *H. pylori* and extragastric manifestations, Suzuki et al. [42] concluded that in the case of diabetes mellitus, the clinical consequences of *H. pylori* infection in terms of metabolic control seems to be low. So this explanation might also fit pre-diabetes. Moreover, Lutsey et al. [43], using data from the Multiethnic Study of Atherosclerosis reported

Table 3 Percent distribution of lifestyle characteristics of participants

	Overall $n = 294$	H. pylori (−) $n = 140$	H. pylori (+) $n = 154$	p-value
Cigarette smoking				
Non Smoker	213 (72.4)	109 (51.2)	104 (48.8)	0.074
Current Smoker	81 (27.6)	32 (39.5)	49 (60.5)	
1–10 cigarettes/day	27 (9.2)	15 (55.6)	12 (44.4)	0.094
11–20 cigarettes/day	37 (12.6)	12 (32.4)	25 (67.6)	
> 20 cigarettes/day	18 (6.1)	5 (27.8)	13 (72.2)	
Duration of smoking (years)	15.74 ± 10.15	15.91 ± 10.14	15.63 ± 10.26	0.904
Waterpipe smoking				
Non Smoker	226 (76.9)	108 (47.8)	118 (52.2)	0.915
Current Smoker	68 (23.1)	33 (48.5)	35 (51.5)	
Daily	28 (9.5)	12 (42.9)	16 (57.1)	0.281
Weekly or monthly	15 (5.1)	10 (66.7)	5 (33.3)	
Occasionally	25 (8.5)	11 (44.0)	14 (56.0)	
Alcohol consumption				
Non drinker	192 (65.3)	92 (47.9)	100 (52.1)	0.984
Current drinker	102 (34.7)	49 (48.0)	53 (52.0)	
One to several times a week	19 (6.5)	12 (63.2)	7 (36.8)	0.144
One to several times a month	83 (28.2)	37 (44.6)	46 (55.4)	
Duration of drinking	11.94 ± 8.04	11.55 ± 7.37	12.30 ± 8.68	0.650
Feeling tense or stressed out				
Not at all	46 (15.6)	21 (45.7)	25 (54.3)	0.455
Occasionally	73 (24.8)	30 (41.1)	43 (58.9)	
A lot of times	57 (19.4)	31 (54.4)	26 (45.6)	
Most of the time	118 (40.1)	59 (50.0)	59 (50.0)	
Sleep per night				
< 7 h per day	136 (46.3)	63 (46.3)	73 (53.7)	0.602
≥ 7 h per day	158 (53.7)	78 (49.4)	80 (50.6)	
Physical activity				
< once per week	227 (77.2)	109 (48.0)	118 (52.0)	0.924
Once per week	31 (10.5)	14 (45.2)	17 (54.8)	
≥ twice per week	36 (12.2)	18 (50.0)	18 (50.0)	
Physical activity intensity				
None	21 (7.1)	11 (52.4)	10 (47.6)	0.090
Light	151 (51.4)	62 (41.1)	89 (58.9)	
Moderate	94 (32.0)	54 (57.4)	40 (42.6)	
Vigorous	28 (9.5)	14 (50.0)	14 (50.0)	

a lower rate of *H. pylori* infection in patients with diabetes, consistent with our results. It remains uncertain how *H. pylori* serostatus affects the pathogenic process leading to metabolic syndrome. This surprising finding might be attributed to the fact that persons with insulin resistance (high glycemia) might be asked to modify their diet upon their diagnosis, and so begin to eat less fatty food items and increase their fruit and vegetable consumption which promotes probiotic populations versus *H. pylori* infection.

Participants with below normal levels of vitamin D were more likely to be infected with *H. pylori* than those having normal vitamin D levels. Few studies have investigated the role of vitamin D in preventing *H. pylori* infection. A case-control study on women aged 70 to 99 years has shown that long-term supplementation of 1

Table 4 Percent distribution of dietary factors of participants

	Overall $n = 294$	H. pylori (−) $n = 140$	H. pylori (+) $n = 154$	p-value
Drinking water during childhood				
Tap water	123 (41.8)	60 (48.8)	63 (51.2)	0.917
Well water	40 (13.6)	18 (45.0)	22 (55.0)	
Mineral or filtered	129 (43.9)	62 (48.1)	67 (51.9)	
Coffee consumption				
No	80 (27.2)	36 (45.0)	44 (55.0)	0.535
Yes	214 (72.8)	105 (49.1)	109 (50.9)	
Coffee cups/day	5.48 ± 3.97	5.59 ± 4.09	5.37 ± 3.87	0.682
Chilli pepper consumption				
No	140 (47.6)	60 (42.9)	80 (57.1)	0.095
Yes	154 (52.4)	81 (52.6)	73 (47.4)	
Eating rate				
Very fast	83 (28.2)	45 (54.2)	38 (45.8)	0.527
Fast	68 (23.1)	29 (42.6)	39 (57.4)	
Normal	102 (34.7)	47 (46.1)	55 (53.9)	
Slow	41 (13.9)	20 (48.8)	21 (51.2)	
Food temperature				
Cooling/warm	141 (48.0)	63 (44.7)	78 (55.3)	0.540
Hot	80 (27.2)	40 (50.0)	40 (50.0)	
Very hot	73 (24.8)	38 (52.1)	35 (47.9)	
Salt status of dishes				
Very salty	41 (13.9)	18 (43.9)	23 (56.1)	0.478
Salty	126 (42.9)	64 (50.8)	62 (49.2)	
Less salty	66 (22.4)	27 (40.9)	39 (59.1)	
Salt free	61 (20.7)	32 (52.5)	29 (47.5)	
Frequency of drinking milk				
None/Less than once per month	167 (56.8)	90 (53.9)	77 (46.1)	**0.030**
1–2 times per month	61 (20.7)	21 (34.4)	40 (65.6)	
Once or more per week	66 (22.4)	30 (45.5)	36 (54.5)	
Frequency of eating yogurt				
None/Less than once per month	36 (12.2)	12 (33.3)	24 (66.7)	0.062
1–2 times per month	167 (56.8)	89 (53.3)	78 (46.7)	
Once or more per week	91 (31.0)	40 (44.0)	51 (56.0)	
Frequency of eating salty cheese				
None/Less than once per month	31 (10.5)	13 (41.9)	18 (58.1)	0.251
1–2 times per month	75 (25.5)	42 (56.0)	33 (44.0)	
Once or more per week	188 (63.9)	86 (45.7)	102 (54.3)	
Frequency of eating red meat				
None/Less than once per month	30 (10.2)	17 (56.7)	13 (43.3)	0.140
1–2 times per month	72 (24.5)	40 (55.6)	32 (44.4)	
Once or more per week	192 (65.3)	84 (43.8)	108 (56.3)	
Frequency of eating ham				
None/Less than once per month	176 (59.9)	83 (47.2)	93 (52.8)	0.774

Table 4 Percent distribution of dietary factors of participants *(Continued)*

	Overall *n* = 294	*H. pylori* (−) *n* = 140	*H. pylori* (+) *n* = 154	*p*-value
1–2 times per month	76 (25.9)	39 (51.3)	37 (48.7)	
Once or more per week	42 (14.3)	19 (45.2)	23 (54.8)	
Frequency of eating sausages				
None/Less than once per month	188 (63.9)	85 (45.2)	103 (54.8)	0.426
1–2 times per month	81 (27.6)	42 (51.9)	39 (48.1)	
Once or more per week	25 (8.5)	14 (56.0)	11 (44.0)	
Frequency of eating hot dogs				
None/Less than once per month	242 (82.3)	117 (48.3)	125 (51.7)	0.746
1–2 times per month	33 (11.2)	14 (42.4)	19 (57.6)	
Once or more per week	19 (6.5)	10 (48.0)	9 (47.4)	
Frequency of eating hamburgers				
None/Less than once per month	102 (34.7)	47 (46.1)	55 (53.9)	0.890
1–2 times per month	107 (36.4)	52 (48.6)	55 (51.4)	
Once or more per week	85 (28.9)	42 (49.4)	43 (50.6)	
Frequency of eating chicken				
None/Less than once per month	13 (4.4)	7 (53.8)	6 (46.2)	0.071
1–2 times per month	48 (16.3)	30 (62.5)	18 (37.5)	
Once or more per week	233 (79.3)	104 (44.6)	129 (55.4)	
Frequency of eating fish				
None/Less than once per month	21 (7.1)	9 (42.9)	12 (57.1)	0.625
1–2 times per month	81 (27.6)	36 (44.4)	45 (55.6)	
Once or more per week	192 (65.3)	96 (50.0)	96 (50.0)	
Frequency of eating green vegetables				
None/Less than once per month	12 (4.1)	6 (50.0)	6 (50.0)	0.801
1–2 times per month	54 (18.4)	28 (51.9)	26 (48.1)	
Once or more per week	228 (77.6)	107 (46.9)	121 (53.1)	
Frequency of eating tuberous vegetables				
None/Less than once per month	61 (20.7)	28 (45.9)	33 (54.1)	0.210
1–2 times per month	81 (27.6)	33 (40.7)	48 (59.3)	
Once or more per week	152 (51.7)	80 (52.6)	72 (47.4)	
Frequency of eating grains				
None/Less than once per month	28 (9.5)	16 (57.1)	12 (42.9)	0.543
1–2 times per month	95 (32.3)	43 (45.3)	52 (54.7)	
Once or more per week	171 (58.2)	82 (48.0)	89 (52.0)	
Consumption of delivery foods or food from outside the house				
Never	79 (26.9)	43 (54.4)	36 (45.6)	0.345
Once per week	164 (55.8)	73 (44.5)	91 (55.5)	
Twice or more per week	51 (17.3)	25 (49.0)	26 (51.0)	

Bolded data are significant

alpha-hydroxyvitamin D-3 as part of osteoporosis treatment significantly inhibited the development of the infection [44]. A cross-sectional study conducted in Iran on patients with end stage renal failure who are on hemodialysis showed an association between serum 25-OH vitamin D and serum *H. pylori* specific IgG antibody titers, suggesting that vitamin D increases the immune response [45]. In fact, a recent article has demonstrated that a decomposition product of vitamin D3 has an antibacterial effect against *H. pylori* bacteria specifically [46]. This area is worth more investigation as vitamin D supplementation might be effective in treatment and

Table 5 Percent distribution of history of digestive diseases gastric neoplasms among participants

	Overall $n = 294$	H. pylori (−) $n = 140$	H. pylori (+) $n = 154$	p-value
Gastroenteritis				
No	260 (88.4)	129 (49.6)	131 (50.4)	0.116
Yes	34 (11.6)	12 (35.3)	22 (64.7)	
Peptic Ulcer				
No	228 (77.6)	126 (55.3)	102 (44.7)	**< 0.001**
Yes	66 (22.4)	15 (22.7)	51 (77.3)	
Esophagitis				
No	278 (94.6)	130 (46.8)	148 (53.2)	0.087
Yes	16 (5.4)	11 (68.8)	5 (31.3)	
Hepatitis C				
No	283 (96.3)	132 (46.6)	151 (53.4)	**0.022**
Yes	11 (3.7)	9 (81.8)	2 (18.2)	
Adenocarcinoma				
No	267 (90.8)	135 (50.6)	132 (49.4)	**0.005**
Yes	27 (9.2)	6 (22.2)	21 (77.8)	
Gastric MALT lymphoma				
No	281 (95.6)	136 (48.4)	145 (51.6)	0.483
Yes	13 (4.4)	5 (38.5)	8 (61.5)	
Stage of Gastric Cancer				
Early	20 (6.8)	7 (35.0)	13 (65.0)	0.456*
Advanced	16 (5.4)	3 (18.8)	13 (81.3)	
Lymph node metastasis				
No	24 (8.2)	8 (33.3)	16 (66.7)	0.711*
Yes	13 (4.4)	3 (23.1)	10 (76.9)	

*p-value of Fischer Exact test
Bolded data are significant

prevention of H pylori infection. In fact, since long time ago, vitamin D deficiency has been suggested to increase the risk for infections, as it was observed that children with rickets were more prone to respiratory infections. This is explained by the modulating role of this vitamin in the immune response, as more recent studies have also shown that the incidence of different infectious diseases, including influenza, respiratory infection and septic shock might be due seasonal variations in vitamin D levels as exposure to solar ultraviolet-B doses is lower during winter [47].

The link between *H. pylori* and a wide range of upper digestive diseases including peptic ulcer and gastric cancers has been well established in the literature. Indeed, peptic ulcer and adenocarcinoma were significantly associated with *H. pylori* infection in this study. Furthermore, a meta-analysis of 52 trials has shown that eradication of *H. pylori* is effective in treating duodenal and gastric ulcers and decreasing their recurrence [48]. *H. pylori* has been found to increase two times the risk of developing gastric adenocarcinoma according to a meta-analysis that included 42 studies [49]. This is consistent with more recent

research showing that patients with *H. pylori*-positive non-atrophic gastritis are at around 10 fold higher risk to develop peptic ulcer and twice higher risk for gastric cancer compared to healthy individuals [50].

None of the food items studied was associated with *H. pylori* infection. The relationship between different food items and *H. pylori* infection remains inconclusive. Consistent with our findings, a recent cross-sectional study conducted in Oman on 100 patients attending Sultan Qaboos University Hospital showed no correlation with the intake of any of the studied food items with the exception of soft drinks [21]. However, meat and fast food consumption were significantly associated with *H. pylori* infection in other studies conducted in Iran and India [11, 22]. Also, while some studies have shown that fruits and vegetables intake decreases the risk for *H. pylori* infection [17, 19, 22], others have not [20]. More randomized controlled trials should be conducted to explore further the effect of different food components on *H. pylori* eradication. Such research would identify healthier alternatives for treating *H. pylori* colonization than

Table 6 Unadjusted and adjusted odds ratios of *H. pylori* infection status with various factors

	Unadjusted OR (95% CI)	Adjusted OR (95% CI)
Age (mean ± SD, years)	1.00 (0.98–1.01)	–
Sex		
Males	1	–
Females	0.80 (0.50–1.29)	–
Marital status		
Non married	1	–
Married	0.93 (0.57–1.53)	–
Education		
Below high school	1	1
High school	1.57 (0.77–3.17)	2.17 (0.84–5.60)
University and higher	1.49 (0.81–2.76)	2.74 **(1.17–6.44)**
Income		
< 660 USD	1	–
≥ 660 USD	0.80 (0.50–1.27)	–
Glycemia		
Normal (≤1.2 g/L)	1	1
Above normal (> 1.2 g/L)	0.26 **(0.08–0.83)**	0.18 **(0.03–0.89)**
Vitamin D level		
Normal (≥20 nanog/L)	1	1
Below normal (< 20 nanog/L)	24.57 **(10.78–56.03)**	29.14 **(11.77–72.13)**
Frequency of drinking milk		
None/Less than once per month	1	–
1–2 times per month	2.23 **(1.21–4.10)**	–
Once or more per week	1.40 (0.79–2.49)	–
Peptic Ulcer		
No	1	1
Yes	4.20 **(2.23–7.90)**	3.80 **(1.80–8.01)**
Hepatitis C		
No	1	1
Yes	0.19 **(0.04–0.92)**	0.18 (0.02–1.43)
Adenocarcinoma		
No	1	1
Yes	3.58 **(1.40–9.15)**	3.99 **(1.35–11.83)**

Bolded data are significant

pharmacological therapy that has side effects and leads to antibiotic resistance [51]. On the other hand, Xia et al. argue that it is important to study dietary patterns and not food items in isolation, since nutrients do not only act independently but may also interact together [52] since *H. pylori* was positively association with a diet rich in carbohydrates and sweets, and negatively associated with a diet high in protein and cholesterol, while no association was found between *H. pylori* and any food items or groups studied in isolation in their cross sectional study.

Some limitations of the study should be considered when interpreting the results. A convenience sampling method was used to select participants, thereby limiting the ability to generalize results to the target population. Potential misclassification bias of the main outcome although minimal is possible, Serological testing, could be improved further by using stains having higher sensitivity and specificity than H&E stain such as Giemsa stain, Warthin-Starry silver stain, Genta stain, and immunohistochemical (IHC) (69–93% and 87–90% respectively, versus 90–100%) [52, 53]. Moreover, the FFQ administered presents some limitations.

Food intake was self-reported with no means of verification, leading to a potential information bias. In addition, intake frequency of specific food items was assessed without specifying quantities or portion sizes. However, it is believed that the variation of portion sizes between different participants is smaller than that of frequency of intake, and thus would have limited impact on the results [54]. Small sample sizes in some of the independent variables might have led to inflated risk estimates and significant results which may be spurious. Finally, the cross-sectional design prevents the inference of inferring causality. This study has several strengths. This is the first study in Lebanon and one of the few in the region to analyze the association between *H. pylori* infection and dietary habits while adjusting for potential confounders. Biopsy has higher specificity than serological testing for assessing infection presence, thereby minimizing misclassification bias [55]. Anthropometric measurements, blood tests results and certain medical conditions were abstracted from patients' charts, eliminating self-report bias. Moreover, an FFQ previously validated by Yassibas et al. [26] was employed to assess general dietary intake; FFQ is considered to be the most appropriate dietary tool for studying the relationship between diet and disease. Finally, as less than 2% refused to participate in the study, non-response bias was negligible.

Conclusion

H. pylori infection is a major public health issue affecting more than half of world population and leading to a range of gastro-intestinal problems. This study is the first in Lebanon and one of the few in the MENA region to examine the dietary correlates of *H. pylori* infection. University education was a risk factor for *H. pylori*. None of the food items or dietary habits was associated with *H. pylori* infection. However, adequate blood level of vitamin D was found to protect against it. Conversely, participants with hyperglycemia were at decreased risk of *H. pylori*, an uncommon association that needs to be investigated further. It is essential to study the treatment potential of dietary substances that appear to have a protective effect against *H. pylori*. This would present a solution with lower cost, higher availability and fewer side effects than medications. Our results, in addition to findings from other studies, suggest that vitamin D supplementation might be one healthy alternative, but more longitudinal studies are needed to confirm its effectiveness. In addition, cohort studies examining the link between *H. pylori* and dietary patterns rather than isolated food items are needed to take into account nutrients interaction. Such studies would help clinicians make better informed decisions based on their patients' dietary and lifestyle habits. It would also allow designing health education interventions that promote general recommendations on healthy eating patterns rather than specific food components intake.

Abbreviations

FFQ: Food frequency questionnaire; *H. pylori*: *Helicobacter pylori*; MENA: Middle East and North Africa; NSAID: Nonsteroidal anti-inflammatory drug; PPI: Proton pump inhibitors

Acknowledgements

The authors would like to thank the support of the Lebanese University, Faculty of Sciences.

Funding

Faculty of Sciences, Lebanese University.

Authors' contributions

SA contributed to hypothesis conception, study design, study logistics, and data collection. CC contributed towards study design, hypothesis conception, data analysis and interpretation, and manuscript drafting; RC contributed to the analysis, interpretation, drafting and write up of the paper; FT contributed to data collection, and study logistics. All authors provided critical insight, and revisions to the manuscript; all authors read and approved the final version of the manuscript submitted for publication.

Competing interests

The authors declare that they have no competing interests.

Author details

[1]Faculty of Sciences, Lebanese University, Beirut, Lebanon. [2]International Committee of the Red Cross, Beirut, Lebanon. [3]Faculty of Sciences, Beirut Arab University, Beirut, Lebanon. [4]School of Kinesiology and Health Science, York University, Toronto, ON M3J1P3, Canada.

References

1. Bardhan PK. Epidemiological features of Helicobacter pylori infection in developing countries. Clin Infect Dis Off Publ Infect Dis Soc Am. 1997;25: 973–8. 9402340
2. Eusebi LH, Zagari RM, Bazzoli F. Epidemiology of Helicobacter pylori infection. Helicobacter. 2014;19: 1–5. 25167938
3. Goh K-L, Chan W-K, Shiota S, Yamaoka Y. Epidemiology of Helicobacter pylori infection and public health implications. Helicobacter. 2011;16:1–9. 21896079
4. Kusters JG, van Vliet AHM, Kuipers EJ. Pathogenesis of Helicobacter pylori infection. Clin Microbiol Rev. 2006;19:449–90. 16847081
5. Crew KD, Neugut AI. Epidemiology of gastric cancer. World J Gastroenterol. 2006;12:354–62. 16489633
6. Raei N, Behrouz B, Zahri S, Latifi-Navid S. Helicobacter pylori infection and dietary factors act synergistically to promote gastric cancer. Asian Pac J Cancer Prev APJCP. 2016;17:917–21. 27039812
7. Graham DY, Malaty HM, Evans DG, Evans DJ, Klein PD, Adam E. Epidemiology of Helicobacter pylori in an asymptomatic population in the United States. Effect of age, race, and socioeconomic status. Gastroenterology. 1991;100:1495–501. 2019355
8. Khalifa MM, Sharaf RR, Aziz RK. Helicobacter pylori: a poor man's gut pathogen? Gut Pathog. 2010;2:2. 20356368

9. Brown LM. Helicobacter pylori: epidemiology and routes of transmission. Epidemiol Rev. 2000;22:283–97. 11218379

10. Hunt RH, Xiao SD, Megraud F, Leon-Barua R, Bazzoli F, van der Merwe S, et al. Helicobacter pylori in developing countries. World gastroenterology organisation global guideline. J Gastrointest Liver Dis JGLD. 2011;299–304: 20. 21961099

11. Mhaskar RS, Ricardo I, Azliyati A, Laxminarayan R, Amol B, Santosh W, et al. Assessment of risk factors of Helicobacter pylori infection and peptic ulcer disease. J Glob Infect Dis. 2013;5:60–7. https://doi.org/10.4103/0974-777X. 112288].

12. Murray LJ, McCrum EE, Evans AE, Bamford KB. Epidemiology of Helicobacter pylori infection among 4742 randomly selected subjects from Northern Ireland. Int J Epidemiol. 1997;26:880–7. 9279623

13. Woodward M, Morrison C, McColl K. An investigation into factors associated with Helicobacter pylori infection. J Clin Epidemiol. 2000;53:175–81. 10729690

14. Ogihara A, Kikuchi S, Hasegawa A, Kurosawa M, Miki K, Kaneko E, et al. Relationship between Helicobacter pylori infection and smoking and drinking habits. J Gastroenterol Hepatol. 2000;15:271–6. 10764027

15. Ozaydin N, Turkyilmaz SA, Cali S. Prevalence and Risk factors of helicobacter pylori in Turkey: a nationally-representative, cross-sectional, screening with the 13C-urea breath test. BMC Public Health. 2013;13:1215. 2435951

16. Fox JG, Dangler CA, Taylor NS, King A, Koh TJ, Wang TC. High-salt diet induces gastric epithelial hyperplasia and parietal cell loss, and enhances Helicobacter pylori colonization in C57BL/6 mice. Cancer Res. 1999;59:4823–8. 10519391

17. Hwang H, Dwyer J, Diet RRM. Helicobacter pylori infection, food preservation and gastric cancer risk: are there new roles for preventative factors? Nutr Rev. 1994;52:75–83. 8015750

18. Tsugane S, Tei Y, Takahashi T, Watanabe S, Sugano K. Salty food intake and risk of Helicobacter pylori infection. Jpn J Cancer Res. 1994;85:474–8. 8014104

19. Shinchi K, Ishii H, Imanishi K, Kono S. Relationship of cigarette smoking, alcohol use, and dietary habits with Helicobacter pylori infection in Japanese men. Scand J Gastroenterol. 1997;32:651–5. 9246703

20. Eslami O, Shahraki M, Shahraki T, Ansari H. Association of Helicobacter pylori infection with metabolic parameters and dietary habits among medical undergraduate students in southeastern of Iran. Journal of research in medical sciences: the official journal of Isfahan University of Medical Sciences 2017;22.

21. Altheeb AlKalbani SR, Naser Al-Shariqi FT, Al-Hinai M, AlMuniri A. Diet and lifestyle factors and the risk of H pylori infection in Omani patients attending SQUH daycare for OGD. J Fam Med Community Health. 2016;3: 1077.

22. Mard SA, Khadem Haghighian H, Sebghatulahi V, Ahmadi B. Dietary factors in relation to Helicobacter pylori infection. Gastroenterol Res Pract. 2014; 2014:826910. 25574164

23. Kalaajieh WK, Chbani-Rima A, Kassab TF, Baghdadi FM. Helicobacter pylori infection in North Lebanon. Cah Détudes Rech Francoph. Santé. 2000;10:31– 5. 10827360

24. Sharara AI, Abdul-Baki H, ElHajj I, Kreidieh N, Kfoury Baz EM. Association of gastroduodenal disease phenotype with ABO blood group and Helicobacter pylori virulence-specific serotypes. Dig Liver Dis Off J Ital Soc Gastroenterol Ital Assoc Study. Liver. 2006;38:829–33. 16931196

25. Naous A, Al-Tannir M, Naja Z, Ziade F, Fecoprevalence E-RM. Determinants of Helicobacter pylori infection among asymptomatic children in Lebanon. J Med Liban. 2007;55:138–44. 17966734

26. Yassibaş E, Arslan P, Yalçin S. Evaluation of dietary and life-style habits of patients with gastric cancer: a case-control study in Turkey. Asian Pac J Cancer Prev APJCP. 2012;13:2291–7. 22901209

27. Ashton-Key M, Diss TC, Isaacson PG. Detection of Helicobacter pylori in gastric biopsy and resection specimens. J Clin Pathol. 1996;49:107–11. 8655673

28. Naja F, Nasreddine L, Hwalla N, Moghames P, Shoaib H, Fatfat M, et al. Association of H. Pylori infection with insulin resistance and metabolic syndrome among Lebanese adults. Helicobacter. 2012;17:444–51. 23066847

29. Khedmat H, Karbasi-Afshar R, Agah S, Taheri S. Helicobacter pylori infection in the general population: a middle eastern perspective. Casp. J Intern Med. 2013;4:745–53. 24294467

30. Abu-Mugesieb RM, Elmanama AA, Mokhallalati MM. Risk factors associated with Helicobacter pylori infection in Gaza, Palestine. 2007; Available from: http://library.iugaza.edu.ps/thesis/74054.pdf

31. Rasheed F, Ahmad T, Prevalence BB. Risk factors of helicobacter pylori infection among Pakistani population. Pak J Med Sci. 2012;28:661–5.

32. Fani A, Rezaei M, Alizade B, Mirzajani P, Shamsikhan S, Rafeie M, et al. Prevalence of Helicobacter pylori infection in arak, Iran during 2011. Govaresh. 2014;19:57–62.

33. Aguemon BD, Struelens MJ, Massougbodji A, Prevalence OEM. Risk-factors for Helicobacter pylori infection in urban and rural Beninese populations. Clin Microbiol Infect Off Publ Eur Soc Clin Microbiol. Infect. Dis. 2005;11:611–7. 16008612

34. Lim SH, Kwon J-W, Kim N, Kim GH, Kang JM, Park MJ, et al. Prevalence and risk factors of Helicobacter pylori infection in Korea: nationwide multicenter study over 13 years. BMC Gastroenterol. 2013;13:104. 23800201

35. Calvet X, Ramírez Lázaro MJ, Lehours P, Mégraud F. Diagnosis and epidemiology of Helicobacter pylori infection. Helicobacter. 2013;18(s1): 5–11. 24011238

36. Dai Y-N, Yu W-L, Zhu H-T, Ding J-X, Yu C-H, Li Y-M. Is Helicobacter pylori infection associated with glycemic control in diabetics? World J Gastroenterol WJG. 2015;21:5407–16. 25954115

37. Vafaeimanesh J, Rajabzadeh R, Ahmadi A, Moshtaghi M, Banikarim S, Hajiebrahimi S, et al. Effect of Helicobacter pylori eradication on glycaemia control in patients with type 2 diabetes mellitus and comparison of two therapeutic regimens. Arab J Gastroenterol Off Publ Pan-Arab Assoc Gastroenterol. 2013;14:55–8 [PMID: 23820501. https://doi.org/10.1016/j.ajg. 2013.03.002.

38. Wada Y, Hamamoto Y, Kawasaki Y, Honjo S, Fujimoto K, Tatsuoka H, et al. The eradication of Helicobacter pylori does not affect glycemic control in Japanese subjects with type 2 diabetes. Jpn Clin Med. 2013;4:41–3 [PMID: 23966817. https://doi.org/10.4137/JCM.S10828].

39. Jafarzadeh A, Rezayati MT, Nemati M. Helicobacter pylori seropositivity in patients with type 2 diabetes mellitus in south-east of Iran. Acta Med Iran. 2013;51:892–6. 24442545

40. Haeseker MB, Pijpers E, Dukers-Muijrers NH, Nelemans P, Hoebe CJ, Bruggeman CA, et al. Association of cytomegalovirus and other pathogens with frailty and diabetes mellitus, but not with cardiovascular disease and mortality in psycho-geriatric patients; a prospective cohort study. Immun Ageing A. 2013;10:30 [PMID: 23880245. https://doi.org/10.1186/1742-4933-10-30.

41. Kamada T, Hata J, Kusunoki H, Ito M, Tanaka S, Kawamura Y, et al. Eradication of Helicobacter pylori increases the incidence of hyperlipidaemia and obesity in peptic ulcer patients. Dig Liver Dis Off J Ital Soc Gastroenterol Ital Assoc Study Liver. 2005;37:39–43 [PMID: 15702858. https://doi.org/10.1016/j.dld.2004.07.017.

42. Suzuki H, Franceschi F, Nishizawa T, Gasbarrini A. Extragastric manifestations of Helicobacter pylori infection. Helicobacter. 2011;16(Suppl 1):65–9.

43. Lutsey PL, Pankow JS, Bertoni AG, Szklo M, Folsom AR. Serological evidence of infections and type 2 diabetes: the MultiEthnic study of atherosclerosis. Diabet Med. 2009;26(2):149–52.

44. Kawaura A, Takeda E, Tanida N, Nakagawa K, Yamamoto H, Sawada K, et al. Inhibitory effect of long term 1 alpha-hydroxyvitamin D3 administration on Helicobacter pylori infection. J Clin Biochem Nutr 2006; 38: 103–106OI: https://doi.org/10.3164/jcbn.38.103].

45. Nasri H, Baradaran A. The influence of serum 25-hydroxy vitamin D levels on Helicobacter pylori infections in patients with end-stage renal failure on regular hemodialysis. Saudi J Kidney Dis Transplant Off Publ Saudi Cent Organ Transplant Saudi Arab. 2007;18:215–9. 17496397

46. Hosoda K, Shimomura H, Wanibuchi K, Masui H, Amgalanbaatar A, Hayashi S, et al. Identification and characterization of a vitamin D3 decomposition product bactericidal against Helicobacter pylori. Sci Rep. 2015;5:8860 [PMID: 25749128. https://doi.org/10.1038/srep08860].

47. Yamshchikov AV, Desai NS, Blumberg HM, Ziegler TR, Tangpricha V, Vitamin D. For treatment and prevention of infectious diseases: a systematic review of randomized controlled trials. Endocr Pract Off J Am Assoc. Clin Endocrinol. 2009;15:438–49. 19491064

48. Ford AC, Delaney BC, Forman D, Moayyedi P. Eradication therapy in Helicobacter pylori positive peptic ulcer disease: systematic review and economic analysis. Am J Gastroenterol. 2004;99:1833–55. 15330927

49. Eslick GD, Lim LL, Byles JE, Xia HH, Talley NJ. Association of Helicobacter pylori infection with gastric carcinoma: a meta-analysis. Am J Gastroenterol. 1999;94:2373–9.

50. Sipponen P, Hyvärinen H. Role of Helicobacter pylori in the pathogenesis of gastritis, peptic ulcer and gastric cancer. Scand J Gastroenterol Suppl. 1993; 196:3–6. 10483994

51. Hołubiuk Ł, Imiela J. Diet and Helicobacter pylori infection. Przeglad
     Gastroenterol. 2016;11:150–4. 27713775
52. Xia Y, Meng G, Zhang Q, Liu L, Wu H, Shi H, et al. dietary patterns are
     associated with Helicobacter pylori infection in Chinese adults: a cross-
     sectional study. Sci Rep. 2016;6:32334 [PMID: 27573193. https://doi.org/10.
     1038/srep32334].
53. Lee JY, Kim N. Diagnosis of Helicobacter pylori by invasive test: histology.
     Ann Transl Med. 2015;3:10. 25705642
54. Shim J-S, Oh K, Kim HC. Dietary assessment methods in epidemiologic
     studies. Epidemiol Health. 2014;36:e2014009. 25078382
55. Taj Y, Essa F, Kazmi SU, Abdullah E. Sensitivity and specificity of various
     diagnostic tests in the detection of Helicobacter pylori. J Coll Physicians
     Surg–Pak JCPSP. 2003;13:90–3. 12685951

19

Efficacy of *Helicobacter pylori* eradication regimens in Rwanda

Jean Damascene Kabakambira[1]* [iD], Celestin Hategeka[2,3], Cameron Page[4], Cyprien Ntirenganya[5], Vincent Dusabejambo[1], Jules Ndoli[5], Francois Ngabonziza[1], DeVon Hale[6], Claude Bayingana[5] and Tim Walker[5,7]

Abstract

Background: Successful *H. pylori* treatment requires the knowledge of local antimicrobial resistance. Data on the efficacy of *H. pylori* eradication regimens available in sub-Saharan Africa are scant, hence the optimal treatment is unknown. Our goals were to determine the efficacy of available regimens in Rwanda as well as evaluate the effect of treatment on health-related quality of life (HRQoL) in patients undergoing esophagogastroduodenoscopy.

Methods: This is a randomized controlled trial conducted from November 2015 to October 2016 at a tertiary hospital in Rwanda. Enrollees were 299 patients (35% male, age 42 ± 16 years (mean ± SD)) who had a positive modified rapid urease test on endoscopic biopsies. After a fecal antigen test (FAT) and HRQoL assessment by the Short Form Nepean Dyspepsia Index (SF-NDI) questionnaire, patients were randomized 1:1:1:1 to either a triple therapy combining omeprazole, amoxicillin and one of clarithromycin/ciprofloxacin/metronidazole or a quadruple therapy combining omeprazole, amoxicillin, ciprofloxacin and doxycycline. All therapies were given for a duration of 10 days. The outcome measures were the persistence of positive FAT (treatment failure) 4 to 6 weeks after treatment and change in HRQoL scores.

Results: The treatment success rate was 80% in the total population and 78% in patients with a history of prior triple therapy. Significant improvement in HRQoL in the total group (HRQoL mean scores before and after treatment respectively: 76 ± 11 and 32 ± 11, $p < 0.001$) and the group with functional dyspepsia (HRQoL mean scores before and after treatment respectively: 73 ± 11 and 30 ± 9, $P < 0.001$) was observed across all treatment groups.
Using clarithromycin based triple therapy (standard of care) as a reference, the group treated with metronidazole had worse HRQoL ($p = 0.012$) and had a trend towards worse treatment outcome ($p = 0.086$) compared to the ciprofloxacin based combination therapies.

Conclusion: Clarithromycin and ciprofloxacin based combination therapies are effective and safe to use alternatively for *H. pylori* eradication and improve HRQoL. Among the regimens studied, metronidazole based triple therapy is likely to be clinically inferior.

Keywords: *H. pylori* eradication, Dyspepsia, Clinical trial, Rwanda

* Correspondence: damaskabakambira@gmail.com
[1]Kigali University Teaching Hospital (CHUK), Kigali, Rwanda
Full list of author information is available at the end of the article

Background

Helicobacter pylori is a known successful human pathogen living on the luminal surface of the gastric epithelium, responsible for various gastro-intestinal pathologies. The prevalence of infection is greatest in countries of the developing world. The most recent Rwandan *H. pylori* prevalence study in 2012 found a prevalence of 75% in an endoscopy population in Southern Rwanda [1]. The prevalence was the same three decades earlier in an endoscopy population in Kigali City, Rwanda [2]. For successful eradication policies in any country, there is need for accurate diagnostic tests and treatment tailored to local antibiotic resistance patterns.

H. pylori diagnosis

There is no single gold standard diagnostic test for *H. pylori*. The choice of a diagnostic test is influenced by the pretest probability of infection, cost, availability, population prevalence of infection and factors such as the previous use of proton pump inhibitors (PPIs) and antibiotics that may alter test results. Several diagnostic tests rely on testing of endoscopy biopsy samples, serum or stools. The urea breath test uses a different technique based on the principle that *H. pylori* hydrolyses urea to produce carbon dioxide and ammonia but it is a nuclear medical technique that requires the use of carbon 13 and 14 isotopes that are not currently available in Rwanda. Major diagnostic challenges exist when it comes to checking eradication after treatment in resource-poor settings. The urea breath test which is the best option to document eradication is not available in most resource limited countries. The Maastricht V/Florence Consensus also suggests bacterial culture for antibiotic resistance testing in those who fail first line therapy [3]. However, *H. pylori* has historically been difficult to culture although techniques are improving. It is also known that *H. pylori* antibiotic sensitivity in vitro may not always predict response in vivo [4]. No laboratory in Rwanda cultures *H. pylori* reliably at present, and resistance testing is also not available.

Fecal antigen assays have been reported in the literature to have sensitivity and specificity above 90% [4–6].

H. pylori treatment

Several studies have been conducted to evaluate efficacy of available *H. pylori* infection combination treatments [7–9]. The common practice is a combination of a PPI and two antibiotics (triple therapy) or the addition of bismuth salts to these three drug agents (quadruple therapy). The choice of antibiotics should be region specific, based on local *H. pylori* resistance to those antibiotics. However, raising antimicrobial therapy resistance to *H. pylori* poses great management challenge worldwide. In

Korea, Byoungrak et al. investigated antibiotic resistance in isolates in two cohorts in 2009–2010 and 2011–2012. Resistance to metronidazole was found to be 45.1% and 56.3% respectively in those two cohorts [10]. In Brazil, Eisig et al. detected *H. pylori* resistance to metronidazole and clarithromycin of 51% and 8% respectively [11]. In Africa, resistance to metronidazole is common. In Cameroon, *H. pylori* resistance was found to be as high as 93% for metronidazole, 85% for amoxicillin, 45% for clarithromycin and 44% for tetracycline in 2008 [12]. In South Africa, marked resistance (96%) to metronidazole was observed. However marked susceptibility to ciprofloxacin (100%), amoxicillin (98%), clarithromycin (80%) and gentamicin (73%) was observed in the same study [13].

No prior studies have assessed *H. pylori* antibiotic resistance in Rwanda. However, data suggest that more than half of patients presenting for endoscopy with a history of prior triple therapy remain positive for *H. pylori* infection, raising concern about potentially high resistance rates to current triple therapies used for *H. pylori* eradication [1]. According to the Rwandan Internal Medicine Clinical Treatment Guidelines, the first choice for *H. pylori* eradication regimen is a triple therapy combining omeprazole 20 mg twice daily, clarithromycin 500 mg twice daily and amoxicillin 1 g twice daily for a 10–14 day duration [14]. While the susceptibility of *H. pylori* to clarithromycin varies widely from 55 to 94% across the world, the efficacy of the clarithromycin-based triple therapy in Rwanda is unknown. Furthermore, the cost of clarithromycin-based regimen is approximately US$18, making it less affordable in a country with a GDP per capita of US$703 and an annual total health spending per capita of US$ 55 [15]. The present study assessed the efficacy of other cheaper *H. pylori* eradication regimens, pragmatically constructed using antibiotics cheaply available in Rwanda.

Health related quality of life

Functional dyspepsia is defined as the presence of one or more of the following: epigastric pain or burning, postprandial fullness and early satiety without evidence of structural disease (including at upper endoscopy) that can explain the symptoms [16]. Whether *H. pylori* improves quality of life among patients with functional dyspepsia, remains controversial. A study by Lane et al. in 2006 failed to detect an improvement in HRQoL after *H. pylori* eradication [17]. A large meta-analysis by Li-Jun revealed contradictory results across 25 randomized controlled trials and recommends individual assessment for clinicians desiring to eradicate *H. pylori* in patients with functional dyspepsia [18]. The American College of Gastroenterology acknowledges the lack of sufficient evidence to show the benefit of treating *H. pylori* in patients with functional dyspepsia but currently recommends testing for and treating *H. pylori* given durable benefit documented in some patients in previous studies [19–21].

The current study examines the efficacy of ciprofloxacin and metronidazole based *H. pylori* eradication therapies compared with clarithromycin based triple therapy, and the observed impact on HRQoL, among patients referred for endoscopy.

Methods

Patients

The study enrolled patients attending the University Teaching Hospital of Butare (CHUB) for esophagogastroduodenoscopy (EGD). CHUB is one of the 4 tertiary level hospitals in Rwanda with approximately 380 beds, located in the Southern Province of Rwanda. Patients are referred for EGD at CHUB by clinicians working in inpatient and outpatient facilities of CHUB, as well as satellite district hospitals and private health facilities in the town. Endoscopies are undertaken by two gastroenterologists or by a trainee physician under the supervision of the gastroenterologists.

The study enrolled patients who were 21 years and older, had a positive modified rapid urease test on endoscopic biopsies and were willing to come back for follow-up. Patients were excluded from the study if they: had used PPIs or a histamine H2 receptor antagonist or antimicrobial therapy in the previous 4 weeks; were allergic to any of the study drugs (omeprazole, amoxicillin, clarithromycin, ciprofloxacin, metronidazole and doxycycline); or had endoscopic or clinical evidence of gastric malignancy. Female patients were not breastfeeding and had a negative pregnancy test prior to randomization.

Randomization and study process

The study required two visits to CHUB, in Huye District in the Southern Province of Rwanda.

At visit 1, patients underwent endoscopy. Biopsies were tested for *H. pylori* infection by the MRU test. Patients provided a stool sample for fecal antigen test and completed a questionnaire about medical history as well as the HRQoL questionnaire. Randomization was done by picking a folded piece of paper under the observation of a study nurse, from a basket containing thoroughly mixed pieces of paper labeled with numbers corresponding to one of the 4 arms of treatment, each in equal quantity.

Patients and the treating clinicians were blinded to treatment. However, given that a high number of patients were unable to read and comprehend drug dosage instructions in English, a different nurse not associated with study analysis, opened envelopes containing medications together with the patients to explain how to take

them. This nurse was not allowed to discuss this information or treatment allocations with the treating clinicians or study staff; neither was she allowed to complete patient assessments at the second visit.

At visit 2 scheduled at 4–6 weeks after treatment completion, patients were clinically evaluated by a study clinician and completed the HRQoL questionnaire again. Patients with an initially positive fecal antigen test (FAT) also provided a stool sample for a post-treatment FAT.

Investigations

H. pylori status was determined by urease activity on 4 (2 antral and 2 fundal) biopsies. MRU test was undertaken by exposing gastric antral/body biopsies to a solution of 1 ml of 10% urea in water to which a drop of 1% phenol red has been added. When *H. pylori* is present, the bacterial urease catalyzes urea to ammonia and carbon dioxide which can be detected by the typical red color change in the solution [22].

A positive reaction, manifested by a color change within 3 h, was necessary for patients to be eligible for the study.

Patients were also required to provide stool samples for FAT. Patients who were unable to provide samples the same day were instructed to return samples the following morning before starting medication. FAT was performed with a rapid antigen test (HEALGEN;-ORIENT GENE;DS; catalog number GCHP-602).

Treatment regimens

Enrollees were randomized to one of the four following regimens:

Group 1: omeprazole 20 mg twice daily + amoxicillin 1 g twice daily + clarithromycin 500 mg twice daily for 10 days (CLARITHRO).

Group 2: omeprazole 20 mg twice daily + amoxicillin 1 g twice daily + ciprofloxacin 500 mg twice daily for 10 days (CIPRO).

Group 3: omeprazole 20 mg twice daily + amoxicillin 1 g twice daily + metronidazole 500 mg three times a day for 10 days (METRO).

Group 4: omeprazole 20 mg twice daily +amoxicillin 1 g twice daily + ciprofloxacin 500 mg twice daily+ doxycycline 100 mg twice daily for 10 days (CIPRO-Plus).

Health related quality of life (HRQoL)

During the first and second visits, the Short Form Nepean Dyspepsia Index (SF-NDI) questionnaire was completed to assess HRQoL before and after treatment.

The SF-NDI questionnaire has been translated and validated for use in a Kinyarwanda speaking population [23]. SF-NDI is a questionnaire with 10 items measured on six-point Likert scales. The instrument assesses five domains namely: tension/anxiety, interference with daily activities, knowledge/control, eating/drinking and work/study. Individual items in each sub-scale are aggregated to obtain a score range from 0 (best HRQoL score) to 100 (worst HRQoL score) as defined by the questionnaire developers [24].Questionnaires were available in English and Kinyarwanda. Adapted questionnaire was availed for illiterate patients to be completed with the help of a literate support person.

H. pylori eradication

Patients with initially positive FAT had a second FAT performed at visit 2. Patients were considered *H. pylori* negative if the second FAT was negative.

Safety considerations

Patients were instructed to report any side effects through a phone hotline to the research group. Symptoms were classified as mild, moderate or severe. Patients with severe symptoms were instructed to cease medication and were assessed by a gastroenterologist who decided on a further treatment regimen. At visit 2, a follow-up with a gastroenterologist was arranged for all patients who were still symptomatic.

Study outcomes
Primary outcome

- Positive fecal antigen test 4 to 6 weeks after treatment (among those with an initially positive fecal antigen test).

Secondary outcome

- Health related quality of life score change by SF-NDI questionnaire.

Statistical analyses

An intention-to-treat analysis was planned and conducted. Data are presented as mean ± standard deviation (SD) for normally distributed continuous variables and frequencies (percentage) for categorical variables. To compare the efficacy of each treatment arm vs standard of care (i.e., CLARITHRO), we performed independent samples t-test for continuous outcome (i.e., mean change in HRQoL score) and Fisher exact test for categorical outcomes. A paired t-test was used to compare pre- and post-treatment HRQoL scores. Statistical analyses were two-tailed and p values of < 0.05 were considered to show statistical significance. Analyses were performed with STATA (v 15, College Station, Texas).

Results

In a period of 1 year, from November 2015 to October 2016, a total of 866 patients underwent EGD. Of the 866 patients, 308 had a negative modified rapid urease (MRU) test for *H. pylori* while 96 patients did not undergo MRU testing.

Therefore, 462 patients had a positive MRU test but 99 patients did not meet inclusion criteria while 134 patients declined to participate to the study. Thus, 229 patients (35% male, age 42 ± 16 (mean ± SD), range 21-81 years) were randomized (Fig.1).

Baseline characteristics

The patient characteristics of the overall study group and each assigned treatment group are presented in Table 1. Access to EGD was generally rapid (mean number of days between endoscopy request by treating physician and endoscopy day: mean 2.2 ± 3.1).The population had a female preponderance at 65%. All patients carried a health insurance: 88% possessed community health insurance (Mutuel de Santé) while 12% had private health insurance. Previous medication use was very common among the study population: 77% had used PPIs or histamine (H2) receptor antagonists, 17% had taken triple therapy before and 14% reported using antibiotics for other illnesses.

The most common presenting symptoms were epigastric pain (96%) and vomiting (30%).

The most common endoscopic diagnoses were gastritis (56%), duodenal ulcer (30%) and gastric ulcers (11%). There was no lesion seen on endoscopy in 37 (16%) patients. These patients with functional dyspepsia had lower baseline HRQoL score compared to the patients with lesions on endoscopy (73 ± 12 and 77 ± 11, $p = 0.027$). Therefore, a post-hoc subgroup analysis was performed after treatment with regards to HRQoL. *H. pylori* testing at endoscopy was positive in 60% of patients who underwent the modified rapid urease test. Only 37% (85/229) patients had a positive FAT. The mean HRQoL score was 76 ± 11 and there was no sex difference in all subdomains, thus men and women were analyzed together after treatment. The previous use of PPIs or H2 blockers was neither associated with negativity of the FAT (OR = 1.1, $p = 0.847$ CI [0.5,2.2]) nor difference in HRQoL among users versus non-users (76 ± 11 and 77 ± 12, $p = 0.354$). Similarly, a previous exposure to triple therapy was neither associated with negativity of the FAT (OR = 1.1, $p = 0.738$ CI [0.5, 2.7]) nor difference in HRQoL among users versus non-users (75 ± 12 and 77 ± 11, $p = 0.549$).

Overall, there was no difference in baseline characteristics with regards to prior exposure to triple therapy except for the presence of duodenal ulcers that were more common among the non-exposed than in the exposed group (70% vs 30%, $p = 0.025$). Therefore, a subgroup

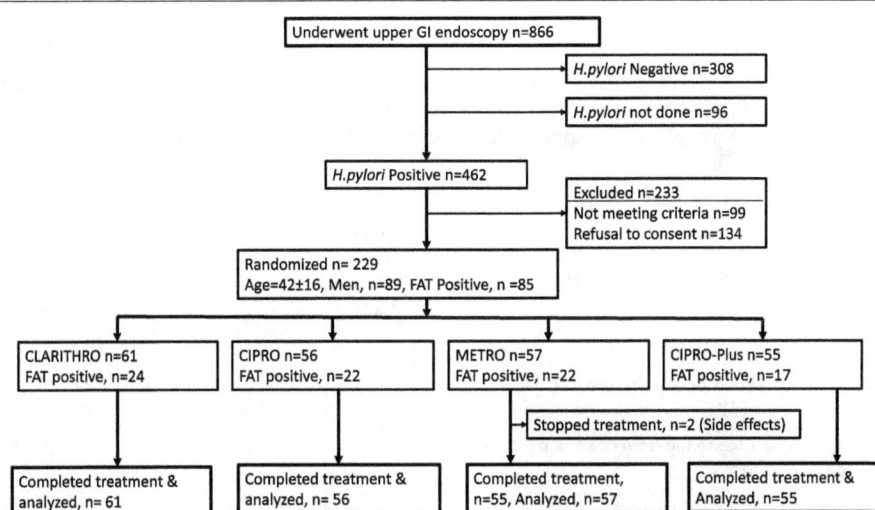

Fig. 1 Flow chart for patient selection and randomization

analysis was undertaken with regards to prior exposure to triple therapy status.

Efficacy of *H. pylori* eradication regimens
Treatment failure
Of the total 85 patients who had an initially positive FAT, 20% (17/85) had a positive test after treatment.

Compared to the treatment success in the overall group, there was a trend towards higher treatment failure in the METRO group although this did not reach statistical significance (36%, *p* = 0.086) (Table 2). Analysis stratified to the group without prior exposure to triple therapy showed a similar trend in treatment failure with the highest proportion in the METRO group (39%, *p* =

Table 1 Baseline population characteristics according to arm of treatment

Characteristics		Total (*n* = 229)	CLARITHRO *n* = 6127%	CIPRO *n* = 5624%	METRO *n* = 5725%	CIPRO-Plus *n* = 5524%
Demographic characteristics	Male (%)	35	43	43	35	35
	Age, years mean ± SD	42 ± 16	40 ± 15	44 ± 16	41 ± 16	41 ± 17
	Married (%)	57	52	68	60	49
	CommunityHealth Insurance (%)	88	85	88	93	87
	Access to endoscopy (days)	2.2 ± 3.1	1.9 ± 0.6	2.8 ± 6	2.3 ± 1.7	1.9 ± 0.6
Medical history	PPI or H2 blocker before (%)	77	74	79	79	78
	Triple therapy before (%)	17	13	23	16	18
	Antibiotics before (%)	14	13	13	13	18
Symptoms	Epigastric pain (%)	96	97	95	95	96
	Vomiting (%)	30	27	38	19	35
	Hematemesis (%)	8	10	9	4	9
	Melena (%)	2	2	4	2	2
Endoscopy finding	Normal endoscopy (%)	16	18	14	21	11
	Gastritis (%)	56	41	55	61	67
	Gastric ulcer (%)	11	10	14	14	7
	Duodenal ulcer (%)	30	41	36	25	16
Initially positive FAT (%)		37	39	39	39	31
Baseline HRQoLtotal group(mean ± SD score)		76 ± 11	77 ± 13	76 ± 12	76 ± 8	78 ± 12
Baseline HRQoLin functional dyspepsia (*n* = 37) (mean ± SD score)		73 ± 12	71 ± 9	70 ± 17	74 ± 10	76 ± 14

Baseline characteristics of the intention to treat population were not significantly different, except for gastritis (CIPRO Plus and METRO were significantly different from CLARITHRO, with *p* = 0.005 and *p* = 0.02, respectively) and for duodenal ulcer (CIPRO Plus was significantly different from CLARITHRO, *p* = 0.004).Abbreviations: *SD* Standard deviation, *FAT* Fecal Antigen Test, *PP* Proton Pump Inhibitors

Table 2 Study outcomes

Outcome		Total N = 229	CLARITHRO n = 61 27%	CIPRO n = 56 24%	METRO n = 57 25%	CIPRO-Plus n = 55 24%	p-value[1]
Treatment failure (Positive FAT) (%)	Total group (n = 85)	20	13	18	36	12	0.191
	No prior exposure to triple therapy (n = 73)	22	14	21	39	14	0.265
HRQoLin total group (mean ± SD)	Score after treatment	32 ± 11	31 ± 10	31 ± 10	36 ± 12**	31 ± 9	0.023
	Mean difference	44 ± 14	46 ± 15	44 ± 15	40 ± 13*	47 ± 13	0.032
HRQoL in functional dyspepsia (n = 37) (mean ± SD)	Score after treatment	30 ± 9	33 ± 13	28 ± 7	32 ± 6	24 ± 5	0.229
	Mean difference	42 ± 15	38 ± 17	42 ± 17	42 ± 10	51 ± 16	0.392
Persistence of symptoms (%)	Total group (n = 229)	22	18	23	26	20	0.715
	No prior exposure to triple therapy (n = 189)	23	19	26	29	18	0.492

*P-value by multiple regression for comparison to the reference group (CLARITHRO), *P ≤ 0.05, **P ≤ 0.01
[1]Student t-test or chi square test as appropriate

0.140). The sample size of the group with prior exposure to triple therapy was too small to establish a statistically sound comparison.

Health-related quality of life

There was a dramatic change in HRQoL scores from 76 ± 11 to 32 ± 11 after treatment ($p = 0.032$) in the total group. A paired t-test showed a significant improvement in HRQoL across all the four arms of treatment ($p < 0.001$) but a group comparison to the standard of care showed a significant difference only with the METRO group (Fig. 2). Infact, the METRO group maintained a higher post-treatment score than the standard of care (36 ± 12 vs 31 ± 10, $p = 0.008$) and registered a lower mean score change than the standard of care (40 ± 13 vs 46 ± 15, $p = 0.012$). In the group with functional dyspepsia, a paired t-test showed significant improvements across all the four arms of treatment. Further analysis

revealed that improvement in HRQoL score was not different in all the four arms of treatment compared to the standard of care (Table 2).

An assessment of clinical evolution after treatment revealed a persistence of symptoms in 22% of the total population. The METRO group had the highest rate of persistence of symptoms (26%) followed by CIPRO (23%), CIPRO-Plus (20%) and CLARITHRO (18%) but no regimen was statistically different from the standard of care.

Patients with persistence of symptoms after treatment had a higher HRQoL than patients who experienced symptom resolution (35 ± 11 vs 31 ± 10, $p = 0.018$) suggesting that persistence of symptoms was associated with worse HRQoL. Stratified analysis within the group of patients with functional dyspepsia ($n = 37$) showed a significant change in HRQoL scores overall (mean difference score: 42 ± 15, $p < 0.001$) but group comparison to

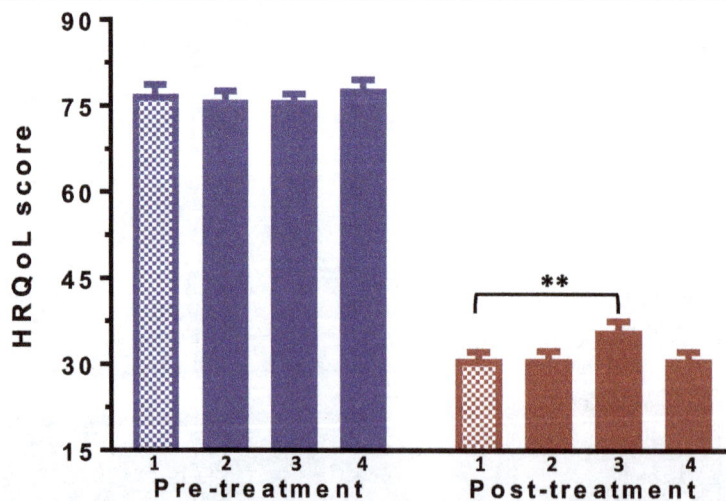

Fig. 2 Health-Related Quality of Life scores before (blue) and 4 to 6 weeks after (red) treatment. Scores were measured by the use of the SF-NDI questionnaire on a range from 0 (best HRQoL) to 100 (worst HRQoL). Arms of treatment: 1: CLARITHRO, 2: CIPRO, 3: METRO, 4: CIPRO-Plus. *p-value by multiple regression for comparison to the reference (REF) group (CLARITHRO), *p ≤ 0.05, **P ≤ 0.01, ***P ≤ 0.001

the standard of care revealed no difference in any arm of treatment. The greatest improvement in HRQoL was observed in "interference with daily activities" ($p = 0.019$) and "eating/drinking" ($p = 0.050$) subdomains.

Drug safety and specific treatment related side effects

A total of 34% (79/229) patients reported treatment related adverse effects. The adverse effects were reported to the investigator and were classified as mild, moderate or severe. The most commonly reported side effects were taste perversion (27%), nausea (18%), dizziness (14%) and vomiting (9%). Some patients had more than one adverse effect. Only two patients in the METRO group had symptoms severe enough to stop medication. These two patients were called back to see a gastroenterologist for further management but they were analyzed in the METRO group. Overall, 99% of patients completed treatment and no patient was lost to follow-up.

Discussion

This study explored the efficacy of pragmatic *H. pylori* eradication regimens available in Rwanda. Our results indicate that treatment success rate was 80% in the total group and 78% in the group without prior exposure to triple therapy. Significant improvement in HRQoL, expressed by decrease in SF-NDI scores, from baseline was observed across all the 4 arms of treatment. Our study results align with eradication success rates found in other studies around the world. The Maastricht IV/ Florence Consensus Report reported that the widely used triple therapy regimen cured 70% of patients [25].

Although there was no statistically significant difference between any of the arms of treatment and the standard of care, the metronidazole (METRO) based triple therapy showed some signals to suggest metronidazole based triple therapy might be inferior to other regimens. Infact, metronidazole based triple therapy registered the highest failure rate (36%) followed by CIPRO (18%), CLARITHRO (13%) and CIPRO-Plus (12%).

Similarly, HRQoL was improved in all the treatment groups but improvement was much less in the metronidazole based triple therapy than in the standard of care. Although the metronidazole based triple therapy was inferior to CLARITHRO group in improving HRQoL, the difference in treatment failure did not reach the level of statistical significance, probably due to lower than expected failure rates overall, and the concomitant reduction in study power. No susceptibility study has ever been conducted particularly in Rwanda but the resistance of *H. pylori* to metronidazole is notoriously high (90–100%) in Africa, which may explain the modest performance of metronidazole based triple therapy that was found [26–28].

On the other hand, ciprofloxacin based triple therapy (omeprazole + amoxicillin+ ciprofloxacin) and quadruple therapy (omeprazole + amoxicillin+ ciprofloxacin+ doxycycline) were not inferior to clarithromycin based triple therapy and presented a very good safety profile. This finding aligns nicely with studies conducted in Nigeria and South Africa which didn't detect any resistance to ciprofloxacin, suggesting that a fluoroquinolone based regimen may be of utility in Africa [12, 27]. Pending more rigorous diagnostic tests for eradication, this finding offers hope that the combination of omeprazole, amoxicillin, ciprofloxacin and doxycycline could be used as a salvage therapy, particularly since bismuth combinations are still unaffordable in Rwanda.

This study shows that *H. pylori* was positive in 60% of the eligible population. This prevalence is lower than other prevalences reported in Africa possibly due to the fact that a portion of our population had previously been treated for *H. pylori* [28].

Although reported to be of high accuracy for initial and post-treatment diagnosis, FAT was only able to detect 37% of patients with *H. pylori*.

The diagnostic performance of FAT shows large variations across the world. Studies assessing the diagnostic accuracy of FAT have concluded to sensitivities and specificities above 90% in Europe and Taiwan [4–6]. A study conducted in Uganda, a neighboring country with Rwanda, found a contrasting sensitivity and specificity of 56% and 74% respectively [29]. In Nigeria, Olufemi et al. reported *H. pylori* prevalence of 68.7% using a serology test but it was only 20.2% using FAT [30]. The poor performance of FAT in this study as well as the two studies in Uganda and Nigeria raise concern about the utility of FAT as a diagnostic test in Rwanda and in Africa in general. Evidence shows that prior exposure to PPIs interferes with diagnostic accuracy of FAT but we had attempted to control this problem by excluding patients who used PPIs or histamine receptor antagonists in the past 4 weeks [31]. The explanation of the diversity in FAT accuracy as a test which uses antigens is most likely to be linked with the diversity of genome and virulence of *H. pylori* strains across the world [32]. Emerging data from studies predominantly conducted in Asian populations unequivocally show large geographical variations in the distribution of *H. pylori* strains [33, 34]. Although extensive work has been done to elucidate how genetic diversity is related to human cancer, little is known about the effect of genetic diversity on the performance of stool antigen test for the diagnosis of *H. pylori* [35].

Our study found significant change in HRQoL scores from baseline across all the 4 arms of treatment. The findings were even true in the sub-group of patients who had normal endoscopy before treatment (functional dyspepsia).

This finding adds to the currently accumulating literature in favor of improvement of HRQoL by treating *H. pylori* in patients with functional dyspepsia. However, we had a small number of patients with functional dyspepsia and we are not statistically powered enough to draw a firm conclusion. Further studies with larger sample sizes are still needed to confirm this finding.

Lastly, although all study participants had health insurance, most (88%) had community health insurance, which is the cheapest and usually the main option accessible to Rwandans with limited financial resources. Community health insurance only gives access to health care and medicine available in public health care facilities. Due to the high cost and low availability in many public facilities, clarithromycin is the least affordable medication for the great majority of patients. It is not available at all in many rural health care facilities. Because of this, clinicians struggle to select appropriate initial and salvage regimens for *H. pylori* eradication. The treatment success rate trend and safety profile from this study make the ciprofloxacin based combination therapies a strong and cost-effective alternative to clarithromycin based therapy.

Strengths and limitations

This is the first ever *H. pylori* eradication clinical trial conducted in Rwanda. By using a multi-arm trial, we were able to study efficacy of various *H. pylori* eradication regimens simultaneously using the same control group, thus saving time and resources to provide locally appropriate evidence to guide clinical practice. Findings are important because they offer chance to clinicians to prescribe affordable treatment regimens with confidence.

Due to financial constraints, this study was conducted in one center and the outcome measurement was limited to the use of FAT, which turned out to be a poorly sensitive diagnostic test in our study population, thus limiting the study's power.

The treatment duration was 10 days across all the four arms of treatment in our study. Infact, earlier studies did not report major differences between short duration treatments (7 days) and long duration treatments (14 days) [36]. Our choice of a 10 day duration was inspired by the Maastricht IV/ Florence Consensus Report which suggested that extending therapies to 10–14 days improves eradication success by 5% [25]. We chose the lower end of the optimal duration due to financial and adverse drug effect considerations. It is important to mention that the weight of recent literature now advocates a long course of treatment (14 days) to optimize outcomes [21, 37].

This study raises awareness in policy makers and paves a path for subsequent studies that will apply more rigorous diagnostic methods such as bacterial culture and urea breath test to better characterize *H. pylori* eradication in sub-Saharan Africa. Further work needs to be done examining other alternatives, including high dose dual therapy, if treatment recommendations are to be optimized.

Conclusion

Given the balance of cost, efficacy and safety profile documented in this study; clinicians should feel confident to use clarithromycin and ciprofloxacin based combination therapies for *H. pylori* eradication in Rwanda. Our findings suggest that metronidazole based triple therapy is likely to be clinically inferior, and make it the worst choice among the four regimens we studied.

Abbreviations

CHUB: Butare University Teaching Hospital; CHUK: Kigali University Teaching Hospital; CIPRO: Omeprazole 20 mg twice daily + amoxicillin 1 g twice daily + ciprofloxacin 500 mg twice daily for 10 days; CIPRO-Plus: Omeprazole 20 mg twice daily + amoxicillin 1 g twice daily+ ciprofloxacin 500 mg twice daily+ doxycycline 100 mg twice daily for 10 days; CLARITHRO: Omeprazole 20 mg twice daily + amoxicillin 1 g twice daily + clarithromycin 500 mg twice daily for 10 days; EGD: Esophagogastroduodenoscopy; FAT: Fecal Antigen Test; GDP: Gross domestic product; HRQoL: Health-related quality of life; METRO: Omeprazole 20 mg twice daily + amoxicillin 1 g twice daily + metronidazole 500 mg three times a day for 10 days; MRU: Modified rapid urease; PPI: Proton Pump Inhibitors; SD: Standard deviation; SF-NDI: Short Form Nepean Dyspepsia Index

Acknowledgements

We thank the clinical staff in the Gastroenterology Unit at CHUB: Dr. Nicaise Nsabimana, Steven Ndayisaba, Leonie Niragire, Fiacre Ngarambe and Samuel Bizimana. Dr. Aimee Nyiramahirwe, Fanny Giraneza and Gladys Uwera have greatly contributed in data collection.

Funding

The study was funded by Butare University Teaching Hospital (CHUB), located in the Southern Province of Rwanda, Huye District. The funding covered study drugs and cost for endoscopy. The funder of the study had no role in study design, data collection, data analysis, data interpretation, or writing of the report.

Authors' contribution

JDK, TW, CB, JN and DH were involved in the conception and design of the study. DH and CB provided laboratory expertise. JDK, TW, CN and FN acquired the data. JDK and CH conducted data analysis. JDK, TW, CP, VD and CH interpreted the data. JDK drafted the manuscript. JDK, TW, CH, CB, JN, DH, VD, CN, CP and FN critically revised the manuscript for intellectual content, approved the final version and agreed to be accountable for all aspects of the work.

Authors' information

JDK: Attending physician at CHUK. Currently undertaking a Research Fellowship at the National Institutes of Health, USA. CH: Vanier Scholar and PhD Candidate, School of Population and Public Health, Faculty of Medicine, University of British Columbia, Vancouver, BC, Canada, CP: Associate Professor of Medicine, University Hospital of Brooklyn, New York, USA, CN: Attending physician at CHUB, VD: Attending physician at CHUK, Academic Head of Medicine, University of Rwanda, JN: Senior anesthesiologist at CHUB, FN: Gastroenterologist at CHUK, DH: Emeritus Professor of Medicine at University of Utah, School of Medicine, CB: Associate Professor of Medical Microbiology, University of Rwanda. TW: Former Chief of Gastroenterology Unit at CHUB, Clinical Dean, Calvary Mater Newcastle, Australia.

Consent for publication
Nota applicable.

Competing interests
The authors declare that they have no competing interests.

Author details
[1]Kigali University Teaching Hospital (CHUK), Kigali, Rwanda. [2]Centre for Health Services and Policy Research, School of Population and Public Health, Faculty of Medicine, University of British Columbia, Vancouver, BC, Canada. [3]Collaboration for Outcomes Research and Evaluation, Faculty of Pharmaceutical Sciences, University of British Columbia, Vancouver, BC, Canada. [4]Department of Medicine, University Hospital of Brooklyn, New York, USA. [5]Butare University Teaching Hospital (CHUB), Huye, Rwanda. [6]Department of Medicine, University of Utah School of Medicine, Salt Lake City, UT, USA. [7]School of Medicine and Public Health, Faculty of Health and Medicine, University of Newcastle, Newcastle, Australia.

References

1. Walker TD, Karemera M, Ngabonziza F, Kyamanywa P. Helicobacter pylori status and associated gastroscopic diagnoses in a tertiary hospital endoscopy population in Rwanda. Trans. R. Soc. Trop. Med. Hyg. 2014; https://doi.org/10.1093/trstmh/tru029.
2. Rouvroy D, Bogaerts J, Nsengiumwa O, Omar M, Versailles L, Haot J. Campylobacter pylori, gastritis, and peptic ulcer disease in central Africa. Br. Med. J. Clin. Res. Ed. 1987;295(6607):1174.
3. Malfertheiner P, et al. Management of Helicobacter pylori infection—the Maastricht V/Florence consensus report. Gut, p. gutjnl–2016. 2016;
4. Vaira D, et al. Diagnosis of helicobacter pylori infection with a new non-in vasive antigen-based assay. Lancet. 1999;354(9172):30–3.
5. Wu DC, et al. Comparison of stool enzyme immunoassay and immunochromatographic method for detecting< i> helicobacter pylori</i> antigens before and after eradication. Diagn Microbiol Infect Dis. 2006; 56(4):373–8.
6. Veijola L, Myllyluoma E, Korpela R, Rautelin H. Stool antigen tests in the diagnosis of Helicobacter pylori infection before and after eradication therapy. World J. Gastroenterol. 2005;11(46):7340.
7. Gatta L, et al. A 10-day levofloxacin-based triple therapy in patients who have failed two eradication courses. Aliment Pharmacol Ther. 2005;22(1):45–9.
8. Gisbert JP, et al. Proton pump inhibitor, clarithromycin and either amoxycillin or nitroimidazole: a meta-analysis of eradication of helicobacter pylori. Aliment Pharmacol Ther. 2000;14(10):1319–28.
9. Fischbach LA, Zanten SV, Dickason J. Meta-analysis: the efficacy, adverse events, and adherence related to first-line anti-helicobacter pylori quadruple therapies. Aliment Pharmacol Ther. 2004;20(10):1071–82.
10. An B, et al. Antibiotic resistance in helicobacter pylori strains and its effect on H. Pylori eradication rates in a single center in Korea. Ann Lab Med. 2013;33(6):415–9.
11. Eisig JN, Silva FM, Barbuti RC, Navarro-Rodriguez T, Moraes-Filho JPP, Pedrazzoli J Jr. Helicobacter pylori antibiotic resistance in Brazil: clarithromycin is still a good option. Arq Gastroenterol. 2011;48(4):261–4.
12. Tanih NF, et al. An African perspective on helicobacter pylori: prevalence of human infection, drug resistance, and alternative approaches to treatment. Ann Trop Med Parasitol. 2009;103(3):189–204.
13. Tanih NF, et al. Marked susceptibility of south African helicobacter pylori strains to ciprofloxacin and amoxicillin: clinical implications. S Afr Med J. 2010;100(1):49–52.
14. "Internal-Medicine-Clinical-Treatment-Guidelines-9-10-2012-1.pdf." [Online]. Available: http://www.moh.gov.rw/fileadmin/templates/Clinical/Internal-Medicine-Clinical-Treatment-Guidelines-9-10-2012-1.pdf. [Accessed: 24-Sep-2015].
15. Farmer PE, et al. Reduced premature mortality in Rwanda: lessons from success. Bmj. 2013;346:f65.
16. Tack J, et al. Functional Gastroduodenal disorders. Gastroenterology. 2006; 130(5):1466–79.
17. Lane JA, et al. Impact of helicobacter pylori eradication on dyspepsia, health resource use, and quality of life in the Bristol helicobacter project: randomised controlled trial. BMJ 2006;332:199.
18. Du L-J, Chen B-R, Kim JJ, Kim S, Shen J-H, Dai N. Helicobacter pylori eradication therapy for functional dyspepsia: systematic review and meta-analysis. World J. Gastroenterol. 2016;22(12):3486.
19. P. Moayyedi et al., "Eradication of helicobacter pylori for non-ulcer dyspepsia," Cochrane Libr., 2006.
20. Suzuki H, Moayyedi P. Helicobacter pylori infection in functional dyspepsia, Nat. Rev. Gastroenterol. Hepatol. 10(3):168, 2013.
21. Chey WD, Leontiadis GI, Howden CW, Moss SF. ACG clinical guideline: treatment of Helicobacter pylori infection. Am. J. Gastroenterol. 2017; 112(2):212.
22. Katelaris PH, Lowe DG, Norbu P, Farthing MJG. Field evaluation of a rapid, simple and inexpensive urease test for the detection of helicobacter pylori. J Gastroenterol Hepatol. 1992;7(6):569–71.
23. Nkurunziza A, Dusabejambo V, Everhart K, Bensen S, Walker T. Validation of the Kinyarwanda-version Short-Form Leeds Dyspepsia Questionnaire and Short-Form Nepean Dyspepsia Index to assess dyspepsia prevalence and quality-of-life impact in Rwanda. BMJ Open. 2016;6(6):e011018.
24. Talley NJ, Verlinden M, Jones M. Quality of life in functional dyspepsia: responsiveness of the Nepean dyspepsia index and development of a new 10-item short form. Aliment Pharmacol Ther. 2001;15(2):207–16.
25. Malfertheiner P, et al. Management of Helicobacter pylori infection—the Maastricht IV/Florence consensus report. Gut. 2012;61(5):646–64.
26. Secka O, et al. Antimicrobial susceptibility and resistance patterns among helicobacter pylori strains from the Gambia, West Africa. Antimicrob Agents Chemother. 2013;57(3):1231–7.
27. Oyedeji KS, Smith SI, Coker AO, Arigbabu AO. Antibiotic susceptibility patterns in helicobacter pylori strains from patients with upper gastrointestinal pathology in western Nigeria. Br J Biomed Sci. 2009; 66(1):10–3.
28. Smith SI, Seriki A, Ndip R, Pellicano R. Helicobacter pylori infection in Africa: 2018 literature update. Minerva Gastroenterol. Dietol. 2018;64(3):222-34.
29. Segamwenge IL, Kagimu M, Ocama P, Opio K. The utility of the helicobacter pylori stool antigen test in managing dyspepsia: an experience from a low resource setting. Afr Health Sci. 2014;14(4):829–34.
30. Olufemi FO, Quadri R, Akinduti PA, Bamiro SA. Potential risk Fcators and prevalence of infection of helicobacter pylori in Nigeria. J Sci Res Rep. 2015; 7(1):42–8.
31. Manes G, et al. Accuracy of the stool antigen test in the diagnosis of helicobacter pylori infection before treatment and in patients on omeprazole therapy. Aliment Pharmacol Ther. Jan. 2001;15(1):73–9.
32. Thorell K, Lehours P, Vale FF. Genomics of Helicobacter pylori. Helicobacter. 2017;22(Suppl. 1):e12409.
33. Gorrell RJ, Zwickel N, Reynolds J, Bulach D, Kwok T. Helicobacter pylori CagL Hypervariable Motif: A Global Analysis of Geographical Diversity and Association With Gastric Cancer. J. Infect. Dis. 2016;213(12):1927–31.
34. Phan TN, et al. Genotyping of helicobacter pylori shows high diversity of strains circulating in Central Vietnam. Infect Genet Evol J Mol Epidemiol Evol Genet Infect Dis. 2017;52:19–25.
35. Hatakeyama M. Anthropological and clinical implications for the structural diversity of the helicobacter pylori CagA oncoprotein. Cancer Sci. Jan. 2011; 102(1):36–43.
36. Kim BG, et al. Comparison of 7-day and 14-day proton pump inhibitor-containing triple therapy for helicobacter pylori eradication: neither treatment duration provides acceptable eradication rate in Korea. Helicobacter. 2007;12(1):31–5.
37. GRAHAM DY. Treating Helicobacter pylori effectively while minimizing misuse of antibiotics. Cleve. Clin. J. Med. 2017;84(4):311.

20

Prevalence of non *Helicobacter pylori* species in patients presenting with dyspepsia

Javed Yakoob[1*], Zaigham Abbas[1], Rustam Khan[1], Shagufta Naz[1], Zubair Ahmad[2], Muhammad Islam[3], Safia Awan[1], Fatima Jafri[1] and Wasim Jafri[1]

Abstract

Background: Helicobacter species associated with human infection include *Helicobacter pylori, Helicobacter heilmannii* and *Helicobacter felis* among others. In this study we determined the prevalence of *H. pylori* and non-*Helicobacter pylori* organisms *H. felis and H. heilmannii* and analyzed the association between coinfection with these organisms and gastric pathology in patients presenting with dyspepsia. Biopsy specimens were obtained from patients with dyspepsia on esophagogastroduodenoscopy (EGD) for rapid urease test, histology and PCR examination for Helicobacter genus specific 16S rDNA, *H. pylori* phosphoglucosamine mutase (*glmM*) and urease B (*ureB*) gene of *H. heilmannii* and *H. felis*. Sequencing of PCR products of *H. heilmannii* and *H. felis* was done.

Results: Two hundred-fifty patients with dyspepsia were enrolled in the study. The mean age was 39 ± 12 years with males 162(65%). Twenty-six percent (66 out of 250) were exposed to cats or dogs. PCR for Helicobacter genus specific 16S rDNA was positive in 167/250 (67%), *H. pylori glmM* in 142/250 (57%), *H. heilmannii* in 17/250 (6%) and *H. felis* in 10/250 (4%), respectively. All the *H. heilmannii* and *H. felis* PCR positive patients were also positive for *H. pylori* PCR amplification. The occurrence of coinfection of *H. pylori* and *H. heilmannii* was 17(6%) and with *H. felis* was 10(4%), respectively. Only one out of 66 exposed to pets were positive for *H. heilmannii* and two for *H. felis*. Histopathology was carried out in 160(64%) of 250 cases. Chronic active inflammation was observed in 53(56%) (p = 0.001) of the patients with *H. pylori* infection alone as compared to 3(37%) (p = 0.73) coinfected with *H. heilmannii* and *H. pylori* and 3(60%) coinfected with *H. felis* and *H. pylori* (p = 0.66). Intestinal metaplasia was observed in 3(3%)(p = 1.0) of the patients with *H. pylori* infection alone as compared to 2(25%) (p = 0.02) coinfected with *H. heilmannii* and *H. pylori* and 1(20%) coinfected with *H. felis* and *H. pylori* (p = 0.15).

Conclusion: The prevalence of *H. heilmannii* and *H. felis* was low in our patients with dyspepsia. Exposure to pets did not increase the risk of *H. heilmannii* or *H. felis* infection. The coinfection of *H. pylori* with *H. heilmannii* was seen associated with intestinal metaplasia, however this need further confirmation.

Keywords: Dyspepsia, gastric biopsies, H. pylori, H. heilmannii, H. felis, coinfection, cats, dogs

Background

Helicobacter species infect the gastrointestinal tracts of many animals from birds through humans. Some of these have been linked to a range of human diseases [1,2] including chronic gastritis, peptic ulcer disease, mucosa-associated lymphoid tissue lymphoma, and gastric adenocarcinoma [1,3]. The principal Helicobacter infection in humans is *Helicobacter pylori*, with infection rates in developing countries reaching 50% to 90% [2,4]. Human gastric biopsy samples, however, have shown to harbor bacteria which were morphologically different from *H. pylori* [5,6]. These include *Helicobacter heilmannii* and *Helicobacter felis* which are primarily pathogens of domestic animals and were later found to infect humans as well [7-9].

Gastric non-*Helicobacter pylori* helicobacters constitute a diverse group of bacterial species that are known to colonize the gastric mucosa of several animals [10]. These include morphologically distinct, typically long spiral shaped bacteria originally referred to as *Gastrospirillum hominis* and later as *H. heilmannii*. The latter was

---

* Correspondence: yakoobjaved@hotmail.com
[1]Department of Medicine, The Aga Khan University, Karachi, Pakistan
Full list of author information is available at the end of the article

further subdivided in two taxa, types 1 and 2 [10]. *H. heilmannii* type 1 are identical to *H. suis* which colonizes the stomachs of pigs. The former *H. heilmannii* type 2 represent a group of species, known to colonize the gastric mucosa of dogs and cats and include *H. felis, H. bizzozeronii, H. salomonis, H. cynogastricus, H. baculiformis* and a bacterium provisionally named in 2004 as "*Candidatus* H. heilmannii" because at that time, it could not be cultured in vitro [10,11]. However, recently, in vitro cultures have been obtained resulting in description of *H. heilmannii*, as a novel Helicobacter species [12]. Sequencing of the 16S or 23S rRNA-encoding genes allows differentiation of *H. suis* from the other gastric non-*H. pylori* helicobacters species, but it cannot distinguish between *H. felis, H. bizzozeronii, H. salomonis, H. cynogastricus, H. baculiformis* and *Candidatus* H. heilmannii [10]. For differentiation between these species, sequencing of the heat shock protein 60 (hsp60) or gyrase B (gyrB) gene is used while sequencing of the urease A and B genes is considered to be the most suitable method since sequences of these genes are available [10,11,13,14].

Dyspepsia describes a variety of symptoms, including abdominal pain, bloating, nausea, and vomiting. In these patients, endoscopy is considered to rule out gastroesophageal reflux disease, peptic or duodenal ulcer and gastric cancer. The role of *H. pylori* infection in dyspepsia remains controversial. This study aims to identify the prevalence of *H. pylori* and non-H. pylori helicobacters, *H. felis* and *H. heilmannii* and to analyze the gastric pathology associated with coinfection of these organisms in patients presenting with dyspepsia.

Results and discussion

Majority of the patients with *H. pylori* infection were in the age range of 18-39 years, while *H. felis* and *H. heilmannii* positive patients did not show this distribution. (Table 1). There was no difference in the gender, ethnicity of patients, crowding index (CI) and source of water distribution among the patients with *H. pylori* and non-*H. pylori* infections (Table 1). All patients had abdominal pain with endoscopic gastritis as the predominant finding. The false positive and false negative results obtained with RUT were 15(36%) and 6(12%), respectively while with histology the false positive and false negative results obtained were 20(30%) and 10(11%), respectively (Table 1-2).

PCR for Helicobacter genus specific *16S rDNA* was positive in 167/250 (67%), *glmM* (*H. pylori*) in 142/250 (57%), *H. heilmanii* in 17/250 (6%) and *H. felis* in 10/250 (4%), respectively (Table 2).

PCR was positive for both *H. pylori* and *H. heilmannii* in 17(6%) and for *H. pylori* and *H. felis* in 10(4%), respectively (Table 2). All the *H. heilmannii* and *H. felis* positive patients were also positive for *H. pylori glmM* PCR amplification (Table 2).

26% (66 out of 250) were exposed to pets either cats or dogs. Most *H. heilmannii* positive patients did not have pet contact. Only one out of 66 exposed to pets was positive for *H. heilmannii* and two for *H. felis* (Table 3).

A higher degree of bacterial density was associated with *H. pylori* infection alone (p < 0.001) (Table 1). Chronic active inflammation was observed in 53(56%) cases with *H. pylori* alone infection (p = 0.001) compared to 3(37%) in *H. heilmannii* (p = 0.73) and 3(60%) in *H. felis* positive patients coinfected with *H. pylori* (p = 0.66) (Table 1). Intestinal metaplasia (IM) was present in 3(3%) out of 94 cases with *H. pylori* infection alone compared to 2(25%) out of 8 cases of *H. Heilmannii* and *H. pylori* coinfection, and 1(20%) out of 5 cases of *H. felis* and *H. pylori* coinfection in which histology has been performed.

PCR product sequences were compared to the sequences of ureaseB of different *H. heilmannii* and *H. felis* strains. The *H. heilmannii* sequences had 100% similarity to '*Candidatus* Helicobacter heilmannii' strains GenBank: AF508012 and L25079; while it was 99% to GenBank: AY139170, AF507996, AY139172, AY139173 and 98% to GenBank: AY139171, respectively. The *H. felis* sequences had 100% similarity to *H. felis* strains GenBank: FQ670179 and X69080; while it was 99% to *H. felis* GenBank: AY368267, AY368261 and 98% to GenBank: DQ865138, respectively.

Among our patients, the cohort exposed to pet animals was limited to 26%. There were more patients with *H. pylori* infection who were in the 18-39 years age range. Such age distribution was not seen in cases with *H. felis* and *H. heilmannii* infection. There was no difference in the gender, ethnicity of patients, crowding index (CI) and source of water distribution among the patients with *H. pylori* and non-*H. pylori* helicobacter species infections. There were no statistically significant differences in the endoscopic findings in patients with *H. pylori* infection alone or with coinfection of *H. pylori* and non-*H. pylori* Helicobacter species. Chronic active inflammation was associated with *H. pylori* infection compared to *H. heilmannii* or *H. felis* coinfections with *H. pylori* (Table 1). However, the histology was not obtained in all the cases that showed *H. heilmannii* and *H. felis* infection. Intestinal metaplasia was present in 2(25%) out of 8 cases of *H. heilmannii* coinfection with *H. pylori* and in 1(20%) out of 5 cases of *H. felis* coinfection with *H. pylori* as compared to 3(3%) of 94 cases with *H. pylori* infection alone who had undergone the histological study. Although it was not possible to draw a conclusion that IM was significantly associated with the coinfection of either of the species and *H. pylori*, a tendency in that way would be likely, as it has also been reported by other authors.

PCR positives at the species level were also positive for the Helicobacter genus specific 16S rDNA and all the *H. heilmannii* and *H. felis* positive patients were also

Table 1 Demography and clinical features of patients enrolled

	PCR for *H. pylori*			PCR for *H. heilmannii*			PCR for *H. felis*		
	Positive n = 142	Negative n = 108	P value	Positive n = 17	Negative n = 233	P value	Positive n = 10	Negative n = 240	P value
Age									
18-39 years	81(57)	55(51)	0.02	8(47)	128(55)	0.82	6(60)	130(55)	0.93
40-55 years	53(37)	35(32)		7(41)	81(35)		3(30)	85(35)	
56-75 years	8(6)	18(17)		2(12)	24(10)		1(10)	25(10)	
Gender									
Male	98(69)	64(59)	0.11	11(65)	151(65)	0.99	5(50)	157(65)	0.33
Female	44(31)	44(41)		6(35)	82(35)		5(50)	83(35)	
Ethnicity									
Karachiite	36(25)	36(33)	0.15	4(24)	68(29)	0.81	2(20)	70(29)	0.75
Quetta resident	47(36)	31(25)		5(29)	73(31)		3(30)	75(31)	
Afghan	55(39)	45(42)		8(47)	92(40)		5(50)	95(40)	
Crowding Index (CI)									
0-1(low)	59(41)	39(36)	0.03	5(29)	93(40)	0.35	5(50)	93(39)	0.59
2-4 (moderate)	82(58)	62(57)		12(71)	132(57)		5(50)	139(58)	
> 4 (crowding)	1(1)	7(7)		0(0)	8(3)		0(0)	8(3)	
Water supply									
Municipal	86(61)	59(55)	0.34	8(47)	137(59)	0.34	7(70)	138(58)	0.52
Boring Water	56(39)	49(45)		9(53)	96(41)		3(30)	102(42)	
EGD									
Gastritis	136(96)	106(96)	0.47	17(100)	225(97)	1	10(100)	232(97)	1
Duodenal ulcer	6(4)	2(4)		0(0)	8(3)		0(0)	8(3)	
Rapid Urease test (n = 90)									
Positive	42(88)	15(36)	> 0.001	4(44)	53(63)	0.28	2(40)	55(63)	0.35
Negative	6(12)	27(64)		5(56)	28(37)		3(60)	30(37)	
Histopathology (n = 160)									
Bacterial density									
Occasional	10(11)	40(61)	> 0.001	3(37)	47(31)	0.27	0(0)	50(32)	0.14
Few in some fields	59(63)	21(32)		2(25)	78(51)		4(80)	76(49)	
Only 1/2 small clusters	25(27)	5(7)		3(38)	27(18)		1(20)	29(19)	
Inflammation type									
Chronic	41(44)	47(71)	0.001	5(63)	83(55)	0.73	2(40)	86(55)	0.66
Chronic active inflammation	53(56)	19(29)		3(37)	69(45)		3(60)	69(45)	
Lymphoid follicles									
Positive	14(15)	8(12)	0.73	0(0)	22(14)	0.30	0(0)	22(14)	0.47
Negative	80(85)	58(88)		8(100)	130(86)		5(100)	133(86)	
Intestinal metaplasia									
Positive	3(3)	2(3)	1.0	2(25)	3(2)	0.02	1(20)	4(3)	0.15
Negative	91(97)	64(97)		6(75)	149(98)		4(80)	151(97)	

Univariate analysis was performed by using the independent sample t-test, Pearson Chi-square or Fisher Exact test where appropriate. A *P*-value of < 0.05 was considered as statistically significant. *All the *H. heilmannii* and *H. felis* PCR positive patients were also positive for *H. pylori* PCR amplification.

Table 2 PCR results for Helicobacter species

	PCR for Helicobacter genus specific *16SrRNA*		
	Positive n = 167	Negative n = 83	P value
H. pylori glmM			
Positive	133(80)	9(11)	< 0.001
Negative	34(20)	74(89)	
H. heilmannii ureB			
Positive	17(10)	0(0)	0.003
Negative	150(90)	83(100)	
H. felis ure A and B			
Positive	10(6)	0(0)	0.03
Negative	157(94)	83(100)	

Univariate analysis was performed by using the independent sample t-test, Pearson Chi-square test or Fisher Exact test where appropriate. A *P*-value of < 0.05 was considered as statistically significant. *All the *H. heilmannii* and *H. felis* PCR positive patients were also positive for *H. pylori* PCR amplification.

positive for *H. pylori* glmM PCR (Table 2). PCR product sequences of ureaseB gene of *H. heilmannii* had shown 100% similarity to '*Candidatus* H. heilmannii strains' GenBank: AF508012 and L25079; while *H. felis* sequences had shown 100% similarity to strains Gen-Bank: FQ670179 and X69080.

In this study, we used urease gene-based PCR method developed by Nieger et al that detected only '*Candidatus* H. heilmannii' DNA from pure in vitro cultures of other non-*H. pylori* helicobacter species [14]. This method was also used by other investigators to demonstrate the presence of *Candidatus* H. heilmannii DNA in gastric biopsies from patients with dyspepsia [11,15,16]. The limitations of our study include the small number of patients who had non-*H. pylori* helicobacter infection and the presence of *H. pylori* co-infection which precluded assessment of the histological effect of these species under consideration. Also, the significance of coinfection in terms of disease development could not be determined. We could have identified few more cases of non-*H. pylori* helicobacter species by other reported methods used to study non *H. pylori* helicobacter species including fluorescent in situ hybridization (FISH), transmission electron microscopy (TEN) and partial 16S ribosomal sequencing for analyses of the amplified products [12,17].

The implications of this study are that non-*H. pylori* helicobacter species infection occurs in patients with abdominal pain or discomfort similar to *H. pylori* infection. Most of our *H. heilmannii* infections were not associated with contact with animals. This is in contrast to a previous analysis of 125 patients with confirmed *H. heilmannii* infection that showed some 70.3% of the 111 patients had a history of contact with one or more animals [17,18]. All of our patients with non-*H. pylori* infection had endoscopic gastritis though their association with peptic ulcer is well known [19,20]. The prevalence of coinfection of *H. felis* with *H. pylori* in our population is less than

what has been reported from South Africa among African population but is certainly higher than that for *H. heilmannii* and *H. pylori* from the northern Europe which showed that only 1.6% had concomitant infection with *H. pylori* [20,21]. The coinfection in our patients demonstrated severe gastric pathology, as intestinal metaplasia was present in 25% of *H. heilmannii* coinfection with *H. pylori* while in 20% of *H. felis* coinfection with *H. pylori*. This was also reported in previous studies [22]. In this study, the difference was not statistically significant due to the number of subjects in each group. The routine transmission of *H. pylori* appears to be human-human whereas non-*H. pylori* helicobacter species are transmitted by cats, dogs, etc [22]. Consequently, the prevalence of *H. heilmannii* is expected to be significantly higher in environment with less hygiene and higher physical exposure to animals. However, in our study there was a negative association with pet contact as the patients reported limited exposure to these animals. There is a need to look into other modes of transmission of these infections.

Conclusion

As non *H. pylori* Helicobacter species are capable of producing complications similar to *H. pylori* so the identification of these species may be of importance in patients with dyspepsia. However, our study fails to show any increased risk of infection with these organisms on exposure to pet animals and any additional complications associated with co-infection in patients infected with *H. pylori*.

Methods
Study population
Between September 2009 and February 2011, a total of 250 patients with abdominal pain or discomfort who attended the gastroenterology outpatient clinic at a tertiary care hospital in Karachi were enrolled. The mean age of these patients was 39 ± 12 years, (range 18-75) with males 162(65%) and females 88(35%). Of these, 136 (54%) were in the age group of 18-39 years, 88(35%) in the group of 40-55 years and 26(10%) in the group of 56-75 years. Ethical approval for the study was obtained from the Aga Khan University Ethics Review Committee. Informed consent was taken for participation in the study. A complete socio-demographic questionnaire including determination of socio-economic status, educational level, ownership of the place of residence, number of rooms in the house, number of people living in the household beside siblings, source of water supply e.g. municipal water pipeline or bore water (ground water) and type of latrine in use, was obtained from the patients. A history of exposure of enrolled patients to cats and dogs was determined and a physical examination was carried out. Inclusion criteria were i) ambulatory adult

Table 3 Association of Helicobacter species with pets

	PCR for H. pylori			PCR for H. heilmannii			PCR for H. felis		
	Positive n = 142	Negative n = 108	P value	Positive n = 17	Negative n = 233	P value	Positive n = 10	Negative n = 240	P value
Pets									
Yes	42(30)	24(22)	0.19	1(6)	65(28)	0.05	2(20)	64(27)	1
No	100(70)	84(78)		16(94)	168(72)		8(80)	176(73)	

Univariate analysis was performed by using the independent sample t-test, Pearson Chi-square test or Fisher Exact test where appropriate. A P-value of < 0.05 was considered as statistically significant. *All the *H. heilmannii* and *H. felis* PCR positive patients were also positive for *H. pylori* PCR amplification.

males and non-pregnant females; ii) age 18 years or older; iii) patients with upper GI symptoms including abdominal/epigastric pain or discomfort, postprandial abdominal distension, postprandial nausea and vomiting. Exclusion criteria included i) receiving treatment for *H. pylori*, concurrent or recent antibiotic use such as metronidazole, clarithromycin, amoxicillin, tetracycline, doxycycline and other cephalosporin, ii) histamine-2 receptor blocker or proton pump inhibitor therapy and bismuth compounds in the last four weeks; iii) patients with regular use of NSAID; iii) patients with severe concomitant disease and iv) patients with upper GI surgery. A crowding index with three categories was constructed by dividing the number of individuals per household by the number of the rooms used as bedrooms [23]. A participant's household crowding was defined as 'low' if they scored an index of 0-1.0, moderately-crowded were '2-4' and > 4 were highly 'crowded'.

On EGD, 242(97%) were found to have endoscopic gastritis (GS) alone while 8(3%) had duodenal ulcer (DU). Biopsy specimens from the gastric corpus and antrum were taken for rapid urease test (RUT) or histopathology for the diagnosis of *H. pylori* and DNA extraction for polymerase chain reaction (PCR) to amplify *H. pylori*, *H. felis* and *H. heilmanii* genes. Ninety patients (36%) out of 250 had a RUT done while 160(64%) out of 250 had histology and provided gastric biopsy specimen for the detection of Helicobacter species.

Histopathology

Biopsy specimens were stained with hematoxylin and eosin. Sections were examined by an experienced gastrointestinal pathologist blinded to the clinical details of the patients and graded according to the updated Sydney classification [24]. The bacterial density was graded from 0 to 3 (0, absent or occasional; 1 to 3, from few and isolated bacteria to colonies). The infiltration of gastric mucosa by mononuclear cells and polymorphonuclear leucocytes, atrophy, and intestinal metaplasia were graded as follows: 0, none; 1, mild; 2, moderate; 3, marked. Chronic inflammation was defined according to an increase in lymphocytes and plasma cells in the lamina propria graded into mild, moderate or marked increase in density. Chronic active gastritis indicated chronic inflammation with neutrophilic polymorph infiltration of the lamina propria, pits or surface epithelium graded as 0 = nil, mild = < 1/3 of pits and surface infiltrated; moderate = 1/3-2/3; and marked = > 2/3. Gastritis was scored by total sum of grade of gastritis (mild = 1, moderate = 2, marked = 3 infiltration with lymphocytes and plasma cells) and activity of gastritis (mild = 1, moderate = 2, marked = 3 infiltration with neutrophilic granulocytes) either in the antrum or in the corpus. Atrophy was defined as the loss of glandular tissue, with or without replacement by intestinal-type epithelium. Criteria for a true positive result was established with positive RUT or histology and 16S rDNA amplification.

DNA Extraction

DNA was extracted from biopsy samples by using a QIAamp DNA mini kit from QIAGEN (Hilden, Germany) according to the manufacturer's protocol. Extracted DNA was stored at -70°C until required.

Polymerase chain reaction

PCR was performed using extracted DNA as the template to identify *H. pylori*, *H. heilmannii* and *H. felis*. Samples that were positive for Helicobacter genus 16S rDNA were subsequently analyzed with different sets of previously published primers (Table 4) which encode *H. pylori* phosphoglucosamine mutase (*glmM*), *H. heilmannii ureB* and *H. felis* internal fragment of the *ureA* and *ureB* genes, respectively [14,21,25,26]. PCR amplification was carried out in a total volume of 25 µl containing 2 µl of 2 mM dNTPs, 1 µl of 50 pmol of each forward and reverse primer used before [14,25-27]. (synthesized by

Table 4 Oligonucleotide primers used in this study to amplify Helicobacter spp. gene fragments

Gene	Sequence (5′ to 3′)	Amplicon size (bp)	Reference
Helicobacter 16S rRNA			
C97	GCT ATG ACG GGT ATC C	400	18
C 98	GAT TTT ACC CCT ACA CCA		
H. pylori glmM			
F	GGATAAGCTTTTAGGGGTGTTAGGGG	294	19
R	GCTTACTTTCTAACACTAACGCGC		
H. heilmannii ureB		580	14
F	GGGCGATAAAGTGCGCTTG		
R	CTGGTCAATGAGAGCAGG		
H. felis ure A and B		241	20
F	GTG AAG CGA CTA AAG ATA AAC AAT		
R	GCA CCAAAT CTA ATT CAT AAG AGC		

MWG Automatic synthesizer, Germany), 2.5 unit of Taq DNA polymerase (Promega, USA), 2.5 μl of 10 × PCR reaction buffer, 3 mM of $MgCl_2$, 2 μl of DNA template containing 0.5 ng of extracted DNA and total volume rounded to 25 μl by double distilled water. The reaction was carried out in a Perkin Elmer 9700 thermal cycler (Massachusetts, USA). The amplification cycles for the different Helicobacter spp. gene fragments were: 94°C for 5 min; 94°C for 1 min, 55°C-58°C for 1 min, 72°C for 60–90 sec (35 cycles); 72°C for 5-7 min. Positive and negative reagent control reactions were performed with each batch of amplifications. After PCR, the amplified PCR products were electrophoresed in 2% agarose gels containing 0.5 × Tris/acetate/ethylenediaminetetraacetic acid, stained with ethidium bromide, and visualized under a short wavelength ultraviolet light source. DNA from *H. pylori* strains ATCC 43504, *H. felis* ATCC 49179 and *H. heilmannii* JF804941.1 was used as a positive control and sterile deionized water as the negative control. Diagnosis of each of the *Helicobacter* species infection was established when Helicobacter genus PCR for 16S rDNA was positive along with a species specific PCR for *H. pylori*, *H. heilmannii* or *H. felis*. PCR product of *H. heilmannii* and *H. felis* were sequenced to further confirm individual infection. The specificity of *H. pylori* phosphoglucosamine mutase (*glmM*) and segment of urease B primers for *H. heilmannii* and *H. felis* has been demonstrated previously [14,21,25-27].

Sequencing of PCR product and BLAST Query

The DNA fragments amplified by *H. felis* and *H. heilmannii* PCRs were purified by Qiagen quick PCR purification kit (Qiagen, USA) and sequenced using both the forward and reverse primers (Table 4) to verify that they represented truly the *H. felis* and *H. heilmannii* ureB gene. Sequence analysis was performed by Macrogen (Seoul, South Korea). ClustalX was used to edit the sequences. The sequences were edited to a length of 488 bp for *H. heilmannii* and 210 bp for *H. felis*. Homology of the DNA sequences to published sequences was determined by using BLAST window on the National Center for Biotechnology Information (NCBI) site at http://www.ncbi.nlm.nih.gov/BLAST.

Nucleotide sequence accession numbers

The sequenced PCR products of *H. heilmannii* and *H. felis* obtained in this study have been deposited in GenBank under the following accession numbers: JF804941, JF804942, JF804943, JF804944, JF804945, JF815095, JF815096, JF815097 and JF815098. PCR product sequences were compared to the sequences of Urease B of *H. heilmannii* sequences GenBank: AF508012, L25079.1, AY139171.0, AY139171.1 and *H. felis* strains ref GenBank: FQ 6701792, AY368267.1 and AY368261.1.

Statistical Method

Using software EPI Info and using 10% prevalence in the study population [21] with 95% confidence level and a bound on error of ± 4% the estimated sample size was 217.

Results are expressed as mean ± standard deviation for continuous variables (e.g., age) and number (percentage) for categorical data (e.g., gender, etc.). Univariate analysis was performed by using the independent sample t-test, Pearson Chi-square test and Fisher Exact test whenever appropriate. A *P*-value of < 0.05 was considered as statistically significant. All p-value were two sided. Statistical interpretation of data was performed by using the computerized software program SPSS version 19.

Acknowledgements

This study was supported by the Higher Educational Commission Grant Ref: 20-1128/R&D/09 to JY. We are grateful to laboratory stuff at the Juma Building at the Aga Khan University for their help during the conduct of this work.

Author details

[1]Department of Medicine, The Aga Khan University, Karachi, Pakistan.
[2]Department of Pathology, The Aga Khan University, Karachi, Pakistan.
[3]Department of Community Health Sciences, The Aga Khan University, Karachi, Pakistan.

Authors' contributions

JY conceived and designed the study, JY, ZAB, RK, WJ coordinated the study, JY, SN, FJ did the work, JY and ZA analyzed the data, ZAH analyzed the histopathology, JY, MI, SA performed the statistical analysis. JY wrote the manuscript. All authors read and approved the final manuscript.

Competing interests

The authors declare that they have no competing interests.

References

1. Fennerty M: *Helicobacter pylori*: why it still matters in 2005. *Clevel Clin J Med* 2005, **72**(Suppl II):S1-S7.
2. Fox J: The non-*H. pylori*: their expanding role in gastrointestinal and systemic diseases. *Gut* 2002, **50**:273-283.
3. Blanchard T, Eisenberg J, Matsumoto Y: Clearance of *Helicobacter pylori* infection through immunization: the site of T cell activation contributes to vaccine efficacy. *Vaccine* 2004, **22**:888-897.
4. Jafri W, Yakoob J, Abid S, Siddiqui S, Awan S, Nizami SQ: *Helicobacter pylori* infection in children: population-based age-specific prevalence and risk factors in a developing country. *Acta Paediatr* 2010, **99**:279-282.
5. Heilmannii KL, Borchard F: Gastritis due to spiral shaped bacteria other than *Helicobacter pylori*: clinical, histological, and ultrastructural findings. *Gut* 1991, **32**:137-140.
6. Debongnie JC, Donnay M, Mairesse J: *Gastrospirillum hominis* (*Helicobacter heilmanii*): a cause of gastritis, sometimes transient, better diagnosed by touch cytology? *Am J Gastroenterol* 1995, **90**:411-416.
7. Bunn J, MacKay W, Thomas J, Reid D, Weaver L: Detection of *Helicobacter pylori* DNA in drinking water biofilms: implications for transmission in early life. *Lett Appl Microbiol* 2002, **34**:450-454.
8. Paster BJ, Lee A, Fox JG, Dewhirst FE, Tordoff LA, Fraser GJ, O'Rourke JL, Taylor NS, Ferrero R: Phylogeny of *Helicobacter felis* sp. nov, *Helicobacter mustelae* and related bacteria. *Int J Syst Bacteriol* 1991, **41**:31-38.
9. Lee A, Hazell SL, O'Rourke J, Kouprach S: Isolation of a spiral-shaped bacterium from the cat stomach. *Infect Immun* 1988, **56**:2843-2850.

10. Haesebrouck F, Pasmans F, Flahou B, Chiers K, Baele M, Meyns T, Decostere A, Ducatelle R: Gastric helicobacters in domestic animals and nonhuman primates and their significance for human health. *Clin Microbiol Rev* 2009, **22**:202-223.

11. O'Rourke JL, Solnick JV, Neilan BA, Seidel K, Hayter R, Hansen LM, Lee A: Description of "*Candidatus Helicobacter heilmannii*" based on DNA sequence analysis of 16S rRNA and urease genes. *Int J Syst Evol Microbiol* 2004, **54**:2203-2211.

12. Smet A, Flahou B, D'Herde K, Vandamme P, Cleenwerck I, Ducatelle R, Pasmans F, Haesebrouck F: *Helicobacter heilmannii* sp. nov., isolated from feline gastric mucosa. *Int J Syst Evol Microbiol* 2011, [doi: 0.1099/ijs.0.029207-0].

13. Kivisto R, Linros J, Rossi M, Rautelin H, Hanninen M-L: Characterization of multiple *Helicobacter bizzozeronii* isolates from a Finnish patient with severe dyspeptic symptoms and chronic active gastritis. *Helicobacter* 2010, **15**:58-66.

14. Neiger R, Dieterich C, Burnens A, Waldvogel A, Corthésy-Theulaz I, Halter F, Lauterburg B, Schmassmann A: Detection and prevalence of *Helicobacter* infection in pet cats. *J Clin Microbiol* 1998, **36**:634-637.

15. van den Bulck K, Decostere A, Baele M, Baele M, Driessen A, Debongnie JC, Burette A, Stolte M, Ducatelle R, Haesebrouck F: Identification of non-*Helicobacter pylori* spiral organisms in gastric samples from humans, dogs, and cats. *J Clin Microbiol* 2005, **43**:2256-2260.

16. Chisholm SA, Owen RJ: Development and application of a novel screening PCR assay for direct detection of '*Helicobacter heilmannii*'-like organisms in human gastric biopsies in Southeast England. *Diagn Microbiol Infect Dis* 2003, **46**:1-7.

17. Trebesius K, Adler K, Vieth M, Stolte M, Haas R: Specific detection and prevalence of *Helicobacter heilmannii*-like organisms in the human gastric mucosa by fluorescent in situ hybridization and partial 16S ribosomal DNA sequencing. *J Clin Microbiol* 2001, **39**:1510-1516.

18. Stolte M, Wellens E, Bethke B, Ritter M, Eidt H: *Helicobacter heilmannii* (formerly *Gastrospirillum hominis*) gastritis: an infection transmitted by animals? *Scand J Gastroenterol* 1994, **29**:1061-1064.

19. Sykora J, Hejda V, Varvarovska J, Stozicky F, Gottrand F, Siala K: *Helicobacter heilmannii*-related gastric ulcer in childhood. *J Pediatr Gastroenterol Nutr* 2003, **36**:410-413.

20. Dieterich C, Wiesel P, Neiger R, Blum A, Corthésy-Theulaz I: Presence of multiple "*Helicobacter heilmannii*" strains in an individual suffering from ulcers and in his two cats. *J Clin Microbiol* 1998, **36**:1366-1370.

21. Fritz EL, Slavik T, Delport W, Olivier B, van der Merwe SW: Incidence of Helicobacter felis and the effect of coinfection with *Helicobacter pylori* on the gastric mucosa in the African population. *J Clin Microbiol* 2006, **44**:1692-1696.

22. Meining A, Kroher G, Stolte M: Animal reservoirs in the transmission of *Helicobacter heilmannii*. Results of a questionnaire based study. *Scand J Gastroenterology* 1998, **33**:795-798.

23. Conde-Glez CJ, Juárez-Figueroa L, Uribe-Salas F, Hernández-Nevárez P, Schmid S, Calderón E, Hernández-Avila M: Analysis of *Herpes simplex* virus 1 and 2 Infection in women with high risk sexual behavior in Mexico. *Int J Epidemiol* 1999, **8**:571-576.

24. Dixon M, Genta R, Yardley J, Correa P: Classification and grading of gastritis-the updated Sydney system. *Am J Surg Pathol* 1996, **20**:1161-1181.

25. Fox JG, Dewhirst FE, Shen Z, Feng Y, Taylor NS, Paster BJ, Ericson RL, Lau CN, Correa P, Araya JC, Roa I: Helicobacter species identified in bile and gallbladder tissue from Chileans with chronic cholecystitis. *Gastroenterology* 1998, **114**:755-763.

26. Lu JJ, Perng CL, Shyu RY, Chen CH, Lou Q, Chong SK, Lee CH: Comparison of five PCR methods for detection of *Helicobacter pylori* DNA in gastric tissue. *J Clin Microbiol* 1999, **37**:772-774.

27. Germani Y, Dauga C, Duval P, Huerre M, Levy M, Pialoux G, Sansonetti P, Grimont P: Strategy for the detection of Helicobacter species by amplification of 16S rRNA genes and identification of *H. felis* in a human gastric biopsy. *Res Microbiol* 1997, **148**:315-326.

21

DPO multiplex PCR as an alternative to culture and susceptibility testing to detect *Helicobacter pylori* and its resistance to clarithromycin

Philippe Lehours[1,2,3], Elodie Siffré[1] and Francis Mégraud [1,2,3]*

Abstract

Background: Macrolide resistance in *Helicobacter pylori* is the major risk factor for treatment failure when using a proton pump inhibitor-clarithromycin containing therapy. Macrolide resistance is due to a few mutations on the 23S ribomosal subunit encoded by the 23S rRNA gene. The present study aimed at investigating the performance of the dual priming oligonucleotide (DPO)-PCR kit named Seeplex® ClaR-*H. pylori* ACE detection designed to detect *H. pylori* and two types of point mutations causing clarithromycin resistance in *H. pylori*.

Methods: The performance of Seeplex® ClaR-*H. pylori* ACE detection was evaluated on 127 gastric biopsies in comparison to conventional bacterial culture followed by the determination of susceptibility to clarithromycin by E-test, as well as by an in-house real-time PCR using a fluorescence resonance energy transfer (FRET) technology.

Results: Considering culture as the reference test, the sensitivity of DPO-PCR and real-time FRET-PCR was 97.7% and 100% while specificity was 83.1% and 80.7%, respectively. However, both PCR were concordant in detecting 14 *H. pylori* positive cases which were negative by culture. Globally, E-test and DPO-PCR were concordant with regard to clarithromycin susceptibility in 95.3% of the cases (41/43), while real-time FRET-PCR and DPO-PCR were concordant in 95% (57/60).

Conclusion: The DPO-PCR is an interesting tool to detect *H. pylori* on gastric biopsies and to study its susceptibility to clarithromycin in laboratories that cannot perform real-time PCR assays.

Background

Macrolide resistance in *Helicobacter pylori* is the major risk factor for treatment failure when using a proton pump inhibitor (PPI)-clarithromycin containing therapy [1]. Macrolide resistance is due to a few mutations on the 23S ribomosal subunit encoded by the 23S rRNA gene [2,3]. These mutations (A2142C, A2142G, A2143G), are easy to detect by numerous molecular methods directly on gastric biopsy specimens and even on stool samples [4-7].

A new PCR format named DPO-PCR for "Dual Priming Oligonucleotide" was recently developed [8]. DPO-PCR is a multiplex PCR assay that increases specificity and sensitivity of detection compared to conventional PCR, by blocking non-specific binding sites therefore eliminating imperfect primer annealing. This new technology can be used for many applications in the field of *in vitro* diagnostics: simultaneous detection of multiple pathogens and of polymorphisms (SNPs), as well as simultaneous genotyping of multiple pathogen subtypes. DPO-PCR is based on a multiplex PCR using a DPO patented technology [8]. The structure of the DPO primers is fundamentally different from that of conventional primers. Indeed, the primer is divided into two parts by a 5 polydeoxyinosine linker which allows a more specific hybridization at temperatures between 55 and 65°C. This linker forms a "bubble-like structure" which itself is not involved in priming, rather it delineates the boundary between two parts. It therefore generates two recognition reactions of the primer on the target sequence. According to the manufacturer (see http://www.seegene.com/en/research/core_020.php), the 5' end (approximately 20 bases) binds preferentially to the matrix and initiates stable annealing acting as a "stabilizer". The 3' end is

* Correspondence: francis.megraud@chu-bordeaux.fr
[1]Université de Bordeaux, Centre National de Référence des Campylobacters et des Hélicobacters, 146 rue Léo Saignat, 33000 Bordeaux, France
Full list of author information is available at the end of the article

shorter (approximately 10 bases) and binds afterwards to the target site but only if the first step has taken place without a mismatch. The 3' end determines a target-specific extension and acts as a "determiner". Therefore, although the longer 5'-segment binds to a non-target site, the shorter segment resists non-specific extension. The short 3'-portion alone fails to make a priming at an annealing temperature. The latter also binds preferentially to the target and avoids non-specific binding. This PCR can be performed in any conventional thermocycler.

The performance of this PCR format for the detection of *H. pylori* 23S rDNA mutations, involved in macrolide resistance was previously evaluated in a study published in 2007 by Woo et al., [9] with a 94.1% concordance between the DPO-based multiplex PCR and culture followed by a phenotypic susceptibility test.

In an article by Cho AR and Lee MK in Korean language, they also compared this method to culture and histology, and concluded that it could be used for the diagnosis of *H. pylori* infection and the determination of clarithromycin resistance [10]. However, they used a disk diffusion method which is not a generally accepted technique for testing *H. pylori* antimicrobial susceptibility. The present study is a retrospective study performed by the National Reference Centre for Helicobacters in France which aimed at investigating the performance of the Seeplex® ClaR-*H. pylori* ACE detection kit (Seegene, Seoul, Korea) in comparison to standard phenotypic tests as well as the real-time fluorescence resonance energy transfer (FRET)-PCR developed and routinely used in our laboratory [7].

Methods
Materials
The Seeplex® ClaR-*H. pylori* ACE detection kit was evaluated retrospectively on DNAs extracted from 127 gastric biopsies received at the French National Reference Centre for Helicobacters (Bordeaux, France) during the year 2009. There was no preselection according to the gastric site. Consecutive biopsies were included until about half of the number of biopsies positive for *H. pylori* was attained.

Methods
The performance of the kit was compared to conventional bacterial culture followed by the determination of susceptibility to clarithromycin by E-test, and an in-house real-time PCR detection using the FRET technology [7].

Culture
H. pylori strains were obtained from the corresponding gastric biopsies, after culture on Wilkins-Chalgren agar plates (Oxoid, Dardilly, France) supplemented with human blood (10% v/v) and antibiotics (10 µg/ml of vancomycin, 10 µg/ml of cefsulodin, 5 µg/ml of trimethoprim, and 10 µg/ml of amphotericin B) under microaerobic conditions, as already described [11,12]. Forty-four culture positive cases were finally included.

Phenotypic susceptibility testing
Susceptibility to clarithromycin was assessed using the E-test method (bioMérieux, Marcy l'Etoile, France) performed as previously described [6] and using the EUCAST breakpoints: S ≤ 0.25 µg/ml; R > 0.5 µg/ml (http://www.eucast.org/clinical_breakpoints/).

DNA extraction from gastric biopsies
Genomic DNA from gastric biopsies was extracted by using the MagnaPure LC DNA Isolation Kit I and the MagnaPure LC Isolation Station (Roche Applied Science, Penzberg, Germany). DNAs were stored at -20°C until required for analysis.

Real-time FRET-PCR
The real-time FRET-PCR is designed to detect clarithromycin susceptible *H. pylori* (wild type) and the mutations responsible for clarithromycin resistance: A4142G and A2143G, without distinguishing between them, as well as A2142C. This test was performed as previously described [7].

DPO-PCR
DPO-PCR was performed using the Seeplex® ClaR-*H. pylori* ACE detection kit according to the manufacturer's recommendations (Seegene distributed by Eurobio Laboratoires, Courtaboeuf, France) and analyzed using a semi-automated system called Screen tape® allowing an ultra rapid migration and analysis of the PCR products in small polyacrylamide gels. 8-methoxysporalen was added during the mix preparation to intercalate between double-stranded nucleic acids generated during amplification, thereby limiting carry-over contamination after UV irradiation and before PCR product analysis. The Seeplex® ClaR-*H. pylori* ACE detection kit includes 3 primer pairs with a DPO structure which allows amplification of the *H. pylori* 23S rDNA (621 bp amplicon) and detection of A2142G and A2143G mutations (194 bp and 475 bp, respectively). The kit also includes a primer pair for internal control.

DPO-PCR is a multiplex PCR that can be performed in any standard thermocycler.

Histology
Briefly, histological preparations were stained with hematoxylin and eosin and Giemsa stains and the presence of *H. pylori* was evaluated according to the Sydney system. Histological results were used only in case of discrepant results obtained between DPO-PCR and FRET-PCR.

Evaluation of Sensitivity and Specificity

The proportion of positives by DPO-PCR among the true positives defined the sensitivity and the proportion of negatives by DPO-PCR among the true negatives defined the specificity.

Results

Concerning the 127 biopsies included in the study, culture was positive for *H. pylori* in 44 cases (34.6%), the real-time FRET-PCR in 60 cases (47.2%), and the DPO-PCR in 57 cases (44.9%). *H. pylori* status obtained from histological diagnosis was available for only 89 patients.

For the 44 biopsies positive by culture, the real-time FRET-PCR and DPO-PCR were also positive, except in one case where DPO-PCR was solely negative. For 67 biopsies, culture, FRET-PCR and DPO-PCR were all negative. Out of 16 biopsies negative by culture, FRET-PCR, DPO-PCR and histology were all positive for 14. For the remaining 2 biopsies, real-time FRET-PCR was solely positive (Tables 1 and 2) and histology confirmed the presence of *H. pylori*.

Using culture as the reference test, the sensitivity of DPO-PCR and real-time FRET PCR was 97.7% and 100%, respectively, and the specificity was 83.1% and 80.7%, respectively.

The concordance between real-time FRET-PCR and DPO-PCR in our study was 95% (57/60) (Table 2). Considering the 44 *H. pylori* strains isolated by culture, clarithromycin susceptibility results were available for 43 (one strain being lost after subculture). Table 2 summarizes the results obtained by the three methods used for determining macrolide susceptibility. For the 17 clarithromycin susceptible isolates, 15 corresponding biopsies contained a wild type isolate in both PCR formats. One biopsy was categorized as wild type by FRET-PCR and as an A2143G mutant by DPO-PCR. The remaining biopsy was considered to be a mixture of wild type and A2142G/A2143G mutant by FRET-PCR whereas DPO-PCR detected an A2143G mutation.

For the 26 macrolide resistant isolates, a 23S rDNA mutation was detected in 25 biopsies by both PCR formats. One biopsy was considered as a wild type by real-time FRET-PCR but was negative by DPO-PCR (histology was also negative).

Globally, E-test and DPO-PCR were concordant in 95.3% of these cases (41/43).

Discussion

We found a good correlation for the detection of *H. pylori* and the detection of clarithromycin susceptibility between the DPO-PCR and the real-time FRET-PCR routinely used in our Reference Centre. Overall, the performance is very good for a non-real-time PCR format. Compared to other PCR formats developed to detect mutations involved in macrolide resistance for *H. pylori*, DPO-PCR requires no investment in additional technical or expensive detection devices. One disadvantage is that users must run the detection of PCR fragments themselves on a 2% agarose gel before analyzing the PCR bands obtained, compared to real-time PCR formats available to date where PCR amplification is monitored automatically. DPO-PCR is therefore more time-consuming. However, in our study the semi-automated system called ScreenTape® was used. ScreenTape® simplifies the analysis of the results of this multiplex PCR assay.

The cost of the test is highly dependent on the activity and equipment of the laboratory in which the test is performed; however, it is significantly higher than the cost of the in-house method tested in parallel in the present study.

DPO-PCR detected more *H. pylori* positive biopsies than culture alone, with an excellent correlation with the FRET-PCR. Woo et al., identified 49 *H. pylori* positive samples among 165 culture-negative specimens using DPO-PCR [9]. This result leads us to believe that there is no specificity problem regarding DPO-PCR, rather a problem of sensitivity regarding culture.

The excellent correlation between DPO-PCR and E-test susceptibility is in line with the previous study published by Woo et al., where they found a 94.1% concordance between both methods [9]. In the work of Woo et al., two strains categorized as susceptible by E-test appeared resistant by DPO-PCR. Cho et al., also described that the results of PCR and E-test on 3 of the 8 mutation-positive biopsies were discrepant [10]. In the present study, DPO-PCR detected resistances missed by E-test also in two cases (Table 2). This could be explained by the detection

Table 1 Global results obtained for different diagnosis tests for the detection of *Helicobacter pylori* in human gastric biopsies

Culture (n = 44)	FRET-PCR (n = 60)	DPO-PCR (n = 57)	Total (n = 127)
(+)	(+)	(+)	43
(+)	(+)	(-)	1
(-)	(-)	(-)	67
(-)	(+)	(+)	14
(-)	(+)	(-)	2

The numbers indicated in parentheses represent the total number of positive samples for each test.

Table 2 Comparison of *Helicobacter pylori* susceptibility to clarithromycin by E-test, real-time FRET-PCR and DPO-PCR on human gastric biopsies

E-test	FRET-PCR	DPO-PCR	Total (n = 60)
R	R*	R[§]	25
WT	WT	WT	15
WT	R[μ]	R	1
WT	WT	R	1
R	WT	NEG	1
ND	R	R	4
ND	WT	WT	11
ND	WT	NEG	2[§]

R: macrolide resistant strain; WT: wild type (macrolide susceptible strain); NEG: negative result; ND: not determined.

* 3 biopsies with a mixture of a wild type and A2142G/A2143G mutants.

μ 1 biopsy with a mixture of a wild type and A2142G/A2143G mutants.

§ 1 double population A2142G + A2143G.

§ positive histology.

limit of the Seeplex® ClaR-*H. pylori* ACE detection kit which is 100 copies/reaction (100 copies/3 μl DNA). According to Woo HY et al., DPO-PCR can detect mutants present among wild-type strains at a level as low as 2% and more than 100 copies/20 μl [9]. For such a low proportion, the E-test method missed a resistant strain.

The Seeplex® ClaR-*H. pylori* ACE detection kit does not allow detection of the A2142C mutation. However, this mutation is less common (usually <5% of resistant isolates) [7,5].

As indicated in the Materials and Methods, the Seeplex® ClaR-*H. pylori* ACE detection kit includes 3 primer pairs with a DPO structure which allows amplification of the *H. pylori* 23S rDNA (621 bp amplicon) and detection of the A2142G and A2143G mutations (194 bp and 475 bp, respectively). The first primer pair is designed to hybridize regardless of the presence of any mutation inside the PCR fragments. In the case of the A2142G mutation, its specific primer hybridizes and generates a 194 bp PCR product with the reverse *H. pylori* 23S rDNA primer. In the case of the A2143G mutation, its specific primer hybridizes and forms a 475 bp PCR product with the forward *H. pylori* 23S rDNA primer. Therefore, it is not possible to distinguish between 1) gastric biopsies containing a mixture of a wild-type strain and a mutated strain and 2) biopsies containing only a mutated strain (the 621 bp band corresponding to amplification of *H. pylori* 23S rDNA is almost always present). It has no practical consequences because the detection of a resistant population is sufficient to exclude macrolides from the eradication therapy to be implemented.

Moreover, for 22 biopsies where A2143G was detected by DPO-PCR, the corresponding 475 bp amplicon was alone in only 4 cases which means that for these corresponding DNAs the reverse *H. pylori* 23S rDNA apparently failed to hybridize and to generate the additional 621 bp amplicon. We believe that this is the reason why, in some rare cases, false negatives by DPO-PCR can occur (a total of 3 in the present study). The primer pairs which allow the amplification of the *H. pylori* 23S rDNA could be slightly modified to avoid this problem.

Conclusion

Users should keep in mind that whenever possible *H. pylori* culture should be performed, and only in cases where standard microbiology fails, the use of molecular methods are really indicated. The rationale behind this is that not only clarithromycin resistance is of interest but also that of other antimicrobials like tetracycline, quinolones, rifamycins and metronidazole. However, the Seeplex® ClaR-*H. pylori* ACE detection kit is an excellent molecular test to detect *H. pylori* in gastric biopsies and to study its sensitivity to clarithromycin, especially in laboratories without expertise in culturing this bacterium and without a real-time PCR apparatus. At a time when clarithromycin resistance is increasing (prevalence is >20% in many countries), clinical laboratories could be enticed by this new PCR format.

Acknowledgements

The authors thank Leila Labadi and Salha Ben Amor (Université de Bordeaux, Centre National de Référence des Campylobacters et des Hélicobacters, Bordeaux, France) for technical assistance.

Author details

[1]Université de Bordeaux, Centre National de Référence des Campylobacters et des Hélicobacters, 146 rue Léo Saignat, 33000 Bordeaux, France. [2]CHU de Bordeaux, Hôpital Pellegrin, Laboratoire de Bactériologie, Place Amélie Raba Léon, 33076 Bordeaux cedex, France. [3]INSERM U853, 33000 Bordeaux, France.

Authors' contributions

PL and FM analyzed the data and wrote the paper. ES performed the research.
All authors read and approved the final manuscript.

Competing interests

The authors declare that they have no competing interests.

References

1. Malfertheiner P, Megraud F, O'Morain C, Bazzoli F, El-Omar E, Graham D, Hunt R, Rokkas T, Vakil N, Kuipers EJ: **Current concepts in the management of Helicobacter pylori infection: the Maastricht III Consensus Report.** *Gut* 2007, **56(6)**:772-781.
2. Occhialini A, Urdaci M, Doucet-Populaire F, Bebear CM, Lamouliatte H, Megraud F: **Macrolide resistance in Helicobacter pylori: rapid detection of point mutations and assays of macrolide binding to ribosomes.** *Antimicrob Agents Chemother* 1997, **41(12)**:2724-2728.
3. Menard A, Santos A, Megraud F, Oleastro M: **PCR-restriction fragment length polymorphism can also detect point mutation A2142C in the 23S rRNA gene, associated with Helicobacter pylori resistance to clarithromycin.** *Antimicrob Agents Chemother* 2002, **46(4)**:1156-1157.

4. Agudo S, Alarcon T, Urruzuno P, Martinez MJ, Lopez-Brea M: **Detection of** *Helicobacter pylori* **and clarithromycin resistance in gastric biopsies of pediatric patients by using a commercially available real-time polymerase chain reaction after NucliSens semiautomated DNA extraction.** *Diagn Microbiol Infect Dis* 2010, **67**(3):213-219.

5. Burucoa C, Garnier M, Silvain C, Fauchere JL: **Quadruplex real-time PCR assay using allele-specific scorpion primers for detection of mutations conferring clarithromycin resistance to** *Helicobacter pylori*. *J Clin Microbiol* 2008, **46**(7):2320-2326.

6. Cambau E, Allerheiligen V, Coulon C, Corbel C, Lascols C, Deforges L, Soussy CJ, Delchier JC, Megraud F: **Evaluation of a new test, genotype HelicoDR, for molecular detection of antibiotic resistance in** *Helicobacter pylori*. *J Clin Microbiol* 2009, **47**(11):3600-3607.

7. Oleastro M, Menard A, Santos A, Lamouliatte H, Monteiro L, Barthelemy P, Megraud F: **Real-time PCR assay for rapid and accurate detection of point mutations conferring resistance to clarithromycin in** *Helicobacter pylori*. *J Clin Microbiol* 2003, **41**(1):397-402.

8. Chun JY, Kim KJ, Hwang IT, Kim YJ, Lee DH, Lee IK, Kim JK: **Dual priming oligonucleotide system for the multiplex detection of respiratory viruses and SNP genotyping of CYP2C19 gene.** *Nucleic Acids Res* 2007, **35**(6):e40.

9. Woo HY, Park DI, Park H, Kim MK, Kim DH, Kim IS, Kim YJ: **Dual-priming oligonucleotide-based multiplex PCR for the detection of** *Helicobacter pylori* **and determination of clarithromycin resistance with gastric biopsy specimens.** *Helicobacter* 2009, **14**(1):22-28.

10. Cho AR, Lee MK: **[A comparison analysis on the diagnosis of** *Helicobacter pylori* **infection and the detection of clarithromycin resistance according to biopsy sites].** *Korean J Lab Med* 2010, **30**(4):381-387.

11. Megraud F: **A growing demand for** *Helicobacter pylori* **culture in the near future?** *Ital J Gastroenterol Hepatol* 1997, **29**(6):574-576.

12. Megraud F, Lehours P: *Helicobacter pylori* **detection and antimicrobial susceptibility testing.** *Clin Microbiol Rev* 2007, **20**(2):280-322.

The effect of *H. pylori* eradication on meal-associated changes in plasma ghrelin and leptin

Fritz Francois[1,2*], Jatin Roper[1], Neal Joseph[1], Zhiheng Pei[1,2], Aditi Chhada[1], Joshua R Shak[1], Asalia Z Olivares de Perez[1], Guillermo I Perez-Perez[1] and Martin J Blaser[1,2]

Abstract

Background: Appetite and energy expenditure are regulated in part by ghrelin and leptin produced in the gastric mucosa, which may be modified by *H. pylori* colonization. We prospectively evaluated the effect of *H. pylori* eradication on meal-associated changes in serum ghrelin and leptin levels, and body weight.

Methods: Veterans referred for upper GI endoscopy were evaluated at baseline and ≥8 weeks after endoscopy, and *H. pylori* status and body weight were ascertained. During the first visit in all subjects, and during subsequent visits in the initially *H. pylori*-positive subjects and controls, blood was collected after an overnight fast and 1 h after a standard high protein meal, and levels of eight hormones determined.

Results: Of 92 enrolled subjects, 38 were *H. pylori*-negative, 44 *H. pylori*-positive, and 10 were indeterminate. Among 23 *H. pylori*-positive subjects who completed evaluation after treatment, 21 were eradicated, and 2 failed eradication. After a median of seven months following eradication, six hormones related to energy homeostasis showed no significant differences, but post-prandial acylated ghrelin levels were nearly six-fold higher than pre-eradication (p = 0.005), and median integrated leptin levels also increased (20%) significantly (p < 0.001). BMI significantly increased (5 ± 2%; p = 0.008) over 18 months in the initially *H. pylori*-positive individuals, but was not significantly changed in those who were *H. pylori*-negative or indeterminant at baseline.

Conclusions: Circulating meal-associated leptin and ghrelin levels and BMI changed significantly after *H. pylori* eradication, providing direct evidence that *H. pylori* colonization is involved in ghrelin and leptin regulation, with consequent effects on body morphometry.

Background

The healthful regulation of energy homeostasis in humans, depends on centrally-acting hormones such as ghrelin and leptin [1,2]. Serum ghrelin concentrations increase during fasting, and decrease after eating [3]; ghrelin decreases energy expenditure and promotes weight gain [4]. In contrast, leptin produced primarily by adipocytes, reduces appetite and increases energy utilization [5]. The gastric epithelium expresses both ghrelin and leptin (and their receptors) [6,7]; inflammation can modify their production [8,9].

Helicobacter pylori, which colonizes the human stomach and interacts with host tissues [10] may affect the regulation of ghrelin and leptin [9]. However, ghrelin and leptin expression in *H. pylori*-colonized hosts has been reported as reduced [11], or increased. Similarly, body mass index (BMI) has been reported to be increased [12] or reduced [13] following *H. pylori* eradication.

We hypothesized that gastric *H. pylori* colonization affects the physiologic regulation of gut hormones involved in food intake, energy expenditure, and body weight maintenance. The hormones that affect overall metabolic function include ghrelin, leptin, amylin, insulin, active glucagon-like peptide-1, gastric inhibitory polypeptide, peptide YY, and pancreatic polypeptide. We used clinically indicated *H. pylori* eradication to evaluate the effect of *H. pylori* on meal-associated changes in ghrelin, leptin, and the other specified insulinotropic and digestive hormones, and to assess post-eradication changes in body mass index.

* Correspondence: Fritz.francois@med.nyu.edu
[1]New York University Langone Medical Center, New York, NY, USA
Full list of author information is available at the end of the article

Methods

Study population

Adults $\geq$ 18 years of age undergoing routine upper endoscopy for any indication at the ambulatory endoscopy unit at the New York campus of the VA New York Harbor Healthcare System were prospectively recruited, as described [9,14]. The Institutional Review Board approved the study protocol, and written informed consent was obtained from all participants.

Clinical evaluation and specimen collection

Each patient had a history and physical examination, and fasted for 12-hours overnight prior to the endoscopy. Demographic and clinical information, including assessment of dyspeptic symptoms (Additional file 1), was collected via a standardized questionnaire administered by trained interviewers at the time of study entry. Ethnic designation was self-reported by participants as White Non-Hispanic, Black Non-Hispanic, Hispanic, or Asian. Participants wore light clothing without shoes; height and weight were measured using the same column scale with a telescopic height rod, and BMI calculated. Between 8 am and 10 am, 15 ml of blood was collected in EDTA-coated tubes from the fasting patients prior to endoscopy. All samples were centrifuged, and stored as serum at -20 C, until examined.

Endoscopy

Complete endoscopic evaluation of the upper gastrointestinal tract was performed in standard fashion to the 2nd portion of the duodenum, after intravenous administration of meperidine and midazolam, as described [14]. Gastric inflammation was graded using the Sydney-Houston system [15]. Using standard forceps, two biopsies each were obtained from the gastric antrum, body, and fundus in accordance with the updated Sydney classification; two additional antral biopsies were used for rapid urease testing.

Histological analysis

One biopsy specimen from each of the three sites was fixed in 10% formalin, embedded in paraffin, and 5 μm consecutive sections obtained for histologic staining. A single experienced GI pathologist (Z.P.) blinded to the data, graded the extent of gastritis and intestinal metaplasia on a scale of 0 to 3+ according to the Sydney classification [16]. Active gastritis refers to the presence of neutrophils in the histopathology, and chronic active reflects both neutrophils and mononuclear cells. For active gastritis, total score < 2 was defined as "low" while $\geq$ 2 was defined as "high". H. pylori was detected using the cresyl violet stain for the identification of spiral or curved-shaped organisms near the mucous layer [17].

H. pylori status determination

Along with histologic evaluation and the rapid urease assays, H. pylori was assessed using one other tissue-based method (bacteriologic culture, as described) [18], and by two serologic methods. Serum samples were examined by ELISA for IgG antibodies to H. pylori whole cell and CagA antigens, with results expressed as OD ratios relative to laboratory standards, as described [19,20]. Subjects were considered H. pylori-positive if positive by histologic examination or culture, or if positive by rapid urease assay, and by IgG antibodies to H. pylori group or CagA antigens. Subjects were considered indeterminate for H. pylori if only the rapid urease test or one serological test was positive, consistent with prior studies [9].

Test meal

Following recovery from endoscopy-related sedation, all patients ate a high-protein non-commercial meal averaging 806 calories. The contents of the meal were selected with the guidance of a trained nutritionist to provide 72 g carbohydrate, 71 g protein, and 26 g fat. Given that the trough that occurs in serum ghrelin levels occurs one hour postprandially [3], 15 ml of blood was collected one hour after completing the meal, and processed as above.

H. pylori eradication therapy

Patients who tested positive for H. pylori were offered a 14-day twice-daily regimen [amoxicillin 1000 mg, clarithromycin 500 mg, and a proton pump inhibitor (PPI; omeprazole 20 mg, rabeprazole or esomeprazole 40 mg)] [21]. Seven patients who had two positive serologic tests were treated to eradicate H. pylori after further confirmation with the 13C Urea Breath Test while off antisecretory medications. One penicillin-allergic patient received metronidazole [500 mg twice a day] instead of amoxicillin. In accordance with current guidelines [22], H. pylori eradication was ascertained using the 13C Urea Breath Test, according to the manufacturer's instructions (Meretek Diagnostics, Rockville, MD) $\geq$8 weeks after treatment ended. At that time blood (15 ml) was again collected after fasting and 1 hour after a standardized meal. Patients who failed eradication were treated for 14 days with bismuth subsalicylate (525 mg four times a day), combined with a twice daily regimen [tetracycline (500 mg), metronidazole (500 mg), and PPI] [21]. The 13C Urea Breath Test was repeated in all patients who completed rescue therapy. If not clinically indicated, antisecretory medications were not continued beyond the treatment period necessary for eradication.

Metabolic tests

A multi-hormone EIA panel (Catalogue HGT-68K; Millipore Corp., Billerica MA) was used to quantify eight gut hormones that are important regulators of food intake [1,3,23], energy expenditure [24], and body weight [25] via the gut-brain axis: acylated (active) ghrelin, leptin, active amylin, insulin, active glucagon-like peptide-1 (GLP-1), total gastric inhibitory polypeptide (GIP), total peptide YY (PYY), and pancreatic polypeptide (PP). We have previously reported a significant correlation between this assay and a standard enzyme linked immunoassay (EIA) for leptin (r = 0.57, p = 0.004). Similarly, we have found the correlation with a standard ghrelin EIA to be significant [r = 0.37; p = 0.018 (data not shown)]. The intra- and inter-assay variabilities ranged between 11% and 19%, respectively, according to the manufacturer, and for the ghrelin assay no cross reactivity exists with desacyl ghrelin. All tests were performed in duplicate on coded samples.

Statistical analysis

Continuous variables were compared using the t-test, or ANOVA method, and pair-wise analyses (e.g. pre-meal vs. post-meal, baseline vs. eradicated) were performed using non-parametric tests (Wilcoxon's signed rank test, Mann-Whitney U test), as appropriate. Data are expressed as mean ± SD, or median and interquartile range (25th- 75th percentile). Categorical variables were compared using the Chi-squared test with Yates' correction or using Fisher's exact test. Spearman correlation coefficients were calculated for the relationship of leptin and ghrelin to BMI. Corrections were made in instances of multiple comparisons using techniques such as Tukey's range test. Based on previous findings showing 75% increase in fasting ghrelin after H. pylori eradication [13], our study was powered to allow for the detection of at least a 30% difference in ghrelin levels following successful eradication of 15 patients. Statistical analysis was performed using SPSS software version 16.0 for Macintosh (SPSS Inc., Chicago, Illinois); a two-tailed p-value of < 0.05 was considered significant.

Results

Patient demographic and clinical characteristics

We enrolled 92 patients who completed the test meal protocol, as shown in Additional file 2, Figure S1. Based on histologic, culture, and serologic results, 38 patients were categorized as H. pylori-negative, 44 as H. pylori-positive, and 10 were indeterminate (Table 1). Compared to H. pylori-negative patients baseline BMI was significantly higher among H. pylori-positive patients. The prevalence of diabetes was also higher among H. pylori-positive compared to H. pylori-negative patients, however this difference did not reach statistical significance. The most common indication for endoscopy in both the H. pylori-negative and H. pylori-positive patients was heme-positive stool, and persistent heartburn in the H. pylori-indeterminate group

(shown in Additional file 3, Table S1); PPI use occurred in 46% of the entire study group. Endoscopic findings did not differ significantly between the groups (Additional file 3, Table S2). There were no significant changes in the maintenance use of antisecretory medications between baseline and follow-up examinations. We excluded the H. pylori-indeterminate group from subsequent analyses.

The H. pylori-negative and -positive groups did not differ significantly in age, ethnicity, PPI use, gender, or prevalence of upper abdominal symptoms, (Table 1), but as expected, they differed in extent of acute gastritis (Additional file 3, Table S3). At baseline, the H. pylori-negative subjects had lower BMI measurements than did the H. pylori-positive group (26.4 ± 4 vs. 29.4 ± 5; p = 0.008). Stratifying the 44 H. pylori-positive hosts according to cagA status of their strain did not reveal any significant differences in baseline demographic and clinical parameters (data not shown).

Energy homeostasis hormones

The study subjects varied substantially in baseline pre-meal (fasting) serum values for the eight studied hormones (Additional file 3, Table S4). As expected, serum leptin values correlated with BMI, for both the H. pylori-negative and H. pylori-positive subjects (Additional file 2, Figure S2). There were no significant differences according to H. pylori status in pre-meal leptin, amylin, insulin, ghrelin, GIP, GLP-1, PP, and PYY levels (Additional file 3, Table S4). As expected, there were hormonal responses to the test meal; post-meal amylin levels rose physiologically [26] in both the H. pylori-negative and H. pylori-positive subjects (Additional file 3, Table S4). Similarly, there were significant post-meal increases in the levels of insulin, GIP, PP, and PYY, in both the H. pylori-negative and H. pylori-positive groups. As expected [3], ghrelin values diminished following the meal, while leptin values rose significantly in both groups. Thus, our observations are consistent with the expected meal-associated hormonal changes, with no significant differences between the H. pylori-positive and -negative subjects, as well as when data were normalized (Additional file 3, Table S5).

Effects of H. pylori eradication

Treatment for H. pylori was accepted by 31 (70.5%) of the 44 subjects in whom it was clinically indicated; 23 completed all of our assessments and eradication was successful in 21 (91%) (Additional file 2, Figure S1). The 21 subjects were representative of the entire group of 44 who were initially H. pylori-positive, with similar meal-associated hormone changes at baseline (compare Table 2, and Additional file 3, Table S4). Following H. pylori eradication, the meal-associated increases in amylin, insulin, GIP, PP, and PYY remained significant (Table 2). Compared to baseline, post-meal levels of the incretin GLP-1 were significantly increased following H. pylori eradication.

Table 1 Demographic and clinical characteristics of the 92 study patients, according to *H. pylori* status

Characteristic	*H. pylori*-negative (N = 38)	*H. pylori*-indeterminate (N = 10)	*H. pylori*-positive (N = 44)	Comparison of *H. pylori*-negative and *H. pylori*-positive subjects (p-value)
Mean age (years) ± SD	65 ± 13	70 ± 6	64 ± 14	0.84[b]
Male, n (%)	36 (95)	10 (100)	43 (98)	0.47[c]
Race/ethnicity, n (%)				0.22[c]
White, non-Hispanic	19 (50)	4 (40)	13 (30)	
Black, non-Hispanic	13 (34)	3 (30)	18 (41)	
Hispanic	5 (13)	3 (30)	12 (27)	
Asian	1 (3)	0 (0)	1 (2)	
Mean BMI (kg/m^2) ± SD	26.4 ± 4	26.0 ± 3	29.4 ± 5	0.008[b]
PPI use, n (%)[a]	15 (40)	9 (90)	18 (41)	0.54[c]
Diabetes, n (%)	7 (18)	3 (30)	14 (32)	0.17[c]

[a]PPI = proton pump inhibitor.

[b] Student's *t*-test; [c]Chi-Squared test.

Pre-meal ghrelin levels did not significantly differ between baseline and post-eradication (Table 2); however, following *H. pylori* eradication, post-meal ghrelin levels did not substantially decrease (Figure 1A). After *H. pylori* eradication, pre-meal, post-meal, and integrated leptin levels rose significantly (Figure 1B), and remained significantly correlated with BMI (r = 0.69, p < 0.01). PPI use did not account for the changes in ghrelin and leptin levels from baseline to follow-up (data not shown). This finding is consistent with other reports that PPI use does not influence ghrelin levels [27,28].

Since the initial measurements were performed on the day of endoscopy while the second measurements were not, we considered that gastric distension might have influenced measurements between the two time-points. We addressed this potential bias by also evaluating seven subjects who were *H. pylori* negative at a second time-point. The same test meal, and metabolic evaluations were repeated in the seven *H. pylori*-negative subjects at baseline and after follow-up (median 14 months). As expected, this control group had no significant changes in the eight measured adipokines between the two time-points (data

Table 2 Levels of eight hormones related to energy homeostasis, and BMI in 21 subjects, according to *H. pylori* eradication status

	Median (IQR) hormone concentration (pg/ml), before and after *H. pylori* eradication						Comparison of values at baseline and after eradication (p-value)	
	Baseline			**Eradicated**				
Hormone	Pre-meal	Post-meal	p[b]	Pre-meal	Post-meal	p[b]	Pre-meal	Post-meal
Amylin	15 (14-43)	19 (15-54)	**0.046**	16 (15-50)	36 (15-106)	**0.008**	0.25	0.16
Insulin	243 (129-414)	584 (462-1,475)	**< 0.001**	265 (139-558)	763 (430-2,100)	**< 0.001**	0.39	0.28
Ghrelin	1,024 (7-3,461)	231 (7-1,329)	**0.004**	1,710 (27-4,573)	1,586 (13-3,360)	0.12	0.51	**0.005**
GIP	15 (5-29)	107 (29-214)	**0.001**	27 (9-54)	82 (41-282)	**0.001**	0.82	0.85
GLP-1	28 (10-56)	16 (9-59)	0.51	36 (12-89)	45 (14-91)	0.95	0.11	**0.04**
Leptin	4,260 (1,890-6,649)	5,690 (1,765-11,350)	**0.02**	6,605 (3,517-14,600)	7,400 (4,120-17,925)	**0.02**	0.001	**< 0.001**
PP	63 (18-113)	107 (44-204)	**0.005**	79 (26-153)	112 (45-172)	**0.001**	0.31	0.23
PYY	39 (27-82)	70 (48-98)	**0.002**	61 (34-90)	70 (47-137)	**0.001**	**0.02**	0.34

[a]p-values < 0.05 are indicated in bold.

[b]Wilcoxon's signed rank test comparing pre-meal and post-meal values.

[c]Paired *t*-test comparing BMI at baseline to after *H. pylori* eradication.

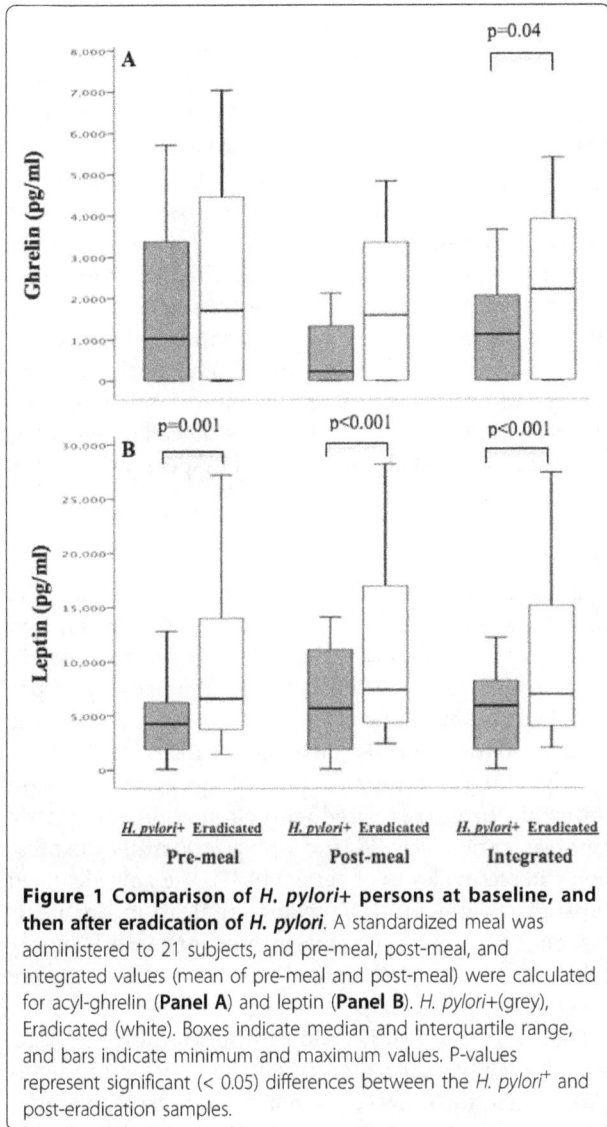

Figure 1 Comparison of *H. pylori+* persons at baseline, and then after eradication of *H. pylori*. A standardized meal was administered to 21 subjects, and pre-meal, post-meal, and integrated values (mean of pre-meal and post-meal) were calculated for acyl-ghrelin (**Panel A**) and leptin (**Panel B**). *H. pylori*+(grey), Eradicated (white). Boxes indicate median and interquartile range, and bars indicate minimum and maximum values. P-values represent significant (< 0.05) differences between the *H. pylori*+ and post-eradication samples.

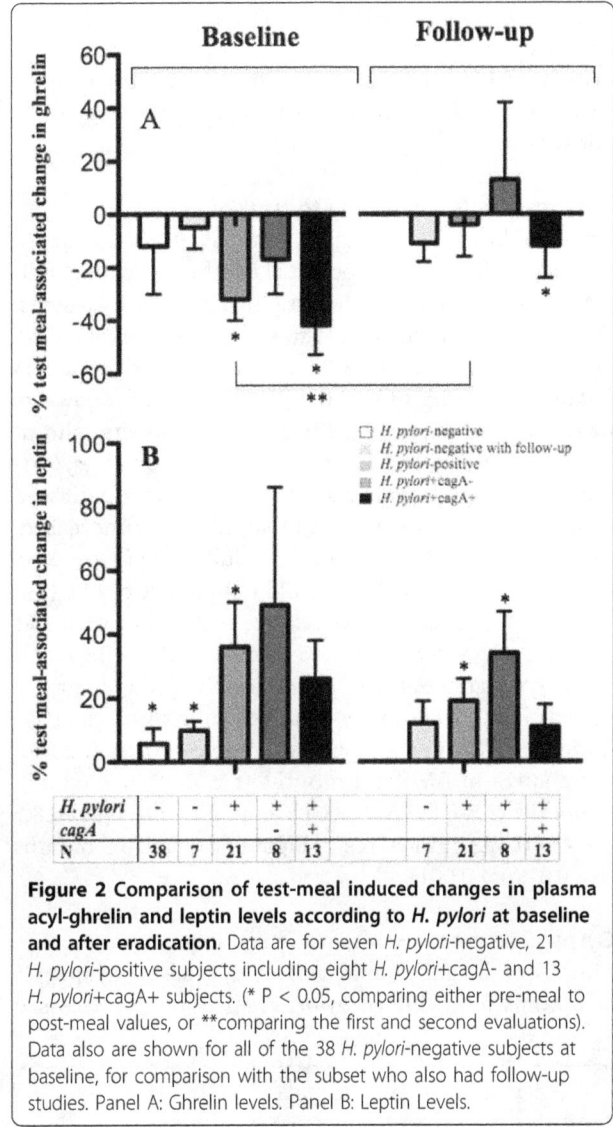

Figure 2 Comparison of test-meal induced changes in plasma acyl-ghrelin and leptin levels according to *H. pylori* at baseline and after eradication. Data are for seven *H. pylori*-negative, 21 *H. pylori*-positive subjects including eight *H. pylori*+cagA- and 13 *H. pylori*+cagA+ subjects. (* P < 0.05, comparing either pre-meal to post-meal values, or **comparing the first and second evaluations). Data also are shown for all of the 38 *H. pylori*-negative subjects at baseline, for comparison with the subset who also had follow-up studies. Panel A: Ghrelin levels. Panel B: Leptin Levels.

not shown), and no changes in meal-associated physiology (Figure 2). In the *H. pylori*-positive subjects at baseline, ingestion of the test meal led to a 32 ± 9% decrease (p = 0.004) in ghrelin with somewhat larger declines in persons with *cagA*-positive strains than in those with *cagA*-negative strains. Data from the 38 *H. pylori*-negative subjects and the subset of seven who had long-term follow-up also showed similar trends (Figure 2A). However, after *H. pylori* eradication, post-meal ghrelin levels only fell minimally (4 ± 12%; p = NS); the difference in meal-associated responses comparing baseline and post-eradication (32% vs. 4%) was significant (p = 0.05). At baseline, leptin levels in both the *H. pylori*-positive and *H. pylori*-negative subjects significantly increased after the test meal (Figure 2B). The meal-associated rise in leptin after eradication (19 ± 7%), remained significant (p = 0.02). Following *H. pylori*-eradication in subjects previously colonized with

cagA-positive strains, the expected meal-associated increase in PP was significantly lower than expected (27% vs. -13%; p = 0.01).

Meal-associated ghrelin physiology in relation to baseline gastric histology

In the group from whom *H. pylori* was eradicated, the severity of histologic inflammation in the fundus at baseline was negatively correlated with pre-meal ghrelin (r = -0.57, p = 0.01), as expected [29,30]. Subjects with more active gastritis had higher pre-meal ghrelin levels at baseline, and greater meal-associated changes post-eradication (Additional file 3, Table S6). Eradication-related changes in ghrelin physiology also correlated with the anatomic location of gastritis; subjects with antral gastritis only showed the largest increases in values obtained pre-meal, post-meal, and across the meal (Additional file 3, Table S7). These data provide evidence that both location and extent of gastric inflammation affects ghrelin secretion, but similar associations were not found with reference to leptin physiology (data not shown).

Body mass index in relation to *H. pylori* status

Since baseline BMI was higher for the *H. pylori*-eradicated group, we addressed this potential bias by comparing individuals to themselves in longitudinal pair-wise analyses. During the six months prior to study initiation, BMI did not change substantially in any of the study subjects (Figure 3). During 18 months (IQR 12, 24) of follow-up, BMI did not change significantly in subjects who at baseline were either *H. pylori*-negative or *H. pylori*-indeterminate. In contrast, in the *H. pylori*-eradicated group, BMI progressively and significantly increased, reaching 105 ± 2% by 18 months of follow-up (p = 0.008); baseline *H. pylori cagA* status did not predict results (p = 0.58). The change in BMI relative to baseline also was significantly greater at 3, 6, and 12 months following eradication compared to the *H. pylori*-negative group (data not shown). The change in pre-meal ghrelin from baseline following *H. pylori* eradication, was positively correlated with the change in BMI at 3 months (r = 0.78; p = 0.005), 6 months (r = 0.86; p = 0.001), and 12 months [r = 0.82; p = 0.001 (Additional file 2, Figure S3)], and 18 months (r = 0.87; p = 0.001).

Dyspepsia symptoms at baseline and follow-up

Since weight gain could reflect decreased dyspeptic symptoms following *H. pylori* eradication, we assessed

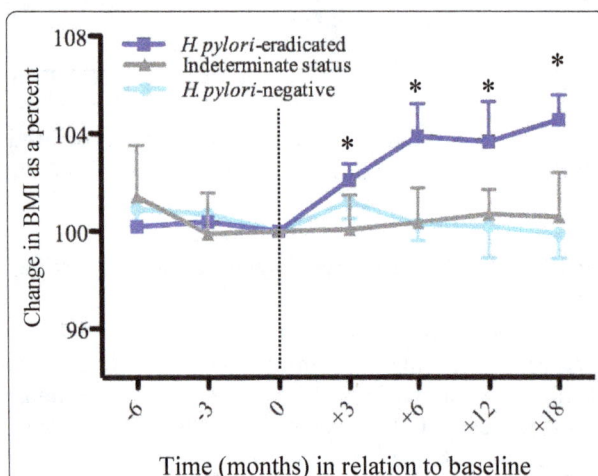

Figure 3 Change in BMI in 69 study subjects over a 2-year period. BMI is calculated relative to the baseline (at time 0), and is shown from 6 months prior to baseline and during 18 months of follow-up in 38 *H. pylori*-negative, 21 *H. pylori*-eradicated, and 10 subjects who were *H. pylori*-indeterminate at baseline (*p < 0.05, comparing time 0 to other follow-up months).

dyspeptic symptoms at baseline and post-eradication. A validated multidimensional assessment tool [31] was used to evaluate three scales: pain intensity, non-pain symptoms, and satisfaction with dyspepsia-related health. At baseline, the 38 *H. pylori*-negative and 44 *H. pylori*-positive subjects did not differ significantly in median pain, non-pain, and satisfaction scores (data not shown). Among the 21 patients from whom *H. pylori* was eradicated, there were no significant differences between baseline and follow-up pain scores [Median (IQR) 9 (2-23) vs. 6 (2-15); p = 0.86], non-pain scores [13 (12-16) vs. 10 (10-18); p = 0.28], or satisfaction scores [13 (10-23) vs. 19 (12-20); p = 0.29]. Thus, the observed increase in BMI following eradication (Figure 3) was not correlated with diminished dyspepsia that could increase appetite.

Discussion

Appetite-reducing hormones, such as amylin, insulin, GIP, GLP-1, PP, and PYY, produced in the small intestine and pancreas are important in mammalian energy homeostasis, [32-35], as is leptin which is produced mostly by adipocytes, but also by gastric chief cells [6]. Importantly, gastric oxyntic endocrine cells [36] account for 65-80% of the body's total ghrelin production. *H. pylori* colonization status has been correlated with circulating and gastric mucosal leptin levels [9], and with gastric mRNA expression and plasma levels of ghrelin [9,37]. We now identified substantial effects of *H. pylori* eradication on meal-associated changes in gastric hormones and energy balance, confirming and extending prior studies in a more rigorous manner [13,38].

That *H. pylori*-positive and *H. pylori*-negative subjects had similar baseline digestive hormonal physiologies (Additional file 3, Table S4) may reflect the highly integrated cross-regulation of energy homeostasis, [39] and the long-term equilibria between *H. pylori* and individual hosts [10,40]. Our observations of high pre-meal levels of acylated (acyl-) ghrelin that then fell post-prandially were as expected [3]. However, several months after *H. pylori* eradication, the extent of physiologic meal-associated reduction in circulating acyl-ghrelin was much diminished. These findings are consistent with other studies of subjects who underwent *H. pylori* eradication and then had increased plasma ghrelin [13,30,38] and gastric ghrelin mRNA levels [29]. Alterations in ghrelin regulation following *H. pylori* eradication may reflect the extent of baseline gastric inflammation [8]. Similarly, plasma levels of acyl-ghrelin may be significantly elevated post-*H. pylori* eradication, and vary reflecting the severity of atrophic gastritis [30], but atrophic gastritis is uncommon in the population we studied (data not shown). Methodological issues across studies, such as the length of follow-up post-*H. pylori* treatment [11,29] and differences in populations examined

[11] may partially account for differing metabolic and anthropometric findings. We now provide evidence that the extent and location of *H. pylori*-induced inflammation at baseline is associated with the differences in ghrelin physiology that develop due to *H. pylori* eradication. Although our data must be considered preliminary with small numbers of subjects, baseline antral gastritis appears to affect responses to eradication.

Although ghrelin is known to induce weight gain, in a study with six weeks of follow-up after *H. pylori* eradication, plasma ghrelin was increased, but median BMI was unchanged [13]. In another study, 12 weeks following *H. pylori* eradication, plasma ghrelin was increased in some subjects and reduced in others [29].

Our study now shows that following *H. pylori* eradication, there is blunting of the meal-associated physiologic reduction in circulating acyl-ghrelin, and there is long-term weight gain; in addition, changes in baseline acyl-ghrelin values and changes in BMI were linked (Additional file 2, Figure S3). Reflecting the observed weight gain, leptin levels pre-meal and post-meal ghrelin levels were significantly elevated after eradication and differed significantly from baseline values. We also observed that *H. pylori* eradication was associated with preservation of the expected [26,41-43] meal-associated increases in amylin, insulin, GIP, PP, and PYY. Post-meal levels of the incretin GLP-1 were significantly increased following eradication compared to baseline, perhaps reflecting the need for a meal-termination signal in the setting of persistently elevated ghrelin levels. We found no evidence that the weight gain associated with *H. pylori* eradication reflected improvement of dyspeptic symptoms as suggested previously [44]. Although in our study group, the *H. pylori*-positive subjects had higher BMIs at baseline compared to *H. pylori*-negative, the study was not designed to compare BMI between *H. pylori*-negative and *H. pylori*-positive groups. Rather, we sought to compare the change in BMI over time within the groups.

Our findings are limited by the study setting at a veteran's hospital where most of the evaluated patients were older men. Measurement of ghrelin is not standardized, [45] and may account for the substantial inter-individual variation that we report. However, comparing each subject to himself before and after the standard test meal, and repeating the same measurements at baseline and during follow-up reduces the effects of inter-individual variation, as well as any potential effect of the endoscopic evaluation performed on all patients. We also verified measurements in the same individuals in duplicate on separate occasions. Since all patients (*H. pylori*-negative and *H. pylori*-positive) had an endoscopic evaluation prior to the first postprandial measurement of hormones, and not prior to the second postprandial measurement, the observed post-eradication changes could not be

explained by the potential effect of the endoscopic examination alone. We measured acyl-ghrelin, which also may be relevant in energy homeostasis following *H. pylori* eradication, as opposed to total ghrelin as others have done [11,29]. We did not address changes in the ratio of circulating active versus inactive ghrelin before and after eradication. Other strengths of the study include the collection of detailed demographic, clinical, and histologic data from a prospectively enrolled group using validated instruments, *H. pylori* status determination using multiple methods for all patients that improve sensitivity and diminish falsely negative categorization [46], measurement of eight gut hormones to ascertain the meal-associated metabolic profile of each subject at baseline, and following up an *H. pylori*-negative group for comparison. We planned to analyze patients who were not successfully treated to eradicate *H. pylori*, however few individuals failed eradication therapy and thus that control group was not sufficiently populated. In addition, our ability to further analyze *H. pylori*-negative patients was limited by the fact that only 7 completed follow-up evaluations.

Conclusions

In conclusion, our study indicates that leptin and ghrelin physiology change and that BMI increases following *H. pylori* eradication. Although the number of subjects is limited, using patients as their own controls and having multiple measurements allowed us to both confirm previous published data, and to use a standard meal technique to extend the findings. This study provides further evidence that gastric *H. pylori* is involved in the physiologic regulation of these hormones, and supports the rationale for randomized controlled *H. pylori* eradication trials to focus on the role of inflammation and endocrine cross-talk in explaining these findings.

Additional material

Additional file 1: Supplemental methods. Provides information regarding exclusion criteria for the study population, symptom evaluation, *H. pylori* evaluation, test meal, and metabolic tests.

Additional file 2: Supplemental figures. Provides information regarding the enrollment and classification of study participants (Figure S1), the relationship of baseline BMI and baseline pre-meal leptin according to *H. pylori* status (Figure S2), and the correlation of changes in ghrelin and BMI post-*H. pylori* eradication (Figure S3).

Additional file 3: Supplemental tables. Provides information regarding the indications for upper GI endoscopy among study subjects (Table S1), findings during upper endoscopy (Table S2), Histologic score at three gastric sites according to *H. pylori* status (Table S3), levels of eight hormones related to energy homeostasis at the baseline evaluation of subjects according to *H. pylori* status and in relation to the test meal (Table S4), test-meal induced change and normalized change in hormone profile according to *H. pylori* status at baseline (Table S5), comparison of baseline and post-eradication meal-associated ghrelin profile in 21 originally *H. pylori*-positive subjects according to severity of baseline histologic gastritis (Table S6), and meal-associated changes in ghrelin profile in 28 subjects[a] who had follow-up evaluation according to anatomical distribution of histologic gastritis at baseline (Table S7).

Acknowledgements

Supported in part by K23CA107123, R01GM63270, R01DK090989, NCRRM01RR0096, and 1UL1RR029893 from the National Institutes of Health, the Michael Saperstein Medical Scholars Program, and the Diane Belfer Program in Human Microbial Ecology. We thank the NYU School of Medicine Division of Gastroenterology, its fellows, and nurses for their support.

Author details

[1]New York University Langone Medical Center, New York, NY, USA. [2]New York Harbor Veteran Affairs Medical Center, New York, NY, USA.

Authors' contributions

All authors read and approved the final manuscript. FF participated in the design of the study, patient recruitment, sample procurement, statistical analysis, and manuscript preparation. JR participated in patient recruitment, sample processing, and manuscript preparation. NJ contributed with patient recruitment and with manuscript preparation. ZP was involved in review of pathology samples and manuscript. AC participated in patient recruitment and manuscript review. JRS participated in sample processing and manuscript preparation. AZO was involved in sample procurement and processing as well as manuscript review. GIP participated in sample processing and manuscript preparation. MJB participated in study design, analysis, and manuscript preparation.

Competing interests

The authors declare that they have no competing interests.

References

1. Shintani M, Ogawa Y, Ebihara K, Aizawa-Abe M, Miyanaga F, Takaya K, Hayashi T, Inoue G, Hosoda K, Kojima M, et al: Ghrelin, an endogenous growth hormone secretagogue, is a novel orexigenic peptide that antagonizes leptin action through the activation of hypothalamic neuropeptide Y/Y1 receptor pathway. Diabetes 2001, 50(2):227-232.
2. Schwartz MW, Seeley RJ, Campfield LA, Burn P, Baskin DG: Identification of targets of leptin action in rat hypothalamus. J Clin Invest 1996, 98(5):1101-1106.
3. Cummings DE, Purnell JQ, Frayo RS, Schmidova K, Wisse BE, Weigle DS: A preprandial rise in plasma ghrelin levels suggests a role in meal initiation in humans. Diabetes 2001, 50(8):1714-1719.
4. Tschop M, Smiley DL, Heiman ML: Ghrelin induces adiposity in rodents. Nature 2000, 407(6806):908-913.
5. Halaas JL, Gajiwala KS, Maffei M, Cohen SL, Chait BT, Rabinowitz D, Lallone RL, Burley SK, Friedman JM: Weight-reducing effects of the plasma protein encoded by the obese gene. Science 1995, 269(5223):543-546.
6. Mix H, Widjaja A, Jandl O, Cornberg M, Kaul A, Goke M, Beil W, Kuske M, Brabant G, Manns MP, et al: Expression of leptin and leptin receptor isoforms in the human stomach. Gut 2000, 47(4):481-486.
7. Gnanapavan S, Kola B, Bustin SA, Morris DG, McGee P, Fairclough P, Bhattacharya S, Carpenter R, Grossman AB, Korbonits M: The tissue distribution of the mRNA of ghrelin and subtypes of its receptor, GHS-R, in humans. J Clin Endocrinol Metab 2002, 87(6):2988.
8. Liew PL, Lee WJ, Lee YC, Chen WY: Gastric ghrelin expression associated with Helicobacter pylori infection and chronic gastritis in obese patients. Obes Surg 2006, 16(5):612-619.
9. Roper J, Francois F, Shue PL, Mourad MS, Pei Z, Olivares de Perez AZ, Perez-Perez GI, Tseng CH, Blaser MJ: Leptin and ghrelin in relation to Helicobacter pylori status in adult males. J Clin Endocrinol Metab 2008, 93(6):2350-2357.
10. Atherton JC, Blaser MJ: Coadaptation of Helicobacter pylori and humans: ancient history, modern implications. J Clin Invest 2009, 119(9):2475-2487.
11. Pacifico L, Anania C, Osborn JF, Ferrara E, Schiavo E, Bonamico M, Chiesa C: Long-term effects of Helicobacter pylori eradication on circulating ghrelin and leptin concentrations and body composition in prepubertal children. Eur J Endocrinol 2008, 158(3):323-332.
12. Azuma T, Suto H, Ito Y, Muramatsu A, Ohtani M, Dojo M, Yamazaki Y, Kuriyama M, Kato T: Eradication of Helicobacter pylori infection induces an increase in body mass index. Aliment Pharmacol Ther 2002, 16(Suppl 2):240-244.
13. Nwokolo CU, Freshwater DA, O'Hare P, Randeva HS: Plasma ghrelin following cure of Helicobacter pylori. Gut 2003, 52(5):637-640.
14. Francois F, Roper J, Goodman AJ, Pei Z, Ghumman M, Mourad M, de Perez AZ, Perez-Perez GI, Tseng CH, Blaser MJ: The association of gastric leptin with oesophageal inflammation and metaplasia. Gut 2008, 57(1):16-24.
15. Tytgat GN: The Sydney System: endoscopic division. Endoscopic appearances in gastritis/duodenitis. J Gastroenterol Hepatol 1991, 6(3):223-234.
16. Dixon MF, Genta RM, Yardley JH, Correa P: Classification and grading of gastritis. The updated Sydney System. International Workshop on the Histopathology of Gastritis, Houston 1994. Am J Surg Pathol 1996, 20(10):1161-1181.
17. Goggin N, Rowland M, Imrie C, Walsh D, Clyne M, Drumm B: Effect of Helicobacter pylori eradication on the natural history of duodenal ulcer disease. Arch Dis Child 1998, 79(6):502-505.
18. Tummuru MK, Cover TL, Blaser MJ: Cloning and expression of a high-molecular-mass major antigen of Helicobacter pylori: evidence of linkage to cytotoxin production. Infect Immun 1993, 61(5):1799-1809.
19. Perez-Perez GI, Dworkin BM, Chodos JE, Blaser MJ: Campylobacter pylori antibodies in humans. Ann Intern Med 1988, 109(1):11-17.
20. Blaser MJ, Perez-Perez GI, Kleanthous H, Cover TL, Peek RM, Chyou PH, Stemmermann GN, Nomura A: Infection with Helicobacter pylori strains possessing cagA is associated with an increased risk of developing adenocarcinoma of the stomach. Cancer Res 1995, 55(10):2111-2115.
21. Egan BJ, Marzio L, O'Connor H, O'Morain C: Treatment of Helicobacter pylori infection. Helicobacter 2008, 13(Suppl 1):35-40.
22. Malfertheiner P, Megraud F, O'Morain C, Bazzoli F, El-Omar E, Graham D, Hunt R, Rokkas T, Vakil N, Kuipers EJ: Current concepts in the management of Helicobacter pylori infection: the Maastricht III Consensus Report. Gut 2007, 56(6):772-781.
23. Zhang F, Chen Y, Heiman M, Dimarchi R: Leptin: structure, function and biology. Vitam Horm 2005, 71:345-372.
24. Zhou H, Yamada Y, Tsukiyama K, Miyawaki K, Hosokawa M, Nagashima K, Toyoda K, Naitoh R, Mizunoya W, Fushiki T, et al: Gastric inhibitory polypeptide modulates adiposity and fat oxidation under diminished insulin action. Biochem Biophys Res Commun 2005, 335(3):937-942.
25. Aaboe K, Krarup T, Madsbad S, Holst JJ: GLP-1: physiological effects and potential therapeutic applications. Diabetes Obes Metab 2008, 10(11):994-1003.
26. Lutz TA: Amylinergic control of food intake. Physiol Behav 2006, 89(4):465-471.
27. Kim BW, Lee BI, Kim HK, Cho YS, Chae HS, Lee HK, Kim HJ, Han SW: [Influence of long-term gastric acid suppression therapy on the expression of serum gastrin, chromogranin A, and ghrelin]. Korean J Gastroenterol 2009, 53(2):84-89.
28. Yamamoto T, Sanaka M, Anjiki H, Hattori K, Ishii T, Kuyama Y: No relationship between plasma desacyl-ghrelin levels and rabeprazole-related delay in gastric emptying: controlled study in healthy volunteers. Drugs R D 2008, 9(5):345-348.
29. Osawa H, Kita H, Ohnishi H, Nakazato M, Date Y, Bowlus CL, Ishino Y, Watanabe E, Shiiya T, Ueno H, et al: Changes in plasma ghrelin levels, gastric ghrelin production, and body weight after Helicobacter pylori cure. J Gastroenterol 2006, 41(10):954-961.
30. Kawashima J, Ohno S, Sakurada T, Takabayashi H, Kudo M, Ro S, Kato S, Yakabi K: Circulating acylated ghrelin level decreases in accordance with the extent of atrophic gastritis. J Gastroenterol 2009, 44(10):1046-1054.
31. Rabeneck L, Cook KF, Wristers K, Souchek J, Menke T, Wray NP: SODA (severity of dyspepsia assessment): a new effective outcome measure for dyspepsia-related health. J Clin Epidemiol 2001, 54(8):755-765.
32. Batterham RL, Cowley MA, Small CJ, Herzog H, Cohen MA, Dakin CL, Wren AM, Brynes AE, Low MJ, Ghatei MA, et al: Gut hormone PYY(3-36) physiologically inhibits food intake. Nature 2002, 418(6898):650-654.

33. Lassmann V, Vague P, Vialettes B, Simon MC: **Low plasma levels of pancreatic polypeptide in obesity.** *Diabetes* 1980, **29(6)**:428-430.
34. Wren AM, Seal LJ, Cohen MA, Brynes AE, Frost GS, Murphy KG, Dhillo WS, Ghatei MA, Bloom SR: **Ghrelin enhances appetite and increases food intake in humans.** *J Clin Endocrinol Metab* 2001, **86(12)**:5992.
35. Baggio LL, Drucker DJ: **Biology of incretins: GLP-1 and GIP.** *Gastroenterology* 2007, **132(6)**:2131-2157.
36. Kojima M, Hosoda H, Date Y, Nakazato M, Matsuo H, Kangawa K: **Ghrelin is a growth-hormone-releasing acylated peptide from stomach.** *Nature* 1999, **402(6762)**:656-660.
37. Isomoto H, Ueno H, Nishi Y, Wen CY, Nakazato M, Kohno S: **Impact of Helicobacter pylori infection on ghrelin and various neuroendocrine hormones in plasma.** *World J Gastroenterol* 2005, **11(11)**:1644-1648.
38. Gunji T, Matsuhashi N, Sato H, Fujibayashi K, Okumura M, Sasabe N, Urabe A: **Helicobacter pylori infection is significantly associated with metabolic syndrome in the Japanese population.** *Am J Gastroenterol* 2008, **103(12)**:3005-3010.
39. Tschop M, Wawarta R, Riepl RL, Friedrich S, Bidlingmaier M, Landgraf R, Folwaczny C: **Post-prandial decrease of circulating human ghrelin levels.** *J Endocrinol Invest* 2001, **24(6)**:RC19-21.
40. Blaser MJ, Kirschner D: **The equilibria that allow bacterial persistence in human hosts.** *Nature* 2007, **449(7164)**:843-849.
41. Adrian TE, Ferri GL, Bacarese-Hamilton AJ, Fuessl HS, Polak JM, Bloom SR: **Human distribution and release of a putative new gut hormone, peptide YY.** *Gastroenterology* 1985, **89(5)**:1070-1077.
42. Feillet CA: **Food for thoughts: feeding time and hormonal secretion.** *J Neuroendocrinol* 2010, **22(6)**:620-628.
43. Stock S, Leichner P, Wong AC, Ghatei MA, Kieffer TJ, Bloom SR, Chanoine JP: **Ghrelin, peptide YY, glucose-dependent insulinotropic polypeptide, and hunger responses to a mixed meal in anorexic, obese, and control female adolescents.** *J Clin Endocrinol Metab* 2005, **90(4)**:2161-2168.
44. Moayyedi P, Soo S, Deeks J, Delaney B, Harris A, Innes M, Oakes R, Wilson S, Roalfe A, Bennett C, *et al*: **Eradication of Helicobacter pylori for non-ulcer dyspepsia.** *Cochrane Database Syst Rev* 2005, , **1**: CD002096.
45. Chandarana K, Drew ME, Emmanuel J, Karra E, Gelegen C, Chan P, Cron NJ, Batterham RL: **Subject standardization, acclimatization, and sample processing affect gut hormone levels and appetite in humans.** *Gastroenterology* 2009, **136(7)**:2115-2126.
46. Cutler AF, Havstad S, Ma CK, Blaser MJ, Perez-Perez GI, Schubert TT: **Accuracy of invasive and noninvasive tests to diagnose Helicobacter pylori infection.** *Gastroenterology* 1995, **109(1)**:136-141.

Diffuse duodenal nodular lymphoid hyperplasia: a large cohort of patients etiologically related to *Helicobacter pylori* infection

Mehnaaz S Khuroo[1], Naira S Khuroo[2] and Mohammad S Khuroo[3*]

Abstract

Background: Nodular lymphoid hyperplasia of gastrointestinal tract is a rare disorder, often associated with immunodeficiency syndromes. There are no published reports of its association with *Helicobacter pylori* infection.

Methods: From March 2005 till February 2010, we prospectively followed all patients with diffuse duodenal nodular lymphoid hyperplasia (DDNLH). Patients underwent esophagogastroduodenoscopy with targeted biopsies, colonoscopy, and small bowel video capsule endoscopy. Duodenal nodular lesions were graded from 0 to 4 based on their size and density. Patients were screened for celiac sprue (IgA endomysial antibody), immunoglobulin abnormalities (immunoglobulin levels & serum protein electrophoresis), small intestine bacterial overgrowth (lactulose hydrogen breath test), and *Helicobacter pylori* infection (rapid urease test, and histological examination of gastric biopsies). Patients infected with *Helicobacter pylori* received sequential antibiotic therapy and eradication of infection was evaluated by ^{14}C urea breath test. Follow up duodenoscopies with biopsies were performed to ascertain resolution of nodular lesions.

Results: Forty patients (Males 23, females 17; mean age ± 1SD 35.6 ± 14.6 years) with DDNLH were studied. Patients presented with epigastric pain, vomiting, and weight loss. Esophagogastroduodenoscopy showed diffuse nodular lesions (size varying from 2 to 5 mm or more) of varying grades (mean score ± 1SD 2.70 ± 0.84) involving postbulbar duodenum. Video capsule endoscopies revealed nodular disease exclusively limited to duodenum. None of the patients had immunoglobulin deficiency or small intestine bacterial overgrowth or positive IgA endomysial antibodies. All patients were infected with *Helicobacter pylori* infection. Sequential antibiotic therapy eradicated *Helicobacter pylori* infection in 26 patients. Follow up duodenoscopies in these patients showed significant reduction of duodenal nodular lesions score (2.69 ± 0.79 to 1.50 ± 1.10; p < 0.001). Nodular lesions showed complete resolution in 5 patients and significant resolution in remaining 21 patients. Patients with resistant *Helicobacter pylori* infection showed no significant reduction of nodular lesions score (2.71 ± 0.96 to 2.64 ± 1.15; p = 0.58). Nodules partially regressed in score in 2 patients, showed no interval change in 10 patients and progressed in 2 patients.

Conclusions: We report on a large cohort of patients with DDNLH, etiologically related to *Helicobacter pylori* infection.

Background

Nodular lymphoid hyperplasia (NLH) of the gastrointestinal tract represents a rare disease that is grossly characterized by the presence of numerous visible mucosal nodules measuring up to, and rarely exceeding, 0.5 cm in diameter [1]. Histologically, hyperplasic lymphoid follicles with large germinal centres are seen in the lamina propria and superficial submucosa [2]. There is enlargement of the mucosal B cell follicles caused by hyperplasia of the follicle centres; surrounded by a normal appearing mantle zone. Disease may involve the stomach, the entire small intestine, and the large intestine [3]. NLH involving the colon can mimic a variety of polyposis syndromes and this may cause difficulties in diagnosis [4]. Disease has been reported to cause pulmonary disease as well [5]. The etiology is unknown. In children, NLH is often associated with viral infection or food allergy; tends to have a benign course and usually regresses spontaneously [6,7]. The disease in adults

* Correspondence: khuroo@yahoo.com
[3]Consultant Gastroenterology, Digestive Diseases Centre, Srinagar, Kashmir, India
Full list of author information is available at the end of the article

is rare and poorly described [8]. It has been suggested that NLH is a risk factor for both intestinal and extra intestinal lymphoma [9-11]. Approximately 20% of adults with common variable immunodeficiency are found to have NLH [12]. Some patients have low or absent IgA and IgM levels, decreased IgG levels, susceptibility to infection, small intestine bacterial overgrowth, diarrhea with or without steatorrhea [13-16]. *Giardia lamblia* is often present in such patients [17-19]. There is also an association with familial adenomatous polyposis and Gardner's syndrome [20]. It has also been reported in patients with human immunodeficiency virus infection [21]. The disease may be associated with other pathologies, especially gastrointestinal malignancies [22]. Except an isolated case of gastric nodular lymphoid hyperplasia, there are no published reports of association of NLH with *Helicobacter pylori* (*H. pylori*) infection [23]. Here, we report on a large cohort of patients with NLH, etiologically related to *H. pylori* infection.

Methods
Study Protocol
From March 2005 till February 2010, we prospectively followed all patients with diffuse duodenal nodular lymphoid hyperplasia (DDNLH). Patients had detailed history and physical examination. Complete blood counts and serum chemistry were done by standard techniques. Stool analysis was done for ova and parasites. Giardia lamblia infection was evaluated by examinations of concentrated, iodine-stained wet stool preparations; duodenal aspirates and duodenal biopsies. IgA endomysial antibodies were detected by indirect immunofluorescence assay. Serum immunoglobulin (IgG, IgA & IgM) were estimated by immunoturbidometry. Serum protein electrophoresis was performed by agarose gel electrophoresis and densitometry. Small intestine bacterial overgrowth was evaluated by lactulose hydrogen breath test. Patient underwent esophagogastroduodenoscopy (EGD), targeted gastric and duodenal biopsies, evaluation of *H. pylori* infection; colonoscopies with ileoscopy and video capsule endoscopy. Patients infected with *H. pylori* received 10 days sequential antibiotic therapy. Eradication of *H. pylori* was evaluated by ^{14}C urea breath Test (^{14}C UBT) 4 to 6 weeks after antibiotic therapy. Patients resistant to sequential therapy received second line antibiotic therapy. Follow up EGD's were performed at/after 6 months of antibiotic therapy to assess the status of the duodenal nodular lesions detected earlier.

Diffuse Duodenal Nodular Lymphoid Hyperplasia (DDNLH)
Nodular lymphoid hyperplasia was diagnosed when numerous mucosal nodules (2 to 5 mm or more) were visible on endoscopic examination of the gut mucosa

and histological examination of the forceps punch biopsies from nodules was reported as NLH [1]. NLH was characterized by presence of well-circumscribed nodes of lymphoid tissue in the lamina propria and/or superficial submucosa. These lymphoid collections showed presence of highly reactive germinal centres, numerous cell types, prominent vascularity and polyclonality as determined immunohistochemically [2]. The extent of nodular lesions was evaluated by various imaging tools including esophagogastroduodenoscopy, colonoscopy with ileoscopy and video capsule endoscopy. Diffuse nodular lesions limited to duodenum were diagnosed as DDNLH.

Esophagogastroduodenoscopy (EGD)
EGD was performed by an experienced endoscopist (MSK 3) with video-esophago-gastro-duodenoscope (Olympus Evis Smartage Gastro GIF V70 Serial, Olympus Japan). Procedures were video-recorded and representative findings documented on high resolution images using software program. Endoscopic findings were recorded on a proforma. Duodenum was carefully examined for nodules (circumscribed elevated mucosal lesions varying in size from 2 mm to 5 mm or more). Nodular lesions in the postbulbar duodenum, second and third part were graded on a scale of 0 to 4, depending upon the size and density of nodules. Grading was done by 2 investigators (MSK 3/NSK), blinded to results, by reviewing EGD images and recorded video. Prior to actual grading, the scoring system was mutually agreed upon and any discrepancies were mutually discussed and sorted out. Normal duodenum (grade 0) showed prominent smooth closely spaced *Valvulae conniventes* (*Kerckring's folds*) without scalloping or nodules. Nodules around 2 to 3 mm in size and less than 20 in number in the region inspected were reported as grade1. Similar size numerous (>20) nodules which had not deformed the duodenal folds were reported as grade 2. Grade 3 nodular disease was seen as numerous large (2 to 5 mm) nodules carpeting the mucosa and causing mucosal fold invasion and deformity. Nodules which were more than 5 mm in size carpeting the whole duodenal mucosa and obscuring the mucosal folds were reported as grade 4. Multiple (6 or more) forceps biopsies were taken from nodules and the intervening mucosa for histology. Biopsy specimens were examined under light microscopy after staining with hematoxylin and eosin; Periodic Acid Schiff (PAS) and reticulin stains. Immunohistochemistry using CD3 & CD20 markers was performed to evaluate the cell (T & B cells) population in the lymphoid nodules. Biopsies were examined for viral inclusions and parasites especially *Giardia lamblia* [24]. *H. pylori* infection was evaluated by rapid urease test (RUT) and at histology. For RUT, 2 forceps punch biopsies were taken from gastric incisura

and embedded in agar gel urea-rich medium (HP test™, Allied Marketing Corporation, Kolkata, India) and read as per manufacturer's instructions. Multiple gastric biopsies (two from antrum; two from body and additional specimens from any visible endoscopic visible lesions, if needed) were taken and stained with Hematoxylin & Eosin to type and grade gastritis; Alcian blue to detect intestinal metaplasia and Giemsa stain for *H. pylori* detection and density [25,26].

Colonoscopy

Colonoscopy with ileoscopy was performed by an experienced endoscopist (MSK) with video-colonoscope (Olympus Evis Smartage Colono CF V70L Serial, Olympus Japan). Forceps biopsies were taken from endoscopic abnormalities as well as terminal ileum.

Video Capsule Endoscopy

Small bowel video capsule endoscopy was performed on capsule endoscopy system, Rapid 5 UPG with help of Pillcam SB2 capsule (Given Imaging, Ltd. Israel). Video images were examined for presence and extent of nodular lesions in the small bowel.

Lactulose Hydrogen Breath Test

Small intestinal bacterial overgrowth was evaluated by analyzing breath hydrogen with Gastrolyzer (Bedfont Scientific Ltd. Rochester, Kent, England) after a challenge dose of lactulose (10 g) and breath samples collected at baseline and subsequent 20 minutes intervals for 3 hours. Positive diagnosis for small intestine bacterial overgrowth was made if the breath hydrogen showed 20 ppm rise above baseline within first 2 hours [27].

H. pylori Eradication

H. pylori eradication was done with sequential antibiotic therapy. Patients received pantoprazole, 40 mg, with amoxillin, 1 g, twice daily for 5 days followed by pantoprazole, 40 mg, clarithromycin, 500 mg, and tinidazole, 500 mg, twice daily for next five days [28]. Following sequential therapy, patients received symptomatic treatment including pantoprazole 40 mg per day for next 4 weeks. Patients with resistant *H. pylori* infection to sequential therapy received 10 days second line therapy (pantoprazole 40 mg twice daily along with levofloxacin 750 mg and doxycycline 100 mg once daily). This antibiotic combination was based on *H. pylori* antibiotic sensitivity in this region (Khuroo et al unpublished data).

^{14}C Urea Breath Test (^{14}C UBT)

Eradication of *H. pylori* infection after antibiotic therapy was evaluated by ^{14}C UBT using Heliprobe™ System 2000 (Kibion AB, Uppsala, Sweden). After an overnight fast, patient swallowed a ^{14}C Urea Capsule (HeliCap™).

After 10 minute wait, patient breathed in to a breath card (BreathCard™) till acid sensitive indicator changed color from orange to yellow suggesting adequate trapping of exhaled breath ^{14}Carbon dioxide as lithium carbonate. Breath Card ^{14}C activity was analyzed in a Geiger Muller Counter (Probe™) and *H. pylori* infection analyzed and presented on the display as Heliprobe TM grade 0 (not infected), 1 (Indeterminate) and 2 (Infected).

Ethics

Written informed consent explaining the indications, adverse affects and alternatives was obtained from all patients before the procedures were carried out. The study protocol was submitted to the ethical committee of Digestive Diseases Centre and was approved. The study protocol conformed to good medical practice as defined in the Helsinki principles.

Statistics

Comparisons of the categorical variables were analyzed using the Fisher's exact test. Comparisons of the continuous variables were analyzed using the Student's t-test. All values are expressed as mean ± SD and frequencies. The statistical analysis was carried out using SPSS for Windows (version 13.0). Two-tailed P values less than 0.05 were considered significant.

Results

From March 2005 till February 2010, 44 patients with NLH of gastrointestinal tract were diagnosed. Two patients had disease limited to distal ileum as visualized at colonoscopy & ileoscopy. Another 2 patients had extensive disease involving duodenum, jejunum and ileum. These 2 patients had common variable immunodeficiency syndrome and one of them presented with superadded recurrent *Giardia lamblia* infection, Remaining 40 patients (Males 23, females 17; mean age ± 1SD 35.6 ± 14.6 years; age range 14 to 62 years) had diffuse nodular disease limited to duodenum and formed the study group (Table 1).

Dominant clinical presentation was epigastric pain, postprandial abdominal distension, vomiting and weight loss. Duration of symptoms varied from 6 months to 5 years (mean ± 1 SD 2.6 ± 1.2 years). Six patients presented with recurrent episodes of diarrhoea, while 4 patients complained of constipation. None of the patients had history suggestive of steatorrhea. Hemoglobin ranged from 6 g/dl to 12.5 g/dl (mean ± 1SD 9.5 ± 2.2 g/dl). Six patients had severe anemia (<6.0 g/dl), 22 patients had moderate anemia (6 to <8 g/dl) and 12 patients had mild anemia (8 to <10 g/dl). Haematological indices revealed iron deficiency anemia in all patients. None of the patients had megaloblastic anemia. Serum albumin ranged from 2.5 g/dl to 4.5 g/dl (mean ± 1SD 3.2 ± 1.1 g/dl). 8 patients had low

Table 1 The clinical profile of 40 patients with diffuse duodenal nodular hyperplasia

Group	All patients	H pylori eradicated group	H pylori persistent group	P value (Eradicated vs. Non-eradicated)
Number of patients	40	26	14	
Age (years ± 1SD)	35.6 ± 14.6	33.6 ± 11.6	37.6 ± 15.6	0.29c
Sex (Male: Female)	23:17	15:11	8:6	0.64a
Symptoms (Number of patients)				
Pain	40	26	14	1.00a
Vomiting	38	24	14	0.41a
Weight loss	35	23	12	0.77a
Diarrhoea	6	4	2	0.65a
Constipation	4	1	3	0.11a
Hemoglobin (g/dl)	9.5 ± 2.2	8.9 ± 3.2	9.7 ± 1.2	0.33c
Serum albumin (g/dl)	3.2 ± 1.1	3.4 ± 1.1	2.9 ± 1.4	0.39c
Immunoglobulins (Number of patients)				
Normal	26	18	8	0.14a
Elevated IgG	6	4	2	0.65a
Elevated IgM	5	4	1	0.41a
Elevated IgA	3	0	3	0.03a
Gastroscopic findings (number of patients)				
No abnormality	8	6	2	0.41a
Antral gastritis	20	11	9	0.16a
Fundic exudative gastritis	6	4	2	0.65a
Atrophic gastritis	4	3	1	0.56a
Ulcerative Nodular antral disease	2	2	0	0.41a
Grade of duodenal nodular disease (Number of patients)				
Grade 1	4	2	2	0.71b
Grade 2	10	7	3	
Grade 3	20	14	6	
Grade 4	6	3	3	
Mean ± 1SD Score	2.70 ± 0.84	2.69 ± 0.79	2.71 ± 0.96	0.94c
Follow up months (mean ± 1SD)	24 ± 12.5 (6-56)	22 ± 14.5 (6-54)	26 ± 12.9 (8-56)	0.65c

a = Fisher's exact test 2 × 2 table; b = Fisher's exact test rxc table; c = students t test.

Key: The profile of 26 patients in whom *H. pylori* infection was eradicated and 14 patients in whom *H. pylori* infection was resistant to eradication therapy are compared.

serum albumin. Serum calcium levels were below normal in 10 patients. Immunoglobulin levels were within normal limits in 26 patients. 14 patients had elevated immunoglobulin levels (IgG in 6 patients, IgM in 5 patients, and IgA in 3 patients). Elevated immunoglobulin levels were less than 1.5 times of the upper limit of normal values. None of the patients had low immunoglobulin level. Serum protein electrophoresis showed normal electrophoretic pattern and none of the patients had M band pattern. None of the patients had small intestine bacterial overgrowth as assessed by lactulose hydrogen breath test. IgA endomysial antibodies were negative in all patients. Stool analysis revealed ova of *Ascaris lumbricoides* in 11 patients. All patients with *Ascaris lumbricoides* infection received anthelmintic therapy namely mebendazole 100 mg twice daily per oral for 3 days. None of the patients had *Giardia lamblia* infection *as* evaluated by examinations of concentrated, iodine-stained wet stool preparations; duodenal aspirates and duodenal biopsies.

EGD showed diffuse nodular duodenal lesions in all patients (Figure 1). Duodenal bulb showed smooth mucosa, devoid of nodules in all patients. Nodular lesions appeared just beyond the apex of the bulb and were prominently seen in the second and third part of the duodenum. Nodular lesions were graded as grade 1 in 4 patients, grade 2 in 10 patients, grade 3 in 20 patients and grade 4 in 6 patients (mean ± 1SD grade 2.7 ± 1.2). All patients showed distensible duodenal lumen and none

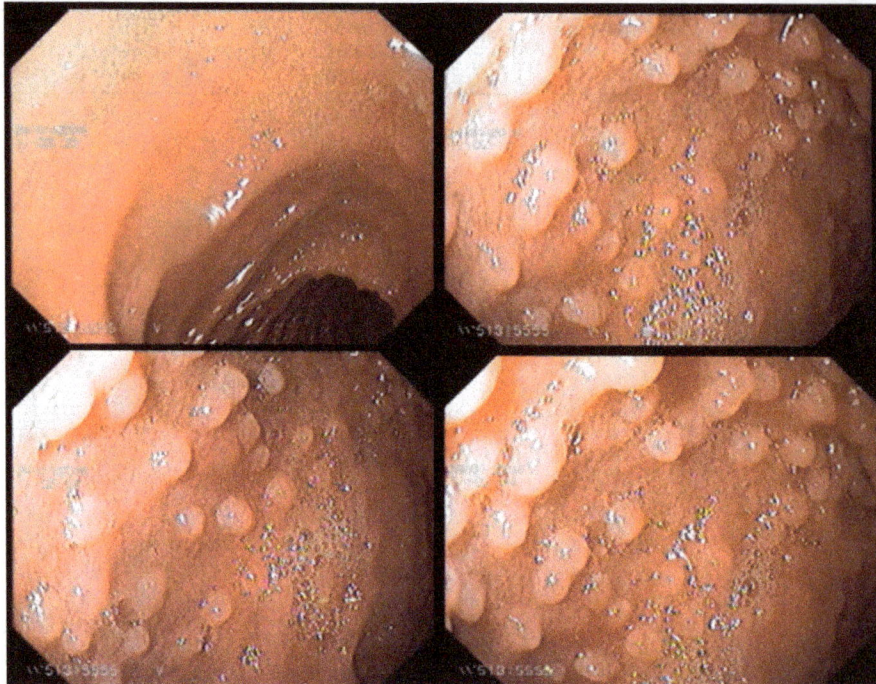

Figure 1 Diffuse Duodenal Nodular Lymphoid Hyperplasia. 35 year male presented with epigastric pain, vomiting and weight loss of 5 kg over the past 6 months. Duodenal composite images. Top left image: Duodenal bulb revealed smooth mucosa without any nodular lesion. Top right and 2 bottom images: post-bulbar region, second and third part of duodenum showed diffuse numerous mucosal nodules (>5 mm size each) scored as grade 4 disease. There was complete loss of *Kerckring's folds*. Duodenal biopsies revealed nodular lymphoid hyperplasia. Immunoglobulin revealed mild elevation of IgG level [IgG 2090 mg/dl (normal 700-1600 mg/dl); IgM. 120 mg/dl (normal = 40-230 mg/dl); IgA 145 mg/dl (normal = 70-400 mg/dl)].

showed luminal narrowing or stricture or stasis or ulcerations. Examination of stomach showed no endoscopic abnormality in 8 patients; linear erythematous antral gastritis in 20 patients; exudative fundic gastritis in 6 patients and atrophic gastritis in 4 patients. Two patients had diffuse ulcerative nodular lesions limited to the antrum. None of the patient had pyloric or duodenal ulcer. RUT was positive in all patients and *H. pylori* were seen in gastric biopsies in all patients. Density of *H. pylori* was moderate in 6 patients and heavy in 34 patients. Histology of gastric biopsies revealed chronic superficial gastritis in 24 patients, and chronic atrophic gastritis with intestinal metaplasia in 14 patients. Two patients with diffuse ulcerative nodular disease of antrum showed histologic features of low grade MALT lymphoma. Duodenal biopsies showed mature nodes of lymphoid follicles in lamina propria (Figure 2). These lymphoid collections showed presence of highly reactive germinal centres. In addition, lamina propria showed mild increase in lymphomononuclear cells. *H. pylori* were infrequently seen on the duodenal mucosa and in small numbers. Duodenal biopsies lacked features of coeliac sprue namely blunted villi, increased crypt depth, increased crypt villous ratio and epithelial cell lymphocytosis. Immunohistochemistry showed polyclonality of the cellular infiltrate which excludes possibility of duodenal lymphoma. There were no viral inclusions or *Giardia lamblia* seen in the tissue specimens.

Video capsule endoscopy showed nodular lesions in the postbulbar duodenum, second and third part of duodenum (Figure 3). There was marked reduction in the

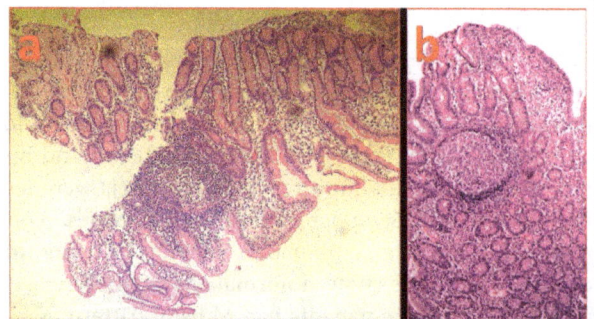

Figure 2 Diffuse Duodenal Nodular Lymphoid Hyperplasia. a) Low power view (H&E 10×) of duodenal biopsy showing a lymphoid follicle. b) High power view (H&E 40×) A mature lymphoid follicle with highly reactive germinal centre and surrounding normal appearing mantle zone is seen. There is mild increase in lymphoid infiltrate in the lamina propria.

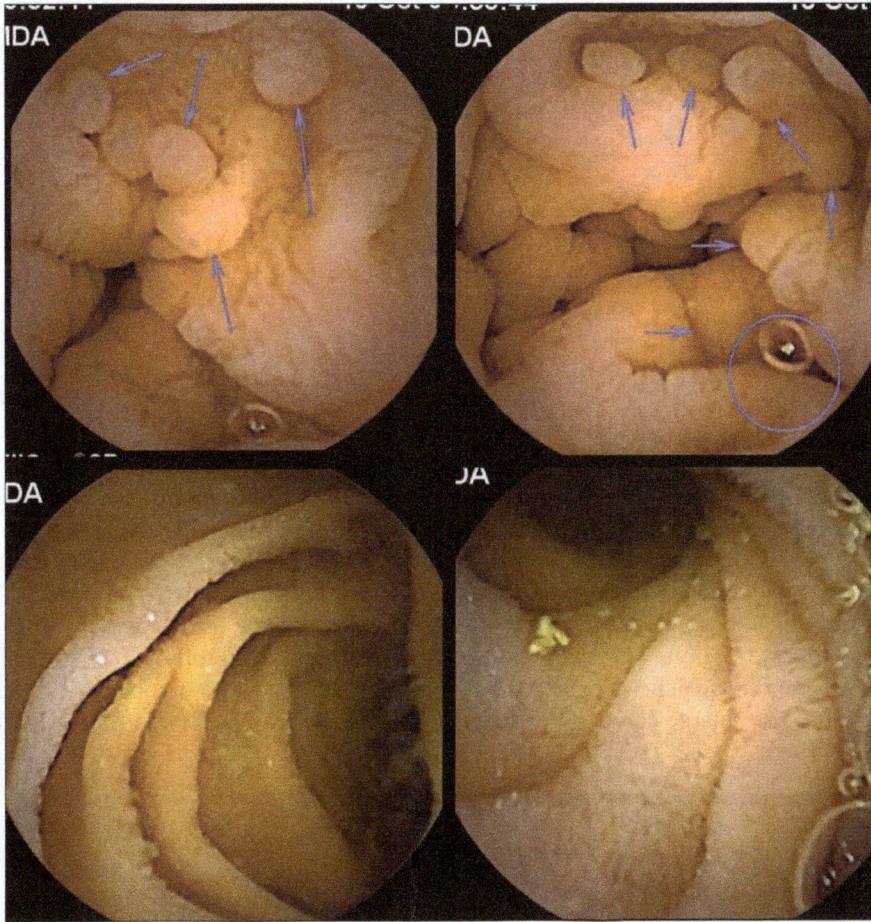

Figure 3 Diffuse Duodenal Nodular Lymphoid Hyperplasia. Video Capsule Endoscopy composite images. Top 2 images: Second and third part duodenum shows carpeting of the mucosa with nodular lesions. Bottom 2 images. Jejunum and ileum showed normal appearing mucosa without any nodular lesions.

number of nodular lesions around the duodeno-jejunal junction. There were no nodular lesions seen in the jejunum and ileum. Colonoscopy and ileoscopy was normal in all cases and biopsies of the terminal ileum did not reveal nodular lymphoid hyperplasia.

All patients received sequential antibiotic therapy. 14C UBT, done 4 to 6 weeks following antibiotic therapy, revealed eradication of *H. pylori* infection in 22 patients. Another 4 patients had *H. pylori* eradication following second line therapy. Remaining 14 patients had persistent *H. pylori* infection. Abdominal pain and vomiting showed improvement in 14 of the 26 patients in whom H pylori had been eradicated (p < 0.001) (Table 2). In contrast only 3 out of 14 patients with persistent *H. pylori* infection had improvement in symptoms (p = 0.22). Follow up duodenoscopies in 26 patients with *H. pylori* eradicated showed significant reduction of duodenal nodular lesions score (2.69 ± 0.79 to 1.50 ± 1.10; p < 0.001). Nodular lesions showed complete endoscopic and histological resolution in 5 patients and significant resolution in

remaining 21 patients (Figure 4). Two patients with low grade MALT lymphoma showed endoscopic and histologic resolution of the disease, after *H. pylori* eradication. Patients with resistant *H. pylori* infection showed no significant reduction of nodular lesions score (2.71 ± 0.96 to 2.64 ± 1.15; p = 0.58). Nodules regressed in 2 patients, showed no interval change in 10 patients and progressed in 2 patients (Figure 5). Histology of nodules which had progressed over the follow up continued to show polyclonality and there was no suggestion of these nodules evolving in to lymphoma.

Discussion

NLH of the gastrointestinal tract is a rare disorder, often reported with immune deficiency disorders and/or recurrent giardiasis [11-13,15,17-19]. The disease may be localized to a segment or may affect longer segments of bowel [13]. In contrast to reported disease in literature, the cohort of patients described in this study had significant differences. Firstly the disease was often

Table 2 The effects of *H. pylori* eradication therapy on 40 patients with diffuse duodenal nodular hyperplasia

Disease severity	All patients (n = 40)		P value	Eradicated group (n = 26)		P value	Not eradicated group (n = 14)		P value
	H. pylori therapy			*H. pylori* therapy			*H. pylori* therapy		
	Before	After		Before	After		Before	After	
Persistent symptoms	40	23	<0.001a	26	12	<0.001a	14	11	0.22a
Grade of nodular disease									
Grade 0	0	5	0.005b	0	5	0.002b	0	0	0.91b
Grade 1	4	12		2	9		2	3	
Grade 2	10	11		7	7		3	3	
Grade 3	20	10		14	4		6	4	
Grade 4	6	2		3	1		3	4	
Mean ± 1SD Score	2.70 ± 0.84	1.83 ± 1.06	<0.001c	2.69 ± 0.79	1.50 ± 1.10	<0.001c	2.71 ± 0.96	2.64 ± 1.15	0.58c

a = Fisher's exact test 2 × 2 table; b = Fisher's exact test rxc table; c = students t test.

encountered and report of 40 cases from one centre in 5 years period is a testimony to that. Second the disease involvement was limited to postbulbar duodenum, second and third part and duodeno-jejunal junction. Duodenal bulb was spared and there was no involvement of jejunum and ileum. Third none of the patients included in this study had immune deficiency or giardiasis. There are several reports of large cohort of patients

similar to described by us from Mexico [16,29]. However, around half of such patients had hypogammaglobinemia.

Diarrhea and weight loss secondary to malabsorption has been the dominant symptom of NLH of small bowel as reported in the literature [1,15,30,31]. Malabsorption is a common symptom in patients with immune deficiency with or without superadded recurrent giardiasis [32]. In contrast our patients with DDNLH presented

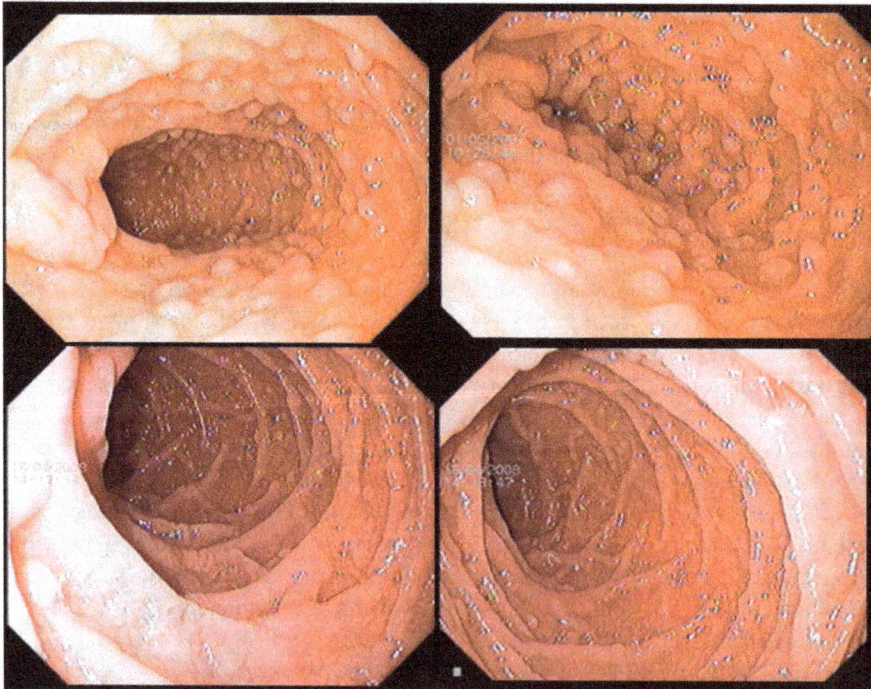

Figure 4 Diffuse Duodenal Nodular Lymphoid Hyperplasia. Duodenal composite images showing effect of *H. pylori* eradication. 25 year woman presented with recurrent epigastric pain, vomiting and weight loss of 10 kg over past 2 years. Immunoglobulin levels were within normal limits [IgG 1460 mg/dl (normal 700-1600 mg/dl); IgM. 190 mg/dl (normal = 40-230 mg/dl); IgA 230 mg/dl (normal = 70-400 mg/dl)]. Patient had *H. pylori* infection with severe fundic exudative gastritis. Top 2 images: Second part of duodenum was carpeted with numerous nodular lesions 3 to 5 mm in size, scored as grade 3 nodular disease. Patient received *H. pylori* sequential therapy and ^{14}C UBT 6 weeks after therapy showed eradication of infection. Bottom 2 images. Follow up duodenoscopic images at one year showed near complete resolution of the nodular lesions (scored as grade 0). Repeat duodenal biopsies failed to show nodular lymphoid follicles.

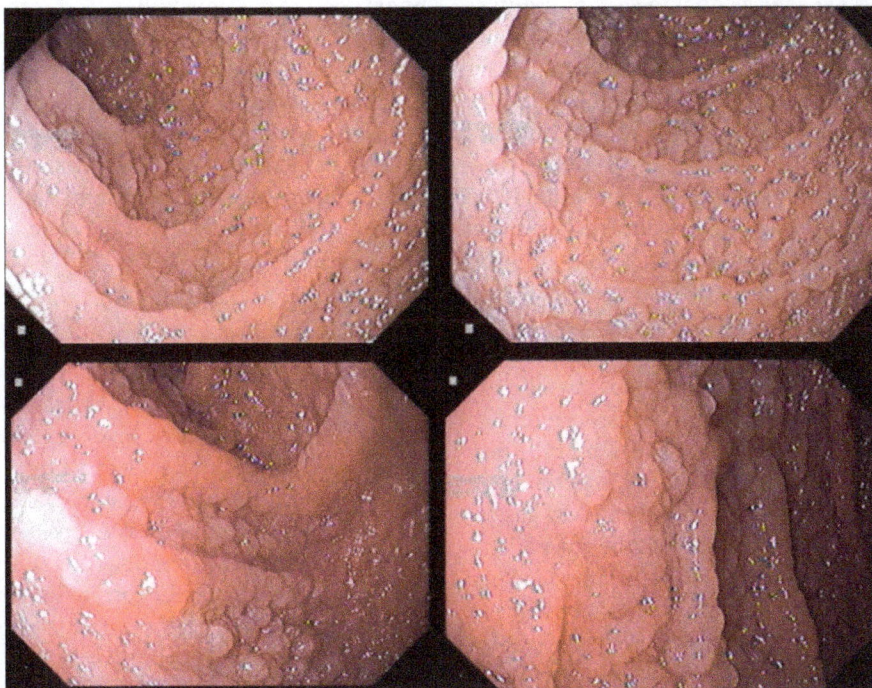

Figure 5 Diffuse Duodenal Nodular Lymphoid Hyperplasia. Duodenal composite images. Progression of disease. 40 year women presented with epigastric pain, vomiting, weight loss and recurrent diarrhoea. IgA levels were elevated [IgG 1400 mg/dl (normal 700-1600 mg/dl); IgM. 220 mg/dl (normal = 40-230 mg/dl); IgA 540 mg/dl (normal = 70-400 mg/dl)]. Patient had *H. pylori* related erythematous antral gastritis. Patient received *H. pylori* eradication sequential therapy followed by Levofloxacin/Doxycycline based second line eradication therapy and ^{14}C UBT showed resistant *H. pylori* infection. Top 2 images. Duodenal mucosa showed diffuse infiltration with nodules of 3 to 5 mm size, scored as grade 3 nodular disease. Bottom 2 images at 2 years follow up. There was significant increase in size (>5 mm) and density of the nodular lesions. *Kerckring's folds* showed infiltration and focal thickening by nodular disease, scored as grade 4 nodular disease. Biopsies showed nodular lymphoid follicles and infiltrate showed polyclonality of the lymphocytes.

with epigastric pain and vomiting, clinically suggesting gastric stasis and obstruction. Only 6 of our patients presented with diarrhea which may suggest co-existent malabsorption. Weight loss, gastric symptoms, iron lack anemia, and hypoalbuminemia in our patients were mostly caused by selective and dominant involvement of the duodenal mucosa [31].

The pathogenesis of nodular lymphoid hyperplasia has been a matter of debate for long. Histology of these lesions demonstrates hyperplasic lymphoid follicles with mitotically active germinal centres. In immune deficiency states, the lymphoid hyperplasia is likely the result of an accumulation of plasma-cell precursors due to maturational defect in the development of B-lymphocytes [2,29]. These cells attempt to compensate for functionally inadequate intestinal lymphoid function. Bacterial contamination of small intestines is often mentioned as an etiological factor for NLH [16]. This is supported by regression of nodules following oral antibiotic therapy in some cases [32]. Some investigators suggest that coeliac disease may be associated with NLH [1]. However, NLH may occur in a whole spectrum of disorders without any abnormalities in immunoglobulins

[33-35]. It is believed that NLH in absence of immune deficiency disorders may be related to immune stimulation of the gut lymphoid tissue.

H. pylori infection is etiologically associated with a number of gastroduodenal disorders. Acute infection causes neutrophilic gastritis with transient hypochlorhydria and subjects complain of epigastric pain and nausea [36]. Chronic infection causes a wide variety of gastritis including chronic superficial gastritis, nodular gastritis and chronic atrophic corpus gastritis with metaplasia [37,38]. *H. pylori* infection is strongly associated with peptic ulceration of duodenum and stomach [39,40]. Chronic corpus atrophic gastritis with intestinal metaplasia caused by *H. pylori* infection is an initiating event in most cases of intestinal type adenocarcinomas stomach. In fact *H. pylori* infection is associated with both diffuse-type and intestinal-type gastric adenocarcinoma [40,41]. Another entity which is etiologically related to *H. pylori* infection is gastric MALT lymphoma. The disease evolves through *H. Pylori* gastritis with mucosa associated lymphoid tissue (MALT), lymphoepithelial lesions, low grade B cell lymphoma and finally diffuse large B cell lymphoma [42-44].

There are no published reports of association of diffuse duodenal nodular lymphoid hyperplasia (DDNLH) with *H. pylori* infection.

A number of findings strongly pointed to *H. pylori* to be etiologically associated with DDNLH in our patients. All patients were infected with *H. pylori* infection. Patients in whom *H. pylori* were eradicated showed significant clinical response and regression/resolution of duodenal events. In contrast patients in whom *H. pylori* could not be eradicated showed persistence of clinical symptoms and persistence of duodenal nodular lesions. A number of earlier studies have suggested *H. pylori* as a possible cause of NLH [16,29], but none has followed this lead and none has substantiated this association.

What could be the pathogenesis of DDNLH in our patients? All patients had heavy *H. pylori* infection with advanced changes in the stomach as evidenced by gastroscopic and histological findings. In fact 2 of our patients had low grade MALT lymphoma. However, the duodenal changes seen were not as a result of direct involvement by *H. pylori*, as the organisms were not consistently present in the duodenal biopsies. A number of nongastrointestinal tract diseases are possibly associated with *H. pylori* infection. Many of these associations are suggested to be related to the effects of *H. pylori* on coagulation and markers of systemic inflammation. We believe the duodenal lesions were as a result of immune stimulation of prolonged and heavy *H. pylori* infection [45]. This was supported by elevated immunoglobulins in a number of patients in our series. Some extragastric disease states are particularly associated with H. *pylori* CagA-positive infections [46,47]. DDNLH seen in our community may be related to high prevalence of such *H. pylori* infections in our community and this need to be explored further. We believe careful examination of post-bulbar and second part of duodenum at EGD and liberal use of duodenal biopsies in patients with heavy *H. pylori* infection in tropical countries is needed to define the impact of this disease.

Two of our patients who failed to eradicate *H. pylori* infection had disease progression. However, biopsies showed prominent lymphoid follicles with active germinal centres located in the mucosa and there was no suspicion of disease evolving in to lymphoma. NLH has special relationship with lymphoma [7-9]. The disease needs to be differentiated from lymphoma. The presence of highly reactive germinal centres, numerous cell types, prominent vascularity, and polyclonality as determined immunohistochemically are the most important features in the differential diagnosis with lymphoma. Lymphoid hyperplasia may be differentiated from follicular lymphoma presenting as lymphomatous polyposis by Bcl-2 immunostaining of follicular germinal centres. NLH may be a manifestation of extraintestinal lymphoma and disease regresses after extraintestinal lymphoma undergoes remission under chemotherapy [48]. May patients with gastrointestinal lymphoma may present with NLH. Moreover, studies have shown that NLH itself may evolve in to lymphoma on long term follow up. The study period in our patients was not enough to define whether disease can evolve in to lymphoma. Long term follow up of these patients needs to be done to evaluate the malignant potential of this entity.

Conclusions

In summary, we report on 40 patients with DDNLH. Patients presented with intractable dyspepsia and esophagogastroduodenoscopy showed diffuse nodular lesions of varying grades involving postbulbar duodenum. None of the patients had immunoglobulin deficiency or small intestine bacterial overgrowth or positive IgA endomysial antibodies. All patients were infected with *H. pylori* infection. Sequential antibiotic therapy eradicated *H. pylori* infection in 26 patients. Follow up duodenoscopies in these patients showed significant reduction of duodenal nodular lesions score. Fourteen patients with resistant *H. pylori* infection showed no significant reduction of nodular lesions score. We believe DDNLH in our patients was etiologically related to *H. pylori* infection.

Acknowledgements
Funding: This work was conducted at Digestive Diseases Centre, Srinagar, Kashmir, India and was supported by funds from "Dr. Khuroo's Medical Trust".

Author details
[1]Lecturer, Department of Pathology, Government Medical college, Srinagar, Kashmir, India. [2]Consultant Radiology, Digestive Diseases Centre, Srinagar, Kashmir, India. [3]Consultant Gastroenterology, Digestive Diseases Centre, Srinagar, Kashmir, India.

Authors' contributions
Contribution by individual authors:
MSK 1 conceived the study; participated in the design of the study; reviewed pathology and performed the statistical work. NSK participated in the design of the study; performed the blind scoring of the endoscopic findings and helped drafting the manuscript. MSK 3 participated in the design of the study; performed the blind scoring of endoscopic findings; and drafted the manuscript. All authors read and approved the final manuscript.

Authors' information
1. Mehnaaz S Khuroo, MBBS, MD (Pathology), Lecturer, Department of Pathology, Government Medical college, Srinagar, Kashmir, India; Formerly Consultant Pathology, Jawahir Lal Nehru Memorial (JLMN) Hospital Rainawari, Srinagar, Kashmir, India. E-mail: mkhuroo@yahoo.com
2. Naira S Khuroo, MBBS, FIMR (KFSHRC Riyadh), Consultant Radiology, Digestive Diseases Centre, Srinagar, Kashmir, India. E-mail: naira_sultan@yahoo.com
3. Mohammad S Khuroo, MBBS, MD, DM, FRCP (Edin), FACP, Master American College of Physicians (MACP, Emeritus), Consultant Gastroenterology, Digestive Diseases Centre, Srinagar, Kashmir, India. E-mail: khuroo@yahoo.com; visit at: http://www.drkhuroo.com

Competing interests

The authors declare that they have no competing interests.

References

1. Ajdukiewicz AB, Youngs GR, Bouchier IAD: Nodular lymphoid hyperplasia with hypogammaglobulinemia. *Gut* 1972, **13**:589-95.

2. Ranchod M, Lewin KJ, Dorfman RF: Lymphoid hyperplasia of the gastrointestinal tract. A study of 26 cases and review of the literature. *Am J Surg Pathol* 1978, **2**:383-400.

3. Molaei M, Kaboli A, Fathi AM, Mashayekhi R, Pejhan S, Zali MR: Nodular lymphoid hyperplasia in common variable immunodeficiency syndrome mimicking familial adenomatous polyposis on endoscopy. *Ind J Pathol Microbiol* 2009, **52**(4):530-3.

4. Schwartz DC, Cole CE, Sun Y, Jacoby RF: Diffuse nodular lymphoid hyperplasia of the colon: polyposis syndrome or normal variant? *Gastrointest Endosc* 2003, **58**:630-2.

5. Abbondanzo SL, Rush W, Bijwaard KE, Koss MN: Nodular lymphoid hyperplasia of the lung: a clinicopathologic study of 14 cases. *Am J Surg Pathol* 2000, **24**:587-97.

6. Colon AR, DiPalma JS, Leftridge CA: Intestinal lymphonodular hyperplasia of childhood: patterns of presentation. *J Clin Gastroenterol* 1991, **13**:163-6.

7. Iacono G, Ravelli A, DiPrima L, Scalici C, Bolognini S, Chiappa S, Pirrone G, Licastri G, Carroccio A: Colonic lymphoid nodular hyperplasia in children: relationship to food hypersensitivity. *Clin Gastroenterol Hepatol* 2007, **5**:361-6.

8. Ersoy E, Gundogdu H, Ugras NS, Aktimur R: A case of diffuse nodular lymphoid hyperplasia. *Turk J Gastroenterol* 2008, **19**(4):268-70.

9. Ryan JC: Premalignant conditions of the small intestine. *Semin Gastrointest Dis* 1996, **7**:88-93.

10. Matuchansky C, Touchard G, Lemaire M, Babin P, Demeocq F, Fonck Y, Meyer M, Preud'Homme JL: Malignant lymphoma of the small bowel associated with diffuse nodular lymphoid hyperplasia. *N Eng J Med* 1985, **313**:1666-71.

11. Castellano G, Moreno D, Galvao O, Ballestin C, Colina F, Mollejo M, Morillas JD, Solis Herruzo JA: Malignant lymphoma of jejunum with common variable hypogammaglobulinemia and diffuse nodular hyperplasia of the small intestine. A case study and literature review. *J Clin Gastroenterol* 1992, **15**:128-35.

12. Washington K, Stenzel TT, Buckley RH, Gottfried MR: Gastrointestinal pathology in patients with common variable immunodeficiency and X-linked agammaglobulinemia. *Am J Surg Pathol* 1996, **20**:1240-52.

13. Crabbe PA, Heremans JF: Selective IgA deficiency with steatorrhea. *Am J Med* 1967, **42**:319-26.

14. Al Samman M, Zuckerman MJ, Mohandas A, Ting S, Hoffpauir JT: Intestinal nodular lymphoid hyperplasia in a patient with chronic diarrhea and recurrent sinopulmonary infections. *Am J Gastroenterol* 2000, **95**:2147-9.

15. Anderson FL, Pellegrino ED, Schaefer JW: Dysgammaglobulinemia associated with malabsorption and tetany. *Am J dig Dis* 1970, **15**:279-86.

16. Castaneda-Romero B, Diaz-Caldelas L, Galvan-Guerra E, Sixtos S, Arista J, Uscanga L: Intestinal lymphoid nodular hyperplasia in a patient with acquired dysgammaglobulinemia, chronic diarrhea, and bacterial overgrowth syndrome. *Rev Gastroenterol Mex* 1993, **58**(3):225-8.

17. Milano AM, Lawrence LR, Horowitz L: Nodular lymphoid hyperplasia of the small intestine and colon with Giardiasis. *Amer J dis Dis* 1971, **16**:735-7.

18. de Weerth A, Gocht A, Seewald S, Brand B, van Lunzen J, Seitz U, Thonke F, Fritscher-Ravens A, Soehendra N: Duodenal nodular lymphoid hyperplasia caused by giardiasis infection in a patient who is immunodeficient. *Gastrointest Endosc* 2002, **55**:605-7.

19. Onbasi K, Gunsar F, Sin AZ, Ardeniz O, Kokuludag A, Sebik F: Common variable immunodeficiency (CVID) presenting with malabsorption due to giardiasis. *Turk J Gastroenterol* 2005, **16**(2):111-3.

20. Shull LN Jr, Fitts CT: Lymphoid polyposis associated with familial polyposis and Gardner's syndrome. *Ann Surg* 1974, **180**(3):319-22.

21. Rosen Y: Nodular lymphoid hyperplasia of gut in HIV infection. *Am J Gastroenterol* 1992, **87**:1200-2.

22. Koren R, Kyzer S, Ramadan E: Nodular lymphoid hyperplasia of the small bowel associated with two primary colonic adenocarcinomas. *Tech Coloproctol* 1999, **3**:161-3.

23. Misra SP, Misra V, Dwivedi M, Singh PA: *Helicobacter pylori* induced lymphonodular hyperplasia: a new cause of gastric outlet obstruction. *J Gastroenterol Hepatol* 1998, **13**:1189-92.

24. Monkemuller KE, Bussian AH, Lazenby A, Wilcox CM: Special histologic stains are rarely beneficial for the evaluation of HIV-related gastrointestinal infections. *Am J Clin Pathol* 2000, **114**:387-94.

25. Genta RM, Robaseon GO, Graham DY: Simultaneous visualization of *Helicobacter pylori* and gastric morphology: A new stain. *Hum Pathol* 1994, **25**:221-6.

26. El-Zimaity HM, Segura AM, Genta RM, Graham DY: Histologic assessment of *Helicobacter pylori* status after therapy: comparison of Giemsa, Diff-Quik, and Genta stains. *Mod Pathol* 1998, **11**:288-91.

27. Bratten JR, Spanier J, Jones MP: Lactulose breath testing does not discriminate patients with irritable bowel syndrome from healthy controls. *Am J Gastroenterol* 2008, **103**(4):958-63.

28. Jafri NS, Hornung CA, Howden CW: Meta-analysis: sequential therapy appears superior to standard therapy for *Helicobacter pylori* infection in patients naive to treatment. *Ann Intern Med* 2008, **148**:923-31.

29. Tapia AR, Calleros JH, Hernandez ST, Uscanga L: Clinical characteristics of a group of adults with nodular lymphoid hyperplasia: a single center experience. *World J Gastroenterol* 2006, **12**:1945-8.

30. Canto J, Arista J, Hernandez J: Nodular lymphoid hyperplasia of the intestine. Clinico-pathologic characteristics in 11 cases. *Rev Invest Clin* 1990, **42**:198-203.

31. Kasirga E, Gülen H, Simşek A, Ayhan S, Yilmaz O, Ellidokuz E: Coexistence of symptomatic iron-deficiency anemia and duodenal nodular lymphoid hyperplasia due to giardiasis: case report. *Pediatr Hematol Oncol* 2009, **26**(1):57-61.

32. Lai Ping So A, Mayer L: Gastrointestinal manifestations of primary immunodeficiency disorders. *Semin Gastrointest Dis* 1997, **8**:22-32.

33. Tomita S, Kojima M, Imura J, Ueda Y, Koitabashi A, Suzuki Y, Nakamura Y, Mitani K, Terano A, Fujimori T: Diffuse nodular lymphoid hyperplasia of the large bowel without hypogammaglobulinemia or malabsorption syndrome: a case report and literature review. *Int J Surg Pathol* 2002, **10**:297-302.

34. Gryboski JD, Self TW, Clemett A, Herskovic T: Selective immunoglobulin A deficiency and intestinal nodular lymphoid hyperplasia: correction of diarrhea with antibiotics and plasma. *Pediatrics* 1968, **42**:833-6.

35. Rambaud JC, De Saint-Louvent P, Marti R, Galian A, Mason DY, Wassef M, Licht H, Valleur P, Bernier JJ: Diffuse follicular lymphoid hyperplasia of the small intestine without primary immunoglobulin deficiency. *Am J Med* 1982, **73**:125-32.

36. Graham DY, Opekun AR, Osato MS, El-Zimaity HM, Lee CK, Yamaoka Y, Qureshi WA, Cadoz M, Monath TP: Challenge model for *H. pylori* infection in human volunteers. *Gut* 2004, **53**:1235-43.

37. Kekki M, Villako K, Tamm A, Siurala M: Dynamics of antral and fundal gastritis in an Estonian rural population sample. *Scand J Gastroenterol* 1977, **12**:321-4.

38. Dwivedi M, Misra SP, Misra V: Nodular gastritis in adults: Clinical features, endoscpic appearance, histological feature and response to therapy. *J Gastroenterol Hepatol* 2008, **23**:943-7.

39. Graham DY, Lew GM, Klein PD, Evans DG, Evans DJ Jr, Saeed ZA, Malaty HM: Effect of treatment of *Helicobacter pylori* infection on the long term recurrence of gastric or duodenal ulcer: A randomized controlled study. *Ann Intern Med* 1992, **116**:705-8.

40. Marshall BJ: *Helicobacter pylori*. *Am J Gastroenterol* 1994, **89**(Suppl):S116.

41. Schistosomes Liver flukes and *Helicobacter pylori*: IARC working group on the evaluation of carcinogenic risks to human. *Lyon, France, 7-14 June, 1994. IARC Monogr Eval Carcinog Risks Hum* 1994, **61**:1.

42. Malfertheiner P, Sipponen P, Naumann M, Moayyedi P, Mégraud F, Xiao SD, Sugano K, Nyrén O, Lejondal , H. pylori-Gastric Cancer Task Force: *Helicobacter pylori* eradication has the potential to prevent gastric cancer: a state-of-the-art critique. *Am J Gastroenterol* 2005, **100**:2100-15.

43. Parsonnet J, Hansen S, Rodriguez L, Gelb A, Warnke R, Jellum E, Orentreich N, Vogelman J, Friedman G: *Helicobacter pylori* infection and gastric lymphoma. *N Engl J Med* 1994, **330**(18):1267-71.

44. Bayerdörffer E, Neubauer A, Rudolph B, Thiede C, Lehn N, Eidt S, Stolte M: Regression of primary gastric lymphoma of mucosa-associated lymphoid tissue type after cure of *Helicobacter pylori* infection. MALT Lymphoma Study Group. *Lancet* 1995, **345**(8965):1591-4.

45. Leontiadis GI, Sharma VK, Howden CW: Nongastrointestinal tract associations of *Helicobacter pylori* infection. *Arch Intern Med* 1999, **159**:925-40.

46. Gasbarrini A, Franceschi F, Armuzzi A, Ojetti V, Candelli M, Torre ES, De
     Lorenzo A, Anti M, Pretolani S, Gasbarrini G: **Extradigestive manifestations**
     of *Helicobacter pylori* gastric infection. *Gut* 1999, **45(S1)**:19-112.
47. Takahashi T, Yujiri T, Shinohara K, Inoue Y, Sato Y, Fujii Y, Okubo M, Zaitsu Y,
     Ariyoshi K, Nakamura Y, Nawata R, Oka Y, Shirai M, Tanizawa Y: **Molecular**
     mimicry by *Helicobacter pylori* **CagA protein may be involved in the**
     pathogenesis of H. pylori-associated chronic idiopathic
     thrombocytopenic purpura. *Br J Haematol* 2004, **124**:91-6.
48. Jonsson OT, Birgisson S, Reykdal S: **Resolution of nodular lymphoid**
     hyperplasia of the gastrointestinal tract following chemotherapy for
     extraintestinal lymphoma. *Dig Dis Sci* 2002, **47**:2463-5.

Permissions

The contributors of this book come from diverse backgrounds, making this book a truly international effort. This book will bring forth new frontiers with its revolutionizing research information and detailed analysis of the nascent developments around the world.

We would like to thank all the contributing authors for lending their expertise to make the book truly unique. They have played a crucial role in the development of this book. Without their invaluable contributions this book wouldn't have been possible. They have made vital efforts to compile up to date information on the varied aspects of this subject to make this book a valuable addition to the collection of many professionals and students.

This book was conceptualized with the vision of imparting up-to-date information and advanced data in this field. To ensure the same, a matchless editorial board was set up. Every individual on the board went through rigorous rounds of assessment to prove their worth. After which they invested a large part of their time researching and compiling the most relevant data for our readers.

The editorial board has been involved in producing this book since its inception. They have spent rigorous hours researching and exploring the diverse topics which have resulted in the successful publishing of this book. They have passed on their knowledge of decades through this book. To expedite this challenging task, the publisher supported the team at every step. A small team of assistant editors was also appointed to further simplify the editing procedure and attain best results for the readers.

Apart from the editorial board, the designing team has also invested a significant amount of their time in understanding the subject and creating the most relevant covers. They scrutinized every image to scout for the most suitable representation of the subject and create an appropriate cover for the book.

The publishing team has been an ardent support to the editorial, designing and production team. Their endless efforts to recruit the best for this project, has resulted in the accomplishment of this book. They are a veteran in the field of academics and their pool of knowledge is as vast as their experience in printing. Their expertise and guidance has proved useful at every step. Their uncompromising quality standards have made this book an exceptional effort. Their encouragement from time to time has been an inspiration for everyone.

The publisher and the editorial board hope that this book will prove to be a valuable piece of knowledge for researchers, students, practitioners and scholars across the globe.

List of Contributors

Andréa BC Fialho, Manuel B Braga-Neto, André MN Fialho, Karine C Fernandes Juliana LM Sun, Cícero IS Silva and Lucia LBC Braga
Clinical Research Unity - Department of Internal Medicine – Federal University of Ceará, Fortaleza, Ceará, Brazil

Christianne FV Takeda and Eder JC Guerra
Laboratory of Bacteriology Research - Federal University of Minas Gerais, Belo Horizonte, Minas Gerais, Brazil

Dulciene MM Queiroz
São José Hospital, F ortaleza, Ceará, Brazil

Min Soo Kim, Nayoung Kim, Sung Eun Kim, Hyun Jin Jo, Cheol Min Shin, Young Soo Park and Dong Ho Lee
Department of Internal Medicine, Seoul National University Bundang Hospital, Seongnam, Gyeonggi-do, South Korea

Young Soo Park, Nayoung Kim and Dong Ho Lee
Department of Internal Medicine and Liver Research Institute, Seoul National University College of Medicine, Seoul, South Korea

Rodrigo Buzinaro Suzuki, Rodrigo Augusto Basso Lopes, George Arouche da Câmara Lopes, Tin Hung Ho and Márcia Aparecida Sperança
Department of Molecular Biology, Marilia Medical School, Marilia, São Paulo, Brazil

Rodrigo Buzinaro Suzuki and Márcia Aparecida Sperança
Center of Natural and Human Sciences, Universidade Federal do ABC, Santo André, São Paulo, Brazil

Amin Talebi Bezmin Abadi, Marc JM Bonten and Johannes G Kusters
Department of Medical Microbiology, University Medical Center Utrecht, Heidelberglaan 100, Utrecht 3584 CX, The Netherlands

Ashraf Mohhabati Mobarez
Department of Medical Bacteriology, School of Medical Sciences, Tarbiat Modares University, Tehran, Iran

Jaap A Wagenaar
Department of Infectious Diseases and Immunology, Faculty of Veterinary Medicine, Utrecht University, Utrecht, Netherlands

Kamran B Lankarani
Health policy Research Center, Shiraz University of Medical Sciences, Shiraz, Islamic Republic of Iran

Mohammad Reza Ravanbod
Bushehr University of Medical Sciences, Bushehr, Islamic Republic of Iran

Aflaki, Mohammad Elham Ali Nazarinia and Akbar Rajaee
Rheumatology Research Center, Shiraz University of Medical Sciences, Shiraz, Islamic Republic of Iran

Fredy Omar Beltrán-Anaya, Tomás Manuel Poblete, Adolfo Román-Román and Gloria Fernández-Tilapa
Clinical Research Laboratory, Academic Unit of Chemical-Biological Sciences, Autonomous University of Guerrero, Chilpancingo, Guerrero C.P. 39090, Mexico

Salomón Reyes
State Institute of Oncology "Dr. Arturo Beltrán Ortega", Acapulco, Guerrero C. P. 39570, Mexico

José de Sampedro
General Hospital "Dr. Raymundo Abarca Alarcón", Chilpancingo, Guerrero C.P. 39090, Mexico

Oscar Peralta-Zaragoza
Department of Chronic Infections and Cancer, Infectious Diseases Research Center, National Institute of Public Health, Av. Universidad No. 655, Cerrada los Pinos y Caminera, Colonia Santa María Ahuacatitlan, Cuernavaca, Morelos C.P. 62100, Mexico

Berenice Illades-Aguiar, Moral-Hernández, Miguel Ángel Rodríguez and Oscar del
Laboratory of Molecular Biomedicine, Academic Unit of Chemical-Biological Sciences, Autonomous University of Guerrero, Chilpancingo, Guerrero C.P. 39090, Mexico

Kazuya Okushin, Yu Takahashi, Nobutake Yamamichi, Kenichiro Enooku, Hidetaka Fujinaga, Takeya Tsutsumi, Yoshizumi Shintani, Yoshiki Sakaguchi, Satoshi Ono, Shinya Kodashima, Mitsuhiro Fujishiro, Kyoji Moriya, Hiroshi Yotsuyanagi and Kazuhiko Koike
Department of Gastroenterology, Graduate School of Medicine, The University of Tokyo, Tokyo, Japan

Takeshi Shimamoto and Toru Mitsushima
Kameda Medical Center Makuhari (CD-2 1–3, Nakase, Mihama-ku, Chiba-city, Japan

Chung-Chuan Chan
Division of Gastroenterology, Department of Internal Medicine, Hsinchu Cathay General Hospital, Hsinchu, Taiwan

Yi-Chen Yang
Committee of Medical Research and Education, Hsinchu Cathay General Hospital, Hsinchu, Taiwan

Chi-Hwa Wu and Chih-Sheng Hung, Chia-Long Lee and Tien-Chien Tu
Division of Gastroenterology, Department of Internal Medicine, Cathay General Hospital, 280, Section 4, Jen-Ai Road, Taipei 10650, Taiwan

Nai-Hsuan Chien
School of Medicine, Fu Jen Catholic University, New Taipei, Taiwan

Chia-Long Lee and Tien-Chien Tu
Department of Internal Medicine, School of Medicine, College of Medicine, Taipei Medical University, Taipei, Taiwan

Yiqiao Xin, Lindsay Govan and Olivia Wu
Health Economics and Health Technology Assessment (HEHTA), Institute of Health and Wellbeing, University of Glasgow, Glasgow, UK

Jan Manson and Robin Harbour
Knowledge and Information, Healthcare Improvement Scotland, Glasgow, UK

Jenny Bennison
Scottish Intercollegiate Guideline Network (SIGN), NHS Education for Scotland, Royal College of General Practitioners (Scotland), Mill Lane Surgery, Edinburgh, UK

Eleanor Watson
Department of gastroenterology, Royal Infirmary of Edinburgh, NHS Lothian, Edinburgh, UK

Kenichi Yamanaka, Hiroyuki Miyatani, Yukio Yoshida, Takehiro Ishii, Shinichi Asabe and Hirosato Mashima
Department of Gastroenterology, Jichi Medical University, Saitama Medical Center, Saitama 330-8503, Japan

Osamu Takada
Department of Surgery, Jichi Medical University, Saitama Medical Center, Saitama 330-8503, Japan

Mitsuhiro Nokubi
Department of Pathology, Jichi Medical University, Saitama Medical Center, Saitama 330-8503, Japan

Ji Young Chang, Ki-Nam Shim, Chung Hyun Tae, Ko Eun Lee, Jihyun Lee, Kang Hoon Lee, Chang Mo Moon, Seong-Eun Kim, Hye-Kyung Jung and Sung-Ae Jung
Department of Internal Medicine, Ewha Womans University School of Medicine, Ewha Medical Research Institute, 1071 Anyangcheon-ro, Yangcheon-gu, Seoul 158-710, South Korea

Cícero ISM Silva, Maria HRB Goncalves, Manuel B Braga-Neto, Andréa BC Fialho and Lucia LBC Braga
Clinical Research Unity – Department of Internal Medicine, University Hospital Walter Cantídio – Federal University of Ceará, Fortaleza, Ceará, Brazil

Dulciene MM Queiroz, André MN Fialho, Gifone A Rocha, Andreia MC Rocha and Sérgio A Batista
Laboratory of Research in Bacteriology, Federal University of Minas Gerais, Belo Horizonte, Minas Gerais, Brazil

Richard L Guerrant
Center for Global Health, University of Virginia, Charlottesville, VA, USA

Aldo AM Lima
Department of Physiology and Pharmacology, Federal University of Ceará, Fortaleza, Ceará, Brazil

Hung-Chieh Lan, Tseng-Shing Chen, Full-Young Chang and Han-Chieh Lin
Division of Gastroenterology, Department of Medicine, Taipei Veterans General Hospital and National Yang-Ming University, #201 Shih-Pai Road, Section 2, Taipei, Taiwan, ROC

Anna Fen-Yau Li
Department of Pathology and Laboratory Medicine, Taipei Veterans General Hospital and National Yang-Ming University, Taipei, Taiwan, ROC

Hung-Chieh Lan
Division of General Medicine, Department of Medicine, Taipei City Hospital, Taipei, Taiwan, ROC

Javed Yakoob, Shahab Abid, Wasim Jafri, Zaigham Abbas Khalid Mumtaz and Saeed Hamid
Department of Medicine, Aga Khan University, Stadium Road, Karachi 74800, Pakistan

Rashida Ahmed
Department of Pathology, Aga Khan University, Stadium Road, Karachi 74800, Pakistan

Seon Hee Lim, Jung Mook Kang, Min Jung Park, Jeong Yoon Yim and Joo Sung Kim
Seoul National University Hospital, Healthcare System Gangnam Center Healthcare Research Institute, Seoul, Korea

Jin-Won Kwon
College of Pharmacy, Kyungpook National University, Daegu, Korea

Nayoung Kim
Department of Internal Medicine, Seoul National University Bundang Hospital, Seongnam, Korea

Joo Sung Kim, Hyun Chae Jung and Nayoung Kim
Department of Internal Medicine and Liver Research Institute, Seoul National University College of Medicine, Seoul, Korea

Gwang Ha Kim
Department of Internal Medicine, Pusan National University School of Medicine, Busan, Korea

Heung Up Kim
Department of Internal Medicine, School of Medicine, Jeju National University, Jeju, Korea

Gwang Ho Baik
Department of Internal Medicine, Hallym University College of Medicine, Chuncheon, Korea

Geom Seog Seo
Department of Internal Medicine, Wonkwang University Hospital, Iksan, Korea

Jeong Eun Shin
Department of Internal medicine, Dankook University College of Medicine, Chonan, Korea

Young-Eun Joo
Department of Internal Medicine, Chonnam National University Medical School, Gwangju, Korea

Takeshi Toyoda, Shinji Takasu and Kumiko Ogawa
Division of Pathology, National Institute of Health Sciences, Tokyo, Japan

Hisayo Ban, Noriko Saito and Takeshi Toyoda
Division of Oncological Pathology, Aichi Cancer Center Research Institute, Nagoya, Japan

Tetsuya Tsukamoto
Department of Pathology, Fujita Health University School of Medicine, Toyoake, Japan

Masami Yamamoto
Faculty of Veterinary Medicine, Nippon Veterinary and Life Science University, Tokyo, Japan

Liang Shi
Chemicals Safety Department, Mitsui Chemicals Inc, Mobara, Japan

Ayumi Saito
Department of Pathology and Matrix Biology, Mie University Graduate School of Medicine, Tsu, Japan

Seiji Ito and Yoshitaka Yamamura
Department of Gastroenterological Surgery, Aichi Cancer Center Hospital, Nagoya, Japan

Akiyoshi Nishikawa
Biological Safety Research Center, National Institute of Health Sciences, Tokyo, Japan

Takuji Tanaka
The Tohkai Cytopathology Institute: Cancer Research and Prevention, Gifu, Japan

Masae Tatematsu
Japan Bioassay Research Center, Hadano, Japan

Verima Pereira and Philip Abraham
Division of Gastroenterology, P D Hinduja Hospital, V S Marg, Mahim Mumbai 400016, India

Sivaramaiah Nallapeta
Bruker Daltonics, Bangalore, India

Anjali Shetty
Division of Microbiology, P D Hinduja Hospital, Mumbai, India

Shafika Assaad
Faculty of Sciences, Lebanese University, Beirut, Lebanon

Rawan Chaaban
International Committee of the Red Cross, Beirut, Lebanon

Fida Tannous
Faculty of Sciences, Beirut Arab University, Beirut, Lebanon

Christy Costanian
School of Kinesiology and Health Science, York University, Toronto, ON M3J1P3, Canada

Jean Damascene Kabakambira Vincent Dusabejambo and Francois Ngabonziza
Kigali University Teaching Hospital (CHUK), Kigali, Rwanda

Celestin Hategeka
Centre for Health Services and Policy Research, School of Population and Public Health, Faculty of Medicine, University of British Columbia, Vancouver, BC, Canada
Collaboration for Outcomes Research and Evaluation, Faculty of Pharmaceutical Sciences, University of British Columbia, Vancouver, BC, Canada

Cameron Page
Department of Medicine, University Hospital of Brooklyn, New York USA

Cyprien Ntirenganya, Jules Ndoli, Claude Bayingana and Tim Walker
Butare University Teaching Hospital (CHUB), Huye, Rwanda

DeVon Hale
Department of Medicine, University of Utah School of Medicine, Salt Lake City, UT, USA

Tim Walker
School of Medicine and Public Health, Faculty of Health and Medicine, University of Newcastle, Newcastle, Australia

Javed Yakoob, Zaigham Abbas, Rustam Khan, Shagufta Naz, Safia Awan Fatima Jafri and Wasim Jafri
Department of Medicine, The Aga Khan University, Karachi, Pakistan

Zubair Ahmad
Department of Pathology, The Aga Khan University, Karachi, Pakistan

Muhammad Islam
Department of Community Health Sciences, The Aga Khan University, Karachi, Pakistan

Elodie Siffré
Université de Bordeaux, Centre National de Référence des Campylobacters et des Hélicobacters, 146 rue Léo Saignat, 33000 Bordeaux, France

Philippe Lehours and Francis Mégraud
CHU de Bordeaux, Hôpital Pellegrin, Laboratoire de Bactériologie, Place Amélie Raba Léon, 33076 Bordeaux cedex, France
INSERM U853, 33000 Bordeaux, France

Fritz Francois, Jatin Roper, Neal Joseph, Zhiheng Pei, Aditi Chhada, Joshua R Shak, Asalia Z Olivares de Perez, Guillermo I Perez-Perez and Martin J Blaser
New York University Langone Medical Center, New York, NY, USA

Zhiheng Pei
New York Harbor Veteran Affairs Medical Center, New York, NY, USA

Mehnaaz S Khuroo
Lecturer, Department of Pathology, Government Medical college, Srinagar, Kashmir, India

Naira S Khuroo
Consultant Radiology, Digestive Diseases Centre, Srinagar, Kashmir, India

Mohammad S Khuroo
Consultant Gastroenterology, Digestive Diseases Centre, Srinagar, Kashmir, India

Index